What the Experts are sayi

THE M Fit
GROCERY SHOPPING GUIDE

"The latest edition of The M-Fit Grocery Shopping Guide *updates one of the most helpful guides to healthy eating available in the United States. Exercise and a good diet are the keys to heart health and this book gives you all the information you need when planning your shopping."*

◆ Stephen P. Fortmann, M.D.
Associate Professor of Medicine
Stanford University
Stanford, California
Chairman (1994-96), Council on Epidemiology and
Prevention, American Heart Association

*"*The M-Fit Grocery Shopping Guide *is an excellent resource for nutrition professionals and consumers. The focus on brand-specific information and choice in an easy to understand format allows the reader to quickly make informed food choices. This is a great addition for everyone's nutrition bookshelf."*

◆ Rebecca M. Mullis, Ph.D., R.D.
Professor and Chair, Department of Nutrition and Dietetics
Georgia State University
President (1995-96), Society for Nutrition Education

"Consumers who need an easy and credible source to make healthy food selections can count on The M-Fit Grocery Shopping Guide. *Our store owners who have been utilizing the M-Fit Guide are receiving high praise for the program from their shoppers."*

◆ Patrick M. Quinn
President & CEO, Spartan Stores, Inc.
Grand Rapids, Michigan
Board Member: National Grocers Association,
National American Wholesaler Grocers Association,
Food Marketing Institute

"This book is the next best thing to having a registered dietitian do your grocery shopping for you!"

◆ Leni Reed, M.P.H., R.D.
Editor/Publisher, *SUPERMARKET SAVVY*™ newsletter
Herndon, Virginia

"A valuable tool for the nutrition-wise shopper. One of the best guides I've seen."

◆ Neil J. Stone, M.D.
Associate Professor of Medicine (Cardiology)
Northwestern University
Chicago, Illinois
(Past Chair) American Heart Association's
Committee on Nutrition

"The M-Fit Grocery Shopping Guide is the most comprehensive and user-friendly manual that I have seen on healthy food choices. By using the Guide to develop their own personalized shopping list of foods and integrating a routine exercise program, consumers will have a recipe for success in minimizing cardiovascular heart disease."

◆ Margaret P. McEwan, M.S., R.D.
Vice President, Consumer Services and Quality Assurance
Shaw's Supermarkets, Inc.
East Bridgewater, Massachusetts
Chairman (1994-95), Consumer Affairs Council
Food Marketing Institute

"This is an excellent investment for people who take food and health seriously. It provides useful guidance on food choices and helps the shopper navigate the difficulties of buying in a market loaded with variety, brands, and confusing claims regarding value (nutritional and other)."

◆ Janice Neville, D.Sc., M.P.H.
Professor of Nutrition, School of Medicine
Case Western Reserve University
Cleveland, Ohio
Former President (1987-88), American Dietetic Association

"Patients frequently ask me to recommend a single book that will provide accurate and helpful advice for a variety of nutritional needs, from weight loss to athletic training to cardiac risk factor reduction. For all these needs, and many more, The M-Fit Grocery Shopping Guide *is the best book I've found!"*

◆ Thomas L. Schwenk, M.D.
Professor and Chair, Department of Family Practice
University of Michigan Medical Center

"This book's Best, Acceptable, and Occasional Choice groupings, based on nutrition criteria, offer uniquely useful guidance to consumers who select foods at different times for different reasons."

◆ Kristen McNutt, Ph.D., J.D.
President, Consumer Choices Inc.
Wheaton, Illinois

"This is an excellent resource for any health-conscious person. This guide really makes shopping for healthy foods very easy and convenient. A must read for anyone interested in serving healthy meals at home."

◆ Jerry Pinney
Vice President, Member Sales
National Grocers Association
Reston, Viriginia

The M*Fit*
Grocery Shopping Guide

Your Guide to Healthier Choices

4th Edition

Nelda Mercer, M.S., R.D.
Director of Preventive and Community Nutrition
The University of Michigan Medical Center

Lori Mosca, M.D., M.P.H.
Assistant Professor of Epidemiology
School of Public Health
Clinical Assistant Professor of Medicine
Division of Cardiology
The University of Michigan

Melvyn Rubenfire, M.D.
Professor of Internal Medicine
Director of Preventive Cardiology
Division of Cardiology
The University of Michigan

Edited By
Cheryl Rock, Ph.D., R.D., FADA
Assistant Professor of Human Nutrition
The University of Michigan

ISBN No. 0-9649656-0-7

Manufactured by Favorite Recipes® Press
P.O. Box 305142
Nashville, Tennessee 37230
1-800-358-0560

First Printing: 1995, 20,000 copies

ABOUT THE AUTHORS

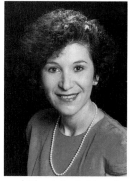

Nelda Mercer, M.S., R.D.

Nelda Mercer is a Registered Dietitian and Director of Preventive and Community Nutrition at the University of Michigan Medical Center. Nelda is a cum laude graduate from North Texas State University, where she received her Bachelor of Science degree in Food and Nutrition. She completed her dietetic internship at University Hospitals of Cleveland and received her Master of Science degree in Clinical Nutrition from Case Western Reserve University. She has authored and co-authored numerous professional articles and abstracts in the areas of hyperlipidemia, diabetes, and maternal and pediatric nutrition, and is co-author of the *Grocery Shopping Guide, High Fit - Low Fat* cookbook, and *Physician's Handbook of Nutrition Support: Maternal and Pediatric*. Nelda's nutrition column, "Eating Well," has appeared weekly for the past two years in *The Ann Arbor News*. She is also past Food & Nutrition co-columnist for *Triathlon Today* magazine. Nelda is an invited commentator for WUOM, the University of Michigan's Public Radio Station. In the late 1980s, Nelda joined the culinary faculty at Schoolcraft College, Continuing Education Services in Livonia, Michigan, where she and a Certified Master Chef co-taught an ACF-accredited nutrition course to students enrolled in the Culinary Arts Program. Nelda is the current chair for marketing and public relations for the Michigan Dietetic Association. Her most recent awards include the 1993 Public Relations Award and the 1994 Registered Dietitian of the Year Award from the Michigan Dietetic Association and the 1994 Recognition of Service Award from the American Dietetic Association.

Nelda is an avid runner. She has completed two marathons and is a Boston Marathon hopeful! A native Texan, she now lives in Ann Arbor, Michigan, with her husband and teenage daughter.

Lori Mosca, M.D., M.P.H.

Dr. Mosca received her medical degree from the State University of New York in Syracuse in 1984. She completed training in Internal Medicine and served on the faculty there until 1990. She then moved to New York City and obtained a Master of Public Health degree from Columbia University while completing fellowships in Preventive Cardiology and Cancer Epidemiology sponsored by the National Institutes of Health. She also served as Research Coordinator for the Children's Cardiovascular Health Center at Columbia-Presbyterian Medical Center.

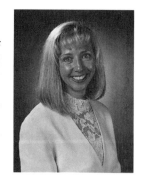

Dr. Mosca came to the University of Michigan in 1992, served as the Director of Preventive Cardiology between 1993 and 1995, and currently is Director of Preventive Cardiology Research and Educational Programs. She holds appointments at the Assistant Professor level in both the Medical School and the School of Public Health. Her major research interests are related to the epidemiology of cardiovascular disease in women, and she is conducting research on the effects of hormone therapy and antioxidant therapy on cardiovascular risk. She is Project Director for the Women's Pooling Project, a national collaborative study to evaluate coronary risk in women. She also chairs the American Heart Association Council on Epidemiology and Prevention Task Force on Women's Issues.

As an interesting aside, Dr. Mosca is an avid triathlete. She has competed in the Hawaii Ironman Triathlon, New York City Marathon, the National Championships and Masters World Cup in cross-country skiing. Her husband is a congenital cardiac surgeon on the faculty of the University of Michigan. They have two small children named Matthew and Michael.

Melvyn Rubenfire, M.D.

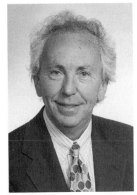

Dr. Rubenfire is a Professor of Internal Medicine and Director of Preventive Cardiology in the Heart Care Program at the University of Michigan. He received his Bachelor of Science degree in Chemistry and Doctor of Medicine degree from Wayne State University, completed a residency at Sinai Hospital and fellowship in Cardiology at Henry Ford Hospital in Detroit, Michigan. In the late 1970s, following the lead and encouragement of Dr. Herman Hellerstein, the father of exercise for cardiac patients, he and colleagues, including Dr. Barry Franklin, developed a model and nationally recognized cardiac rehabilitation program at Sinai Hospital. Recognizing the importance of nutrition and the need for reducing blood cholesterol in coronary disease, he established the first Lipid Clinic and Lipid Research Laboratory in a Cardiology Division in the United States. He joined the Cardiology Division of the University of Michigan in 1991 to pursue his clinical and investigative interests in the early detection and prevention of coronary arteriosclerosis. He has authored many scientific publications on exercise, nutrition, management of lipids, lipid chemistry, and designed and participated in several research trials on the effects of treatment modalities for coronary heart disease and its complications. Current research and clinical interests are to develop cost-effective methods of determining persons at risk for arteriosclerosis and alternatives to by-pass and angioplasty in the management of coronary heart disease. He is married, has two children and three grandchildren. He feels his personal prevention program is enhanced by his passion for golf. "It affords hours of relaxation if you don't let your ego get in the way, stress reduction when you're not putting, great exercise for those who walk, and little time for eating."

Cheryl L. Rock, Ph.D., R.D., FADA

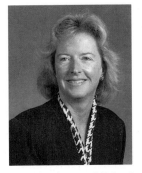

Dr. Rock received her Bachelor of Science degree in Dietetics from Michigan State University, a Master of Medical Science degree in Clinical Nutrition from Emory University, and her doctorate degree in Nutritional Sciences from UCLA. She currently holds the position of Assistant Professor in the Program in Human Nutrition, with a joint appointment in the Comprehensive Cancer Center, at the University of Michigan. Dr. Rock is a full and active member of several recognized scientific and professional associations, including the American Dietetic Association, the American Institute of Nutrition, the American Society for Clinical Nutrition, and the American Federation for Clinical Research. She has published numerous reports, review articles, and book chapters in the areas of carotenoids, micronutrients, and clinical nutrition.

CONTRIBUTING AUTHORS

To Your Health!
Amy

Amy Therese Longcore, M.S.

Amy Longcore received her Bachelor of Science degree in Movement Science at the University of Michigan's School of Kinesiology and her Master of Science degree in Clinical Human Nutrition, also at the University of Michigan. Amy joined the Community Nutrition staff at the University of Michigan Medical Center in 1993. She currently serves as the chief research assistant, responsible for maintaining the food product database for the M-Fit Supermarket Program and *The M-Fit Grocery Shopping Guide*.

Amy organized and directed the focus groups that were conducted to give content and design input for the fourth edition of *The M-Fit Grocery Shopping Guide*. She provided valuable assistance in incorporating the numerous editing changes for the text, interpretation of the new government labeling regulations, and served as the team leader for the criteria task force that was assembled to write the current criteria used to evaluate food products.

Katherine Sigal Rhodes, Ph.D., R.D.

Katherine Rhodes completed her undergraduate work in Botany at Indiana University and received her master and doctorate degrees in Biological Sciences from the University of Michigan. She then entered the field of dietetics and joined the nutrition staff at the University of Michigan Medical Center Preventive Cardiology Services at MedSport in 1988. Kathy is a registered dietitian and counsels patients individually and in groups on cardiovascular risk reduction. Kathy helps each client develop an individualized eating plan to fit personal goals.

Kathy's contributions to this and previous editions of *The M-Fit Grocery Shopping Guide* have been significant. Kathy served on the criteria task force for writing the current criteria used to evaluate food products. She devoted many hours to proofreading the food product sections, and she consulted on the many text edits.

Kathleen Jordan Pompliano, M.S., R.D.

Kathleen Pompliano received her Bachelor of Science degree in Food Science and Nutrition from the University of Massachusetts and her Master of Science degree in Human Nutrition from Eastern Michigan University. Kathy joined the Community Nutrition staff at the University of Michigan Medical Center in 1993. Kathy is a registered dietitian and manager of the M-Fit Supermarket Program, directing the day-to-day operations for sales and marketing. She is the recipient of the 1995 Michigan Dietetic Association Public Relations Award.

Kathy directed the data collection, computer inputting and proofing of the food product section and also served on the criteria task force for writing the current criteria used to evaluate food products for the fourth edition of *The M-Fit Grocery Shopping Guide*.

Chavanne B. Hanson, M.P.H., R.D., L.D.

Chavanne Hanson received her Bachelor of Science degree in Dietetics from Baylor University in Waco, Texas, and her Master of Public Health degree in Human Nutrition from the University of Michigan. She is the Director of Nutrition Services for the University Hospitals Synergy Preventive Cardiology Program in Cleveland, Ohio. Chavanne is a registered dietitian and works in coordination with physicians, exercise physiologists, behavioral specialists, and culinary professionals to establish personalized lifestyle recommendations for clients, so that they may achieve optimal health. She oversees the day-to-day operations of the Synergy program, which includes a state-of-the-art culinary school dedicated to teaching low-fat cuisine.

Chavanne served on the advisory panel and assisted in the development of section criteria for the fourth edition of *The M-Fit Grocery Shopping Guide*.

Lisa C. Bookstein, M.S., R.D.

Lisa Bookstein received her Bachelor of Science degree in Exercise Physiology from the University of California, Los Angeles, and her Master of Science degree from Tufts University School of Nutrition in Boston. She is a registered dietitian and Clinical Research Associate at Children's Memorial Medical Center in Chicago. Lisa specializes in individualized nutrition counseling for lipid disorders, diabetes mellitus, and weight management. She has authored and co-authored professional articles and abstracts and is a contributing author of the *American Diabetes Association Family Cookbook Volume III*. Lisa is a recipient of the 1994 American Dietetic Association Recognized Young Dietitian of the Year Award.

Lisa served on the advisory panel and assisted in the development of section criteria for this and previous editions of *The M-Fit Grocery Shopping Guide*.

ADVISORY PANEL

Chair–Adam Drewnowski, Ph.D.
Professor of Human Nutrition and of Psychology in Psychiatry
Director of the Human Nutrition Department
The University of Michigan School of Public Health

Judith Anderson, Dr.P.H., R.D.
Nutrition Consultant for the Center for Health Promotion
Michigan Department of Public Health

Karen Bremenstul, M.P.H., R.D.
Health Promotion Coordinator for M-CARE
The University of Michigan

Stella Cash, M.Ed., M.S., R.D.
Professor, Foods Program Director, Dietetics
Michigan State University

LaVaughn Palma-Davis, M.A.
Associate Hospital Administrator
The University of Michigan Medical Center

Penny Kris-Etherton, Ph.D., R.D.
Professor of Nutrition
Pennsylvania State University

Cecilia Fileti, M.S., R.D.
President, C. P. Fileti Associates, Inc.
Ann Arbor, Michigan

Lynn Glazewski, M.P.H, R.D.
Nutrition Counseling Center
Food & Nutrition Services
The University of Michigan Hospital

Debi Silverman, M.S., R.D., L.D., FADA
Assistant Professor of Nutrition and Dietetics
Eastern Michigan University

Shari Steinbach, M.S., R.D.
Consumer Affairs and Public Relations
Spartan Stores, Inc.
Grand Rapids, Michigan

Judith Tomer, R.D.
Nutrition Counseling Center
Food & Nutrition Services
The University of Michigan Hospital

Evelyn Tribole, M.S., R.D.
Consulting Nutritionist
Beverly Hills, California

ACKNOWLEDGEMENTS

The authors wish to express their sincere appreciation to John Forsyth, Executive Director, University of Michigan Hospitals, and Patricia A. Warner, Associate Hospital Director, for their enthusiastic support of this book.

The authors also wish to recognize the direction and help given by LaVaughn Palma-Davis, Associate Hospital Administrator, for facilitating our efforts.

We are especially grateful to Adam Drewnowski and other members of the advisory panel for their thoughtful review and professional critique of the manuscript.

Many devoted individuals worked on the preparation of this *Guide*. We especially wish to thank the contributing authors Amy Longcore, Kathy Rhodes, Kathy Pompliano, Chavanne Hanson, and Lisa Bookstein for their dedication and the standard of excellence they maintained throughout the production of this book. We are particularly grateful to Amy Longcore for her extraordinary effort in preparing the manuscript for publication, from data collection, computer inputting of data, interpretation of the new government labeling regulations, organizing and directing the focus groups, serving as team leader for the criteria task force, and assisting with the numerous editing changes for the final text. *That's my girl - she is really special.....*

The contributions of Robin Shear, Jennifer Schill, and Becky Buchanan, along with many other devoted volunteers, were significant for the long hours they endured in the grocery store aisles reviewing food products. We also wish to recognize Janet Simpson for her help in proofing the food product section. The artistic talents of Debbie Cremering enhanced the design and layout of the book.

A special note of thanks goes to the professional staff of USDA's Center for Nutrition Policy and Promotion and The U.S. Food and Drug Administration, who reviewed the sections of the manuscript covering the *Dietary Guidelines for Americans* and food labeling regulations to ensure content accuracy.

Finally, the authors wish to acknowledge the expert editorial contribution by Cheryl Rock for her guidance in the interpretation of nutrition science as it relates to making dietary recommendations. Her contribution was invaluable in preparing this book for publication.

Amy said this book would be a wonderful guide and assist you in maintaining maximum health! God Bless your family & have a grand Holiday and New Year.

Sharon

P.S. Amy's a new age woman - she kept her maiden name when she married my son. Also she didn't want to cause confusion between their two careers. He is a doctor.

TABLE OF CONTENTS

Preface 10
Introduction 11
How to Use The M-Fit Grocery Shopping Guide 13
    Figure 1 - Sample Page from Fats and Oils 14
    Color Coding 15
    Definition of Colors 15
    Typical American Diet 16
    Heart-Healthy American Diet 17
    Symbol Key 18
How to Use The M-Fit Grocery Shopping Guide To: *Follow The Dietary*
Guidelines For Americans 19
    DIETARY GUIDELINES FOR AMERICANS 19
    ❖ Eat a Variety of Foods 20
        Figure 2 – Food Guide Pyramid and How to Use the Daily Food Guide . 21
        How To Use The M-Fit Grocery Shopping Guide To: *Eat A Variety Of Foods* . 23
        Table 1 – Food Guide Pyramid / The M-Fit Grocery Shopping Guide
            Category Comparisons 23
    ❖ *Balance the Food You Eat with Physical Activity; Maintain or Improve Your Weight* . 24
        Table 2 – Suggested Weights for Adults 25
        How To Use The M-Fit Grocery Shopping Guide To: *Balance the Food You Eat*
    with Physical Activity; Maintain or Improve Your Weight. 26
        Why is it Important to Decrease Calories from Fat? 26
    ❖ *Choose a Diet with Plenty of Grain Products, Vegetables and Fruits* 27
        What Are Antioxidants? 27
        What Are Carbohydrates? 28
        Dietary Fiber—What is it and Why is it Good for You? 28
        Table 3 – Food Sources of Antioxidants 29
        How To Use The M-Fit Grocery Shopping Guide To: *Choose a Diet with*
    Plenty of Grain Products, Vegetables and Fruits 31
        Table 4 – Vitamin C, Vitamin A, and Fiber Content of Fruits 32
        Table 5 – Vitamin C, Vitamin A, and Fiber Content of Vegetables . . . 33
    ❖ *Choose a Diet Low in Fat, Saturated Fat, and Cholesterol* 34
        What is the Recommendation for Amount of Fat in the Diet? 34
        Table 6 – Upper Limits of Fat and Cholesterol Recommended 35
        What is Cholesterol and How Does it Affect Your Health? 35
        Table 7 – Cholesterol and Saturated Fat Contents of Selected Foods . . 36
        What are HDL and LDL Cholesterol and Triglycerides? 37
        How Do Fats Affect Cholesterol? 38
        What Is Saturated Fat? 39
        What Is Monounsaturated Fat? 39
        What Is Polyunsaturated Fat? 40
        Table 8 – Sources Of Fat and Effect on Blood Cholesterol Levels . . . 42
        What About Hydrogenated Oils: Are They Good or Bad Fats? 43
        Table 9 – Effect of Hydrogenation on Fatty Acid Content 43
        How To Use The M-Fit Grocery Shopping Guide To: *Choose A Diet Low*
    in Fat, Saturated Fat, and Cholesterol 44
    ❖ *Choose a Diet Moderate in Sugars* 45
        Table 10 – Where are the Added Sugars? 46
        How To Use The M-Fit Grocery Shopping Guide To: *Choose a Diet*
    Moderate in Sugars 47
    ❖ *Choose a Diet Moderate in Salt and Sodium* 48

How To Use The M-Fit Grocery Shopping Guide To: *Choose a Diet*
    Moderate in Salt and Sodium 49
❖ *If You Drink Alcoholic Beverages, Do So In Moderation* 50
Learn to Use the New Food Label to Select a Healthful Diet 51
    What's New About The New Food Label? 51
        Serving Sizes 51
        Mandatory Nutrients 52
        Daily Value and % Daily Value 52
        Nutrient Content Claims 52
        Health Claims 54
    Figure 3 – The New Food Label at a Glance (Nutrition Facts Label) 55
    Figure 4 – The New Food Label at a Glance (nutrient content claims
        and health claims) 56
Still Confused About the New Food Label? 57
Food Products
    Baking Mixes (Pancakes, Muffins, Biscuits) 59
    Baking Mixes (Desserts) 65
    Bread 71
    Bread Products 83
    Cereal 93
    Chips, Pretzels, Popcorn, and Other Snacks 103
    Cookies, Bars, and Snack Cakes 121
    Crackers 139
    Pasta, Potatoes, Stuffing, and Grains 149
    Vegetables 167
    Fruits 179
    Cheese and Cheese Products 187
    Milk and Milk Alternatives 197
    Yogurt and Non-Dairy Alternatives 203
    Beef, Lamb, Pork, Veal 207
    Poultry and Game 213
    Fish 219
    Lunchmeats, Cured Meats, and Canned Meats, Fish, Poultry 227
    Egg Substitutes and Egg Products 241
    Legumes and Meat Alternatives 245
    Meals and Main Dishes 255
    Soups 277
    Nut and Seed Butters 289
    Butter and Margarine 293
    Cream, Cream Substitutes, and Toppings 299
    Fats and Oils 305
    Salad Dressing 311
    Desserts 319
    Beverages 335
    Dips and Salsas 353
    Entrée Sauces 361
Appendix A: Body Mass Index 369
Appendix B: Waist-To-Hip Ratio 370
Appendix C: Nutrient Content Claims and Definitions 371
Appendix D: Fat Substitutions Suggestions 373
References 374
Index 379
Order Form 397

PREFACE

by Kim A. Eagle, M.D.

Director, Clinical Cardiology
Co-Director, Heart Care Program
Associate Chief, Division of Cardiology
Associate Professor of Internal Medicine
University of Michigan

Despite major advances in understanding the cause of coronary heart disease and its treatment, and despite health care expenditures measured in billions of dollars annually for this problem, coronary artery disease continues to kill more American citizens than any other disease process. In 1996, more than 500,000 Americans will have heart attacks, and several hundred thousand individuals will suffer sudden, unexpected cardiac death due to the same disease. Yet, despite these discouraging observations, new research in the role of lifestyle modification and aggressive treatment of abnormal cholesterol profiles (with diet, exercise, and, when appropriate, cholesterol lowering medications) has Americans facing a far more optimistic future than might have been imagined just several years ago. Recent studies strongly suggest that preventive measures not only work, but have **profound** results, lowering heart attack and death rates as much as 30 to 40 percent in patients with known coronary heart disease.

The ability to prevent, delay, and, for some patients, reverse the atherosclerotic process that ultimately leads to coronary heart disease begins with the diet. In this regard, The M-Fit Grocery Shopping Guide is a wonderfully practical tool for helping people understand and achieve a heart-conscious diet. First, it introduces the interrelationship of exercise, body weight, and diet. Next, it helps you understand, in broad terms, heart-healthy goals for total intake of fats, cholesterol, vegetables, grain products, vitamins, and proteins. Then, after reviewing concepts of how foods and their ingredients are labeled, the Guide walks you through the grocery store, aisle by aisle, brand by brand, to identify those products that contain healthful ingredients and those that are less heart-healthy. For example, do you know which cuts of red meat are the leanest? Do you know which snack foods are the best choices? Are you aware that you can now choose among dozens of fat-free ice creams and frozen yogurts? Let this book guide you to the many choices you can make to achieve the kind of diet that is not only heart-healthy, but also very enjoyable for you and your loved ones.

The M-Fit Grocery Shopping Guide has already benefitted thousands of individuals. By combining the talents of professionals in nutrition and preventive medicine, the authors and editor have achieved just the right balance between current medical science, real-life practicality, and range-of-product review to help virtually anyone interested in heart-healthy eating.

Isn't it great to know that "eating right" for the heart allows a wide choice of foods, yet achieves so much benefit in improving and prolonging life?

Bon appetit!!

Kim A. Eagle

Introduction

Why is this book important for you?

Cardiovascular disease is the No. 1 killer in America. To help put the startling consequences of this disease into perspective, here are a few potent facts:[1]

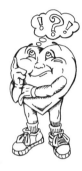

FACT: More than two out of every five Americans die of cardiovascular disease.

FACT: Of the current U.S. population of about 252 million, more than 56 million people—*greater than one in five Americans*—suffer from some form of cardiovascular disease.

FACT: The most current statistics released by the American Heart Association state that heart and blood vessel disease kills more than 923,000 Americans yearly—*this accounts for one death every 32 seconds.*

Heart disease remains the leading cause of death in both men and women. An increased blood cholesterol level has been implicated as an important risk factor for the development of coronary artery disease. It is estimated that 55% (139 million) of Americans have cholesterol levels greater than 200 mg/dL and are therefore at an increased risk for the development of coronary artery disease. Furthermore, only 3% of middle-aged American men (35 to 57 years of age) are considered at low risk for cardiovascular death. Low risk is defined by non-smoking, normal blood cholesterol, normal blood pressure, and no family history of heart attack.[2]

Eating better is important for all people, regardless of risk factor status. Prevention strategies work! There has been a dramatic reduction in deaths from heart attacks in the United States during the past 40 years. Fifty-four percent of the 630,000 heart disease deaths prevented over a 10-year period in the 1970s were considered to be due to lifestyle changes related to the reduction of blood cholesterol levels and smoking cessation, while only 3.5% of the deaths prevented were attributable to coronary by-pass operations and 10% to other medical treatments. It has been estimated that 75% of the premature deaths from cardiovascular disease may be preventable by simple changes in food choices and amounts.[3]

The population and adult treatment panel for blood cholesterol reduction of the National Institutes of Health predicts that the future incidence and mortality from coronary disease will be reduced through modifications of our current dietary habits.[4] Dietary measures appear to contribute to a reduction in mortality and re-occurrence rates in heart attack survivors, and a reduction in dietary saturated fats has been associated with a decrease in the rate of progression, fewer new blockages, and reversal of coronary heart disease.[5-7]

Did you know that a powerful tool for preventing heart disease is in your grocery store? But, you first have to know how to find it! The purpose of *The M-Fit Grocery Shopping Guide* is to assist you in making wise food selections that are appropriate for controlling the intake of total fat, saturated fat, cholesterol, sodium, calories, and increasing dietary fiber.

Scientific studies have shown that diets high in saturated fat and cholesterol may adversely affect health by predisposing people to heart diseases, obesity, and certain types of cancer.[8] On the other hand, it has been shown that diets *lower* in fat and *higher* in dietary fiber reduce blood cholesterol and blood pressure, lower elevated blood sugar levels in persons with diabetes, lower risk for coronary heart disease, and may improve health and well-being.[9]

Our goal is to teach you to make better food choices so that you can lower your risk for heart disease. We recognize that adherence to nutrition guidelines can't guarantee health or well-being; however, good eating habits based on wise food selections can help you stay healthy and may even improve your health.

The University of Michigan Medical Center has a strong commitment to prevention. We emphasize the importance of assessing each individual's risk for coronary heart disease, as well as a community-approach to lowering risk factors for disease.

To optimize prevention through nutrition, our health experts at the University of Michigan Medical Center Preventive Cardiology Programs have developed *The M-Fit Grocery Shopping Guide* to help you modify your risk for heart disease through wise food choices.

Initially, the *Guide* was developed as an educational tool for University of Michigan cardiology patients who suffered from heart disease, high cholesterol, and high blood pressure. We soon realized that many people concerned about their risk for heart disease would benefit from the information contained in this *Guide*, and we are now pleased to offer it to those interested in maximizing prevention through nutrition. Health professionals will also benefit from the more technical information contained in this *Guide*.

Some of the most important steps you can take towards healthier eating habits are those taken behind the grocery cart. *The M-Fit Grocery Shopping Guide* is a comprehensive and convenient "map" guiding you to the best nutritional choices for you and your family.

Bon appetit, and good shopping!

HOW TO USE THE M-FIT GROCERY SHOPPING GUIDE

The *M-Fit Grocery Shopping Guide* is an aisle-by-aisle listing of brand name foods designating those that are **"BEST"** choices for healthy eating and those foods that should be consumed **less often** in order to maintain an overall healthy diet.

The *Guide* is organized into 31 major food categories (see table of contents). Individual criteria for classifying foods have been established for each category: **"BEST CHOICE," "ACCEPTABLE CHOICE,"** or **"OCCASIONAL CHOICE."**

Because of the unique nature of foods, certain criteria established for one type of food may not apply to another. For example, in the Fats and Oils section, all products are high in fat and should be used in moderation. However, choosing the appropriate **type** of fat is equally as important as monitoring the **amount** of fat. There are three criteria columns for this category: green "BEST CHOICE," yellow "ACCEPTABLE CHOICE," and red "OCCASIONAL CHOICE." Refer to Figure 1, page 14, for pictorial representation.

BEST CHOICE

ACCEPTABLE CHOICE

OCCASIONAL CHOICE

In this example, the "BEST CHOICE" classification is given to the oils that are predominantly monounsaturated fat. Oils that are predominantly polyunsaturated are classified as "ACCEPTABLE CHOICE." Oils that are predominantly saturated may significantly elevate blood cholesterol levels, which, in turn, can increase the risk for heart disease. For this reason, saturated fats are classified in the "OCCASIONAL CHOICE" category.

Foods that provide a significant amount of fat such as butter, margarine, salad dressing, snack foods, dairy foods, nut butters, meats, desserts, and entrée meals will be evaluated using fat as a major criterion. Alternatively, foods that provide small amounts of fat to the diet such as grain products, cereals, breads, fruits, vegetables, legumes, and some beverages will be evaluated using other nutritional criteria, such as fiber, sodium, and added sugar (which contributes extra calories), in addition to fat as the major criterion. For example, *The M-Fit Grocery Shopping Guide* does not evaluate Cereals (p. 93) in the same manner as Fats and Oils (p. 305). Whereas Fats and Oils provide a significant amount of fat to our diets, Cereals may provide a significant amount of fiber to the diet. Therefore, in addition to fat, fiber is added to the evaluating criteria of the Cereal category.

In all cases, criteria have been written to comply with the new food labeling regulations of the Food and Drug Administration (FDA) as specified by the ***Nutrition Labeling and Education Act*** (NLEA) of 1990.[10] For an explanation on how to use the new food label to select a healthful diet, see pages 55 and 56.

FIGURE 1

SAMPLE PAGE FROM FATS AND OILS

BRAND	BEST CHOICE	ACCEPTABLE CHOICE	OCCASIONAL CHOICE
	Predominantly Monounsaturated Fat	Predominantly Polyunsaturated Fat	Predominantly Saturated Fat
OILS			
Alessi	∇ Extra Vergine Di Oliva		
All Brands	∇ Avocado Oil ∇ Canola Oil ∇ High Oleic Safflower ∇ High Oleic Sunflower ∇ Olive Oil ∇ Peanut Oil	∇ Corn Oil ∇ Safflower Oil ∇ Sesame Oil ∇ Soybean Oil ∇ Sunflower Oil	∇ Coconut Oil
Arrowhead Mills		∇ Flax Seed Oil	
Bella	∇ Olive Oil		
Bellino	Olive Oil: ∇ Extra Virgin		

Bertolli	Olive Oil:
	  ∇ Classico
	  ∇ Extra Light		

Calavo	∇ Avocado Oil		
California Naturals	∇ Fra Diavalo Hot Oil ∇ Pesto Pasta Oil		
Colavita	∇ Extra Virgin Olive Oil ∇ Limonolio ∇ Olive Oil ∇ Pepperolio		
Crisco	∇ Corn and Canola Oil Blend ∇ Natural Blend Oil ∇ Pure Vegetable Oil ∇ Puritan Canola Oil		
DaVinci	∇ 100% Pure Olive Oil ∇ Extra Virgin Olive Oil		
Delallo	∇ Olive Oil		
Dell' Alpe	∇ Extra Virgin Olive Oil ∇ Olive Oil		
Ferrara	∇ 100% Extra Virgin Olive Oil		

∇ Low Sodium, 140 mg. or less per serving

2   Fats and Oils

COLOR CODING

Color coding has been added in an attempt to make the book more user-friendly. The colors green, yellow, and red are used to give the criteria for evaluating foods an added dimension, further aiding the consumer in making wise food selections within each food category. Criteria for evaluating foods and classifying them into **"BEST CHOICE," "ACCEPTABLE CHOICE,"** and **"OCCASIONAL CHOICE"** categories are explained at the beginning of each product section. Color triangles next to each criteria statement correspond to the colored heading at the top of the product columns.

DEFINITIONS OF COLORS

▲ **GREEN**: "BEST CHOICE" — Products coded green are the best selections within each food category. These selections are usually the lowest in fat (total fat or saturated fat). In some sections, amounts of sodium, fiber or sugar may be used in addition to fat to determine the most desirable food selections. Although foods in this column are identified as the best choice within a particular food category, it **does not** mean that these food choices should be consumed indiscriminately. Variety and moderation are important in all product categories.

▲ **YELLOW**: "ACCEPTABLE CHOICE" — Products coded yellow are acceptable food choices. Most products in these categories contain greater amounts of total fat or saturated fat and in some cases are higher in sodium or sugar or are lower in fiber than those coded "green."

▲ **RED**: "OCCASIONAL CHOICE" — Products coded red are higher in total fat or saturated fat than products in the green or yellow categories. Red **does not** mean a person should never eat a particular food in this listing. Instead, the red color is meant to alert the consumer that these foods should be eaten less often than comparable foods within the same category. The reason for this is that regular consumption of "red" labeled foods without limitation, over the course of several years, may contribute to added risk for heart disease. Red-coded products may be incorporated into the diet by using smaller serving sizes.

The intent of *The M-Fit Grocery Shopping Guide* is to help consumers identify foods that are the best choices in each product category. The intent is not to suggest that only green-coded or yellow-coded foods should be consumed in order to maintain a healthful diet. On the contrary, foods listed in all three color-coded columns can be included in the overall diet while still maintaining the recommended amounts of nutrients. The key is **Balance, Variety,** and **Moderation**. For example, higher-fat food products listed in the red "Occasional Choice" column can be balanced with lower-fat foods in the green "Best Choice" and yellow "Acceptable Choice" columns so that the average amount of fat consumed over several days falls within the recommended limits (i.e., less than 30% calories from fat). The goal is not to minimize fat intake, but to reduce consumption to recommended levels which are lower than what the typical American consumes. The following examples illustrate this point.

TYPICAL AMERICAN DIET

(34% calories from fat, 12% calories from saturated fat, 2400 Calories)

Meal	Serving Size	Color Designation
Breakfast		
Puffed Rice Cereal	1 cup	Yellow
2% Milk	3/4 cup	Yellow
Orange Juice	8 fl oz	Green
Coffee	12 fl oz	————
Cream (Half-and-Half)	1 Tbsp	Red
Morning Snack		
Doughnuts (plain)	1 item	Red
Coffee	12 fl oz	————
Non-Dairy Powdered Creamer	1 tsp	Red
Lunch		
Ham and Cheese Sandwich	1 item	
w/Regular Ham	1 oz	Yellow
w/Cheddar Cheese	1 oz	Red
w/Mayonnaise	1 Tbsp	Red
w/White Bread	2 slices	Yellow
Potato Chips	1 oz	Red
Carrot Sticks	1 cup	Green
Cola	12 fl oz	Yellow
Afternoon Snack		
Chocolate Bar	1 bar	Red
Dinner		
Chicken Breast, fried	5 oz	Red
Mashed Potatoes	3/4 cup	Green
Canned Peas & Carrots	3/4 cup	Green
Brown & Serve Roll	1 roll	Yellow
Margarine (corn oil)	1 tsp	Yellow
Salad		
(iceberg lettuce, tomatoes, carrots)	1 cup	Green
w/Ranch Dressing	2 Tbsp	Red
Evening Snack		
Vanilla Ice Cream	1 cup	Red

HEART-HEALTHY AMERICAN DIET

(26% calories from fat, 7% calories from saturated fat, 2300 Calories)

Meal	Serving Size	Color Designation
Breakfast		
Ready-to-eat Oat Cereal	1 1/4 cups	Green
Skim Milk	1 cup	Green
Orange Juice	8 fl oz	Green
Coffee	12 fl oz	———
Creamer (Half-and-Half)	1 Tbsp	Red
Strawberries	3/4 cup	Green
Morning Snack		
Blueberry Muffin	1 muffin	Red
Coffee	12 fl oz	———
Fat-Free Creamer	1 tsp	Green
Lunch		
Grilled Chicken Sandwich	1 item	
Grilled Chicken Breast	4 oz	Green
w/Swiss Cheese	1 oz	Red
w/Mayonnaise	1 Tbsp	Red
w/Lettuce	2 leaves	Green
w/Tomatoes	1 slice	Green
w/Wheat Bun	1 bun	Yellow
Carrot Sticks	1 cup	Green
Instant Tea (unsweetened)	12 fl oz	Green
Afternoon Snack		
Pretzels	1 oz	Green
Apple	1 medium	Green
Diet Cola	12 oz can	Green
Dinner		
Spaghetti (cooked)	1 1/2 cups	Green
w/Meatballs	1 oz	Red
w/Tomato & Mushroom Sauce	3/4 cup	Green
Salad		
(romaine lettuce, tomatoes, carrots)	1 cup	Green
w/Light Ranch Salad Dressing	2 Tbsp	Green
Whole Wheat Roll	1 roll	Yellow
w/Margarine (corn oil)	1 tsp	Yellow
Evening Snack		
Low-Fat Vanilla Ice Cream	1 cup	Yellow

**The following symbols will be used throughout the book
to identify certain food choices:**

Symbol	Key
▲	High sodium, 480 milligrams or greater per serving [20% or more of the Daily Value (2400 milligrams per day)].
▽	Low sodium, 140 milligrams or less per serving.
★	High fiber, 5 grams or higher per serving [20% or more of the Daily Value (25 grams per day)].
☆	Good Source of fiber, between 2.5 and 5.0 grams per serving [contains between 10-19 % of the Daily Value (25 grams per day)].
●	Fish and Veal containing greater than 95 milligrams cholesterol per 3.5 ounce serving.

Authors' Note
Individuals have different nutrient and caloric requirements. It is beyond the scope of this book to prescribe actual amounts of certain foods that should be eaten to promote good health. The purpose of this book is to identify those foods that are the best choices for healthy eating and those that may need to be limited by most people who are concerned about their risk for cardiovascular disease. Individual requirements need to be assessed by a registered dietitian or other qualified health professional.

HOW TO USE THE M-FIT GROCERY SHOPPING GUIDE TO:
FOLLOW THE
"DIETARY GUIDELINES FOR AMERICANS"

The *Dietary Guidelines for Americans*[11] is the most up-to-date advice from nutrition scientists and is the basis of federal nutrition policy. These guidelines are considered to be the foundation for formulating all nutrition recommendations. They are not individualized to meet each person's specific requirements, however, they give a basis from which to work. For this reason, the authors have used the Dietary Guidelines as the "nutritional standard" from which to base their product and diet recommendations. *The M-Fit Grocery Shopping Guide* is designed to help individuals make food choices that will help them meet the *Dietary Guidelines For Americans* as they aim for heart-healthy eating.

DIETARY GUIDELINES FOR AMERICANS

- ❖ Eat a variety of foods
- ❖ Balance the food you eat with physical activity; maintain or improve your weight
- ❖ Choose a diet with plenty of grain products, vegetables and fruits
- ❖ Choose a diet low in fat, saturated fat, and cholesterol
- ❖ Choose a diet moderate in sugars
- ❖ Choose a diet moderate in salt and sodium
- ❖ If you drink alcoholic beverages, do so in moderation

These guidelines are jointly developed by the U. S. Department of Agriculture (USDA) and the U.S. Department of Health and Human Services (USHHS) and are revised every five years.[11,12] These guidelines are for healthy Americans ages 2 years and over and are not intended for younger children and infants, whose dietary needs are different. The guidelines reflect the recommendations of nutrition authorities and are based on publications such as *The Surgeon General's Report on Nutrition and Health,*[8] *Diet and Health: Implications for Reducing Chronic Disease Risk,*[13] *Recommended Dietary Allowances,*[14] and *Healthy People 2000.*[15]

Nutrition authorities agree that there is sufficient knowledge about diet's effect on health to encourage the adoption of certain dietary practices by Americans. Although food alone cannot make you healthy, a diet based on these guidelines can help keep you healthy and may improve your health. Many factors can influence your health, such as your genetics, your environment, and the health care you receive. Your lifestyle, such as how much you exercise and whether you smoke, drink alcohol in excess, or abuse drugs, is also an important factor that affects your health.

By following the *Dietary Guidelines for Americans,* you can enjoy better health and may lower your chances of getting certain diseases, such as heart disease, high blood pressure, stroke, certain cancers, and the most common type of diabetes (Type II diabetes mellitus). These guidelines call for moderation with an emphasis on avoiding extremes in diet. In other words, either eating too much or eating too little of a particular food or nutrient can be harmful.

The discussion that follows will explain each of these dietary guidelines and give suggestions on how to implement them using the food product selections in *The M-Fit Grocery Shopping Guide*. Sections of this discussion were taken in part from: Dietary Guidelines for Americans[11] and Using Food Labels to Follow the Dietary Guidelines for Americans: A Reference.[16]

EAT A VARIETY OF FOODS

Eating a variety of foods is the key to a healthful diet. The average person needs more than 40 nutrients to maintain good health. Essential nutrients include vitamins, minerals, amino acids from protein, certain fatty acids from fat, and sources of energy or calories (protein, carbohydrates and fat).

No single food can supply all the nutrients in the amounts you need for good health. Certain foods may be good sources of some nutrients but are lacking in others. For example, milk supplies calcium but little iron; meat supplies iron but little calcium. To ensure a nutritious diet, it is necessary to eat a variety of foods.

It is easy to eat a variety of foods by following the recommendations of The *Food Guide Pyramid*[17] (See Figure 2). The *Food Guide Pyramid* suggests a range of servings from five major food groups (1) bread, cereal, rice, and pasta group; (2) vegetable group; (3) fruit group; (4) milk, yogurt, and cheese group; and (5) meat, poultry, fish, dry beans, eggs, and nuts group. Fats, oils, and sweets are located at the tip of the *Pyramid*. While there is no suggested servings established for this group, it is okay to include selections from the tip of the *Pyramid*. However, individuals are cautioned to use these foods sparingly, especially those who are sedentary or trying to lose weight. Each of the food groups provides some, but not all, of the 40 or more nutrients needed for good health. Foods in one group cannot replace those in another. In other words, no one food group is more important than another. To ensure adequate nutrition for good health, you need to incorporate them all. When planning a healthful diet, remember these key words: **Balance, Variety,** and **Moderation**.

FIGURE 2

Food Guide Pyramid
A Guide to Daily Food Choices

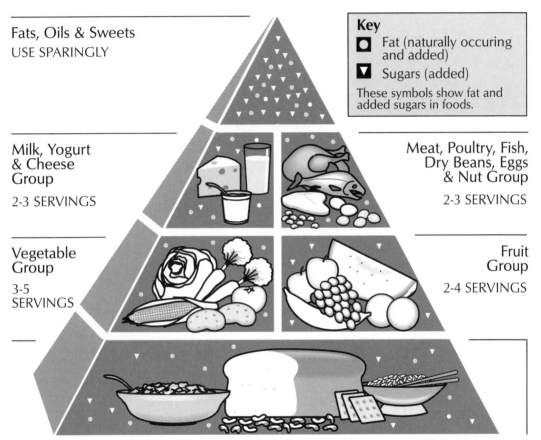

Fats, Oils & Sweets
USE SPARINGLY

Key
◻ Fat (naturally occuring and added)
▼ Sugars (added)

These symbols show fat and added sugars in foods.

Milk, Yogurt & Cheese Group

2-3 SERVINGS

Meat, Poultry, Fish, Dry Beans, Eggs & Nut Group

2-3 SERVINGS

Vegetable Group

3-5 SERVINGS

Fruit Group

2-4 SERVINGS

Source: U.S. Department of Agriculture/U.S. Department of Health and Human Services

Bread, Cereal Rice & Pasta Group

6-11 SERVINGS

Use the Food Guide Pyramid to help you eat better every day . . . the Dietary Guidelines Way. Start with plenty of Breads, Cereals, Rice, and Pasta; Vegetables; and Fruits. Add two to three servings from the Milk Group and two to three servings from the Meat Group.

Each of these food groups provides some, but not all, of the nutrients you need. No one food group is more important than another—for good health you need them all. Go easy on fats, oils, and sweets, the foods in the small tip of the Pyramid.

To order a copy of "The Food Guide Pyramid" booklet, send a $1.00 check or money order made out to the Superintendent of Documents to: Consumer Information Center, Department 159-Y, Pueblo, Colorado 81009.

U.S. Department of Agriculture, Human Nutrition Information Service, August, 1992, Leaflet No. 572.

How to Use The Daily Food Guide

WHAT COUNTS AS ONE SERVING?

Breads, Cereals, Rice, and Pasta
1 slice of bread
1/2 cup of cooked rice or pasta
1/2 cup of cooked cereal
1 ounce of ready-to-eat cereal

Vegetables
1/2 cup of chopped raw or cooked vegetables
1 cup of leafy raw vegetables

Fruits
1 piece of fruit or melon wedge
3/4 cup of juice
1/2 cup of canned fruit
1/4 cup of dried fruit

Milk, Yogurt, and Cheese
1 cup of milk or yogurt
1 1/2 to 2 ounces of cheese

Meat, Poultry, Fish, Dry Beans, Eggs, and Nuts
2 1/2 to 3 ounces of cooked lean meat, poultry, or fish
Count 1/2 cup of cooked beans, or 1 egg, or 2 tablespoons of peanut butter as 1 ounce of lean meat (about 1/3 serving)

Fats, Oils, and Sweets
LIMIT CALORIES FROM THESE especially if you need to lose weight

> The amount you eat may be more than one serving. For example, a dinner portion of spaghetti would count as two or three servings of pasta.

How many servings do you need each day?

	Women & some older adults	Children, teen girls, active women, most men	Teen boys & active men
Calorie level*	about 1,600	about 2,200	about 2,800
Bread group	6	9	11
Vegetable group	3	4	5
Fruit group	2	3	4
Milk group	**2-3	**2-3	**2-3
Meat group	2, for a total of 5 ounces	2, for a total of 6 ounces	3, for a total of 7 ounces

*These are the calorie levels if you choose lowfat, lean foods from the 5 major food groups and use foods from the fats, oils, and sweets group sparingly.

**Women who are pregnant or breastfeeding, teen-agers, and young adults to age 24 need 3 servings.

A Closer Look at Fat and Added Sugars

The small tip of the Pyramid shows fats, oils, and sweets. These are foods such as salad dressings, cream, butter, margarine, sugars, soft drinks, candies, and sweet desserts. Alcoholic beverages are also part of this group.

These foods provide calories but few vitamins and minerals. Most people should go easy on foods from this group.

Some fat or sugar symbols are shown in the other food groups. That's to remind you that some foods in these groups can also be high in fat and added sugars, such as cheese or ice cream from the milk group, or french fries from the vegetable group. When choosing foods for a healthful diet, consider the fat and added sugars in your choices from all the food groups, not just fats, oils, and sweets from the Pyramid tip.

HOW TO USE THE M-FIT GROCERY SHOPPING GUIDE TO:
EAT A VARIETY OF FOODS

The M-Fit Grocery Shopping Guide is sectioned into 31 food categories which can be matched up with each of the major groups in the *Food Guide Pyramid* (see Table 1).

TABLE 1

Food Guide Pyramid / The M-Fit Grocery Shopping Guide Comparisons

FOOD GUIDE PYRAMID	THE M-FIT GROCERY SHOPPING GUIDE
Bread, Cereal, Rice, & Pasta Group 6 – 11 servings	Baking Mixes (pancake, muffins, biscuits), p. 59 Breads, p. 71 Bread Products, p. 83 Chips, Pretzels, Popcorn, Snacks, p. 103 Cereals, p. 93 Cookies, Bars, and Snack Cakes, p. 121 Crackers, p. 139 Pasta, Suffings & Grains, p. 149
Vegetable Group 3 – 5 servings	Potato and Potato Mixes, p. 149 Vegetables, p. 167 Vegetable Juices, p. 335
Fruit Group 2 – 4 servings	Fruits, p. 179 Fruit Juices, p. 335
Milk, Yogurt, & Cheese Group 2 – 3 servings	Cheese and Cheese Products, p. 187 Milk and Milk Alternatives, p. 197 Yogurt and Non-Dairy Alternatives, p. 203

Meat, Poultry, Fish, Dry Beans,
    Eggs, & Nuts Group
2 – 3 servings
	Beef, Lamb, Pork, Veal, p. 207
	Poultry and Game, p. 213
	Fish, p. 219
	Lunchmeats, Cured Meats and
	    Canned Meat, Fish and Poultry, p. 227
	Egg Substitutes and Egg Products, p. 241
	Legumes and Meat Alternatives, p. 245
	Meals and Main Dishes, p. 255
	Soups, p. 277
	Nut and Seed Butter, p. 289

Fats, Oils, & Sweets USE SPARINGLY	Cream, Cream Substitutes and Toppings, p. 299 Fats and Oils, p. 305 Butter and Margarine, p. 293 Salad Dressing, p. 311 Desserts (sorbet, gelatins, sherbet), p. 319 Baking Mixes (desserts), p. 65 Beverages, p. 335

The food choices listed in the **"BEST CHOICE"** and **"ACCEPTABLE CHOICE"** categories will help guide you to the lower fat, lower saturated fat, lower cholesterol, lower sodium, lower sugar (and thus, calories) and higher fiber food selections. The food choices listed in the "**OCCASIONAL CHOICE**" category will help you to identify foods that should be consumed less often in order to maintain an overall healthy diet. Follow the recommended serving for each food group in order to ensure a nutritionally-complete diet.

BALANCE THE FOOD YOU EAT WITH PHYSICAL ACTIVITY; MAINTAIN OR IMPROVE YOUR WEIGHT

Managing your weight plays a vital role in maintaining good health while enhancing the quality of your life. The key is to maintain or improve your weight through proper food choices and exercise habits. Making permanent lifestyle changes that include balancing the amount of energy in food with the amount of energy the body uses through physical activity is critical to the successful achievement of long-term weight management.

A variety of factors, including your genetic makeup, your physical activity level and dietary practices, influence your weight. Obesity is one of the most prevalent diet-related problems in the United States. One-third of American adults over the age of 18 are overweight and nearly one-tenth are obese, according to reports published by government health agencies.[8,13,18] Government survey data defines overweight as having a Body Mass Index (BMI) greater than or equal to 27.8 for men and 27.3 for women, and severe overweight as having a BMI greater than or equal to 31.1 for men and 32.3 for women.[18] Refer to Appendix A, page 369, to determine your own BMI.

Being overweight increases a person's risk for high blood pressure, heart disease, stroke, some types of diabetes, certain cancers and gallbladder disease.[8,13] Although less common, being too thin is also linked with health problems such as anorexia nervosa, osteoporosis in women, and early death in both women and men.

To date, researchers have yet to determine a precise way to describe a "healthy" weight. In the meantime, you can use the guidelines on Table 2, page 25, to help judge if your weight is within the range suggested for persons of your height.[11] The table applies to adult men and women of all ages. The health risks due to excess weight appear to be the same for older as for younger adults. The weight ranges given in the table may change, based on research in progress.

Ranges of weights are given in the chart because people of the same height may have equal amounts of body fat but differ in amounts of muscle and bone. The higher weights in the range apply to people with more muscle and a larger frame, while those with less muscle and a smaller frame will fall at the lower end of the range.

Weights above the range are believed to be unhealthy for most people. Weights slightly below the range may be healthy for some small-boned people, but are sometimes linked to health problems, especially if sudden, unplanned weight loss has occurred.

The distribution of fat may be an important determinant of cardiovascular risk. Research suggests that, for adults, body shape (i.e. Waist–to–Hip ratio) as well as total weight is important to health. Excess fat in the abdomen (apple-shape) is believed to be a greater health risk than that in the hips and thighs (pear-shape).[19,20.] To calculate your Waist–To–Hip ratio see Appendix B, page 370.

Managing your weight plays a vital role in maintaining good health while enhancing the quality of your life. The key is to achieve and maintain your "healthy" weight through proper food choices and exercise habits. By making permanent lifestyle changes, long-term weight management can be achieved.

TABLE 2

Healthy Weight Ranges for Men and Women

Height[1]	Weight (in pounds)[2]
4"10"	91-119
4'11"	94-124
5'0"	97-128
5'1"	101-132
5'2"	104-137
5'3"	107-141
5'4"	111-146
5'5"	114-150
5'6"	118-155
5'7"	121-160
5'8"	125-164
5'9"	129-169
5'10"	132-174
5'11"	136-179
6'0"	140-184
6'1"	144-189
6'2"	148-195
6'3"	152-200
6'4"	156-205
6'5"	160-211
6'6"	164-216

[1]Without shoes
[2]Without clothes

Source: Derived from National Research Council, 1989, for adults.

HOW TO USE THE M-FIT GROCERY SHOPPING GUIDE TO:
BALANCE THE FOOD YOU EAT WITH PHYSICAL ACTIVITY; MAINTAIN OR IMPROVE YOUR WEIGHT

In addition to exercise, the most effective way to maintain a healthy weight range is to achieve a moderate caloric intake, which can be facilitated by monitoring the total fat content in your diet. *The M-Fit Grocery Shopping Guide* will help you select foods that are lower in fat. Each food category lists the fat-free or low-fat food choices in the "green" or "yellow" columns. The foods listed in the green "BEST CHOICE" columns are generally lower in fat than those listed in the yellow "ACCEPTABLE CHOICE" columns. The only exception to this is in the category: Fats and Oils. These products are evaluated by **type** of fat. Choices that contain primarily monounsaturated fats are identified as the green "BEST CHOICE" and choices that contain primarily polyunsaturated fats are identified as yellow "ACCEPTABLE CHOICE." The products listed in this category are high in **total** fat and should be consumed sparingly, especially by those persons who are trying to lose weight or who have sedentary lifestyles.

Why is it important to decrease calories from fat?

Fat is an essential nutrient, but one that is needed in only very small amounts. Fat is very dense in calories. In fact, the caloric content of one gram of fat is greater than two times the caloric content of one gram of carbohydrate or protein. For example:

Fat	=	9 calories per gram
Protein	=	4 calories per gram
Carbohydrate	=	4 calories per gram
Alcohol	=	7 calories per gram

Therefore, eating a high-fat diet makes it easy to consume excessive calories, so that weight gain is much more likely to occur. As an example, in one study, researchers provided eight healthy non-obese young men with different 'buffets' of food, and instructed them to eat until they were satisfied. When high-fat food choices were offered, the subjects' daily intake averaged 4,135 calories per day (with 53% from fat). When these foods were replaced with low-fat food choices, the subjects' daily intake averaged 2,998 calories per day (with 22% from fat).[21]

Therefore, decreasing your total fat intake can help achieve a significant reduction in total calories, facilitating weight loss. There is no question that in addition to increasing your physical activity, reducing your intake of fat can be an effective way to reduce weight. However, it is important to remember that the indiscriminate use of fat-free or low-fat foods can contribute as many, if not more, calories than normally consumed. Excess intake of calories from any source, whether it be from protein, carbohydrate, fat or alcohol will lead to weight gain.

CHOOSE A DIET WITH PLENTY OF
GRAIN PRODUCTS, VEGETABLES, AND FRUITS

As the relationship between diet and health has become more clearly understood, nutrition authorities have recognized the importance of increasing consumption of fruits, vegetables and grain products. Federal health agencies and scientific advisory bodies[8,11,13,22] all recommend that Americans should eat a balanced diet lower in fat that includes lots of fruits and vegetables. The rationale for emphasizing vegetables, fruits, and grain products is to provide the recommended amounts of vitamins and minerals, to increase dietary fiber intake, and to replace calories from fat with calories from carbohydrates. Vegetables, fruits and grain products are good sources of complex carbohydrates, dietary fiber, vitamins, and minerals.

Epidemiological studies (studies of large population groups that examine the relationship between certain behaviors and risk of disease) have found that people consuming diets rich in fruits and vegetables have a significantly lower risk of developing cancer and other chronic diseases.[23-25] To encourage increased consumption of fruits and vegetables, the *5-a-Day for Better Health!* national project, between the Produce for Better Health Foundation and the National Cancer Institute, was launched in the early 1990s. The program was designed to encourage consumption of at least five servings of fruits and vegetables every day as part of a low-fat, high-fiber diet. Eating a variety of fruits and vegetables is recommended for different reasons. Some fruits and vegetables are high in vitamins, while others are full of minerals or fiber that the body needs. In addition, many fruits and vegetables contain compounds called phytochemicals which are not nutrients but may have a long-term beneficial effect in cancer prevention. Yet another reason for this recommendation is that fruits and vegetables contain protective micronutrients including antioxidants.

What are antioxidants?

Antioxidant micronutrients, including vitamin C, vitamin E, Beta-carotene (and related plant pigments), and selenium, may help to protect cells from damage caused by unstable chemicals called free radicals. Free radicals are highly reactive chemical substances that are produced during normal body metabolism. The changes that occur to body cells as a result of these oxidation reactions are analogous to oxidative reactions that cause vegetable oil to turn rancid, fruit to turn brown, and metal to rust. Antioxidants, however, may protect the cells from damage by neutralizing these free radicals.

Free radicals can be formed by normal cellular processes and external sources such as cigarette smoke and other carcinogens, pollution and environmental toxins, radiation, excessive sunlight and certain medications. If free radical formation is left unchecked, the process can lead to a damaging chain-reaction in which the free radicals damage the body's cells by attacking their membranes and genetic material and altering biochemical compounds. This cellular damage is believed to be a contributing cause of certain types of cancer, heart disease, premature aging and cataract formation.

Antioxidants protect cells by protecting against damage from free radicals. Antioxidants are also responsible for repairing the cellular damage caused by oxidation. Some of these antioxidants are manufactured by the cells themselves, but others are in the foods we eat. (See Table 3, page 29.) In addition to antioxidants, there are many other micronutrients that are required for the body's defense system. These nutrients (e.g., copper, iron, zinc) are provided by a variety of foods that are included in a well-balanced and diverse diet.

What are carbohydrates?

Diets that supply adequate servings of fruits, vegetables and grains also supply liberal amounts of carbohydrates. However, not all carbohydrates are created equal. Carbohydrates in foods come in two forms, simple and complex. Simple carbohydrates (often referred to as sugars) consist of single or double sugar molecules. They are classified as monosaccharides (glucose, fructose, galactose), and disaccharides (maltose, sucrose, lactose). Simple carbohydrates are found in foods such as table sugar (sucrose), milk (lactose and galactose), fruit and fruit juice (fructose), and malt (maltose). Foods containing large quantities of simple sugars, such as table sugar, honey, molasses, corn syrup, fructose and/or other nutritive sweeteners, are often low in nutrients. Additionally, many foods high in refined sugars are also high in added fat. Such foods include candy bars, cakes, pastries, cookies, and other sweet desserts. Most people should use these foods sparingly.

Complex carbohydrates (often referred to as "starch") consist of hundreds or even thousands of glucose molecules joined end to end. Complex carbohydrates are classified as polysaccharides. Food sources of complex carbohydrates include grains and grain products (cereals, breads, pasta, rice) and starchy vegetables (potatoes, corn, dried beans and peas). These foods are typically good sources of vitamins and minerals, generally low in fat, and can also be high in dietary fiber.

Dietary fiber—what is it and why is it good for you?

Fiber only comes from plant sources. It forms part of the outer structure of each cell. Dietary fiber is that portion of fruit, vegetables, whole grain cereals and other plant foods which is not broken down by the body during digestion. Diets without an adequate amount of fiber have been linked to a number of diseases, including heart disease, stroke, diabetes, obesity and certain types of cancer.[13,22] Preliminary studies indicate that some types of fiber may help to lower elevated blood cholesterol levels and thus may help to reduce the risk of coronary heart disease.[26,27]

TABLE 3

Food Sources of Antioxidants

	Vitamin C	Beta Carotene (and related plant pigments)	Vitamin E	Selenium
Fruits	cantaloupe, grapefruit, kiwi, mango, orange, papaya, strawberries, tangerine, blackberries, raspberries	apricots, cantaloupe, mango, papaya, peach, persimmon	mango, avocado	
Vegetables	broccoli, cabbage, cauliflower, dark green leafy vegetables (kale, collards, mustard greens, turnip greens), peppers (red and green), potatoes, tomatoes, kohlrabi, Brussels sprouts	broccoli, carrots, dark green leafy vegetables (spinach, kale, mustard greens, collard greens, Swiss chard), arugula, pumpkin, sweet potatoes, winter squash (butternut, hubbard), tomatoes, watercress	dark green leafy vegetables (spinach, kale, collard greens), asparagus	
Grains			whole grains (wheat, rye, oats, barley, brown rice), whole grain cereals and breads, wheat germ	all whole grains
Oils			sources of monounsaturated oils (canola, olive, peanut), avocado; and sources of polyunsaturated oils (corn, safflower, soybean, sunflower, sesame)	
Nuts & Seed Butters			all nuts and nut butters, all seeds	Brazil nuts
Meat & Seafood				seafood, meat

29

Not all fibers are created equal. Dietary fiber is often classified as two general types:

◆ Water Insoluble
❖ Water Soluble

Water *insoluble* fibers are found in plant cell walls. They include cellulose, hemicellulose and lignin. Water *insoluble* fiber adds bulk to the diet, holding water and decreasing the time it takes food to move through the digestive system. This swift passage helps to prevent constipation. As a result, this type of fiber may be useful in the prevention and treatment of diverticular disease and hemorrhoids. Research also indicates a link between high fiber diets and the prevention of some types of cancer.[13,22] By increasing the intestinal bulk, *insoluble* fiber may help to dilute any cancer-causing agents present in the lower bowel, giving them less time to do harm.

Foods that are sources of water insoluble fiber	
Whole Grains	buckwheat, millet, oats, rice, rye, wheat
Whole Grain Products	low-fat bread, cereal (especially wheat bran-containing cereals), low-fat crackers, pasta
Fresh Fruits and Vegetables	with peel
Nuts and Seeds	all types

Water *soluble* fiber is another type of dietary fiber. The fibers in this category include gums, psyllium and pectins, which are found in varying amounts in plants. While these fibers are useful in promoting bowel regularity and increasing bulk, they also slow stomach emptying and therefore delay the absorption of carbohydrates in the body. Research studies have shown possible beneficial effects of diets rich in water *soluble* fiber in the management of certain types of diabetes.[28,29] Water *soluble* fiber is also effective in lowering previously elevated blood cholesterol, particularly if consumed along with a low-cholesterol, low-fat diet.[26,27]

Foods that are sources of water soluble fiber	
Whole Grains	oat bran, oatmeal, barley
Legumes (dry beans and peas)	garbanzo, kidney, lentil, navy, pinto, soy, black, split peas, etc.
Fruits	citrus, apples, pears, plums
Vegetables	broccoli, Brussels sprouts, cabbage, okra, onion

The typical American diet provides approximately 16 grams of dietary fiber per day for men and 12 grams for women.[30] The National Cancer Institute recommends that Americans double their intake of fiber to 20-30 grams per day, with an upper limit of 35 grams.[31] Fiber should be consumed by eating a variety of whole grains, fresh fruits and vegetables, and dry beans and peas.

HOW TO USE THE M-FIT GROCERY SHOPPING GUIDE TO:
CHOOSE A DIET WITH PLENTY OF
GRAIN PRODUCTS, VEGETABLES AND FRUITS

The M-Fit Grocery Shopping Guide identifies those Vegetables (p. 167) and Fruits (p. 179) that are lowest in fat in the green "BEST CHOICE" categories. Foods meet the FDA definition of "Good Source" by providing 10 to 19 percent of the Daily Value of the nutrient described per reference amount and per labeled serving. Those fruits and vegetables that are a "Good Source" of vitamin C, dietary fiber, and vitamin A are identified on Tables 4 and 5. Many of these foods may also meet FDA's definition for "High," in which case they provide at least 20 percent of the Daily Value of the specified nutrient. These labeling requirements are as follows:

	GOOD SOURCE	HIGH
Dietary fiber	2.5 - 4.9 grams	5 grams or more
Vitamin A	500 - 950 IUs	1000 IUs or more
Vitamin C	6 - 11 milligrams	12 milligrams or more

Grain products are found in several food categories throughout the book, which include: Baking Mixes (pancake, muffins, biscuits), page 59; Breads, page 71; Bread Products, page 83; Chips, Pretzels, Popcorn, Snacks, page 103; Cereals, page, 93; Crackers, page 139; Grain and Grain Mixes, page 149; Pasta and Pasta Mixes, page 149; and Stuffing Mixes and Croutons, page 149.Those products that are the lowest in fat and saturated fat are listed in the green "BEST CHOICE" columns. Food products higher in fat and/or saturated fat are listed in the yellow "ACCEPTABLE CHOICE" columns. Grain products meeting the FDA definition for "Good Source of Fiber" (greater than or equal to 2.5 but less than 5 grams fiber per serving) are marked with a ☆ symbol. Grain products meeting the FDA definition for "High Fiber" (5 grams or more fiber per serving) will be marked with a ★ symbol.

TABLE 4

Vitamin C, Vitamin A, and Fiber Content of Fruits
☆ = Good Source
★ = High

Fruits	Vitamin C	Vitamin A	Fiber
Apple with skin	☆		☆
Apricots (3)	☆	★	☆
Banana	☆		
Blueberries (½ cup)	☆		
Cantaloupe (½ cup)	★	★	
Figs (2)			☆
Grapefruit (½)	★		
Kiwifruit	★		☆
Mango	★	★	
Nectarine	☆	★	
Orange	★		☆
Papaya	★	★	☆
Peach	☆		
Pear			☆
Pineapple (½ cup)	★		
Plum	☆		
Prunes (10 pc)			★
Raisins (¼ cup)			☆
Raspberries (½ cup)	★		★
Strawberries (½ cup)	★		☆
Watermelon (1 cup)	★		

Source: United States Department of Agriculture, Handbook #8.[32a]
Plant Fiber in Foods, Anderson J. 1990.[33]
Bowes & Church's Food Values of Portions Most Commonly Used, ed. Pennington J., 1994.[34]

TABLE 5

Vitamin C, Vitamin A, and Fiber Content of Vegetables
☆ = Good Source
★ = High

Vegetables	Vitamin C	Vitamin A	Fiber
Artichoke (1 medium)	★		★
Asparagus (¹/₂ cup, cooked)	★	☆	
Broccoli (¹/₂ cup, cooked)	★	★	☆
Brussels Sprouts (¹/₂ cup, cooked)	★	☆	☆
Cabbage (¹/₂ cup, cooked)	★		☆
Carrots (1 medium, raw)	☆	★	
Cauliflower (¹/₂ cup)	★		
Corn (¹/₂ cup)			☆
Dried Beans & Peas (¹/₂ cup)			★
Green Peppers (¹/₂ cup)	★		
Lettuce (1 cup fresh)			
Spinach	☆		
Romaine	★	★	
Red and Green Loose-leaf	☆	★	
Iceberg			
Onions	☆		
Pumpkin		★	
Red Peppers	★		
Summer Squash (yellow or zucchini, ¹/₂ cup)	☆		
Sweet Potato (¹/₂ cup)	★	★	☆
Tomato	★	★	
Winter Squash (¹/₂ cup)	☆	★	☆

Source: United States Department of Agriculture, Handbook #8.[32b]
Plant Fiber in Foods, Anderson J. 1990.[33]
Bowes & Church's Food Values of Portions Most Commonly Used, ed. Pennington J., 1994.[34]

CHOOSE A DIET LOW IN FAT, SATURATED FAT, AND CHOLESTEROL

Fat is an essential nutrient needed to maintain good health. Without adequate fat in our diets we would suffer from essential fatty acid deficiencies, and conceivably, from fat-soluble vitamin (A, D, E, K) deficiencies.

However, in today's society the risk for these deficiencies is rare. The major health problem facing the American population today is not that of deficiency, but rather, of overconsumption. There is little disagreement in the scientific community that fat is a contributor to the incidence of heart disease and other chronic diseases.

What is the recommendation for amount of fat in the diet?

The National Cholesterol Education Program,[35] along with the American Heart Association[36] and other health organizations, recommend reducing total fat in the diet to less than 30% of total daily calories. It is important to remember that this recommendation applies to the amount of fat for the entire day or an average over several days, and not to a single food or meal.

Fats should be distributed in the diet as follows:

Saturated fat— less than 10% of total calories

Polyunsaturated fat — up to 10% of total calories

Monounsaturated fat — up to 10 - 15% of total calories

Cholesterol — 300 milligrams or less

Your goal for total fat depends on your calorie needs. In certain situations, however, further restriction of *saturated* fat may be recommended. For example, a further reduction in saturated fat intake to less than 7% of calories may be suggested for individuals with high blood cholesterol, if they are not responding to the initial recommendations. These added restrictions, however, should be individualized and based on recommendations from your physician or registered dietitian. Table 6 will help you determine the maximum number of total grams of fat you should include in your daily diet in order to stay within the basic recommendations.

TABLE 6

Upper Limits of Fat and Cholesterol Recommended

Calories per Day	Grams Total Fat (30%)	Grams Saturated Fat (7-10%)	Grams Poly-unsaturated Fat (Up to 10%)	Grams Mono-unsaturated Fat (10-15%)	Milligrams Cholesterol
1200	40	9-13	13	13-20	<300
1500	50	11-16	16	16-25	<300
1800	60	14-20	20	20-30	<300
2000	66	15-22	22	22-33	<300
2400	80	18-26	26	26-40	<300

What is cholesterol and how does it affect your health?

Cholesterol is a waxy substance used by the body to manufacture: (1) certain hormones which control the body's metabolism, (2) bile acids which aid in fat digestion, and (3) cell membranes, the outer boundaries of each cell of the body which help to maintain the delicate chemical balance required for normal bodily functions. Although cholesterol is essential for life, our bodies produce sufficient quantities to meet our physiological needs. In other words, if we never ate a single milligram of cholesterol we would not suffer from an inadequacy!

There are two approaches to discussing cholesterol

Dietary Cholesterol is cholesterol that is in the food you eat. It is present only in foods of animal origin (e.g., meat, poultry, fish, dairy products), and *not* in foods of plant origin (e.g., vegetables, vegetable oil, fruits, grains). Dietary cholesterol, like saturated fat, tends to raise blood cholesterol, but to a lesser degree, and individuals appear to vary in responsiveness.

Perhaps there has been too much emphasis on dietary cholesterol. Reducing dietary cholesterol by itself may have little impact on blood cholesterol. A significant lowering of blood cholesterol can occur when we restrict dietary choices high in cholesterol because most are also high in saturated fat, which is the major food substance responsible for elevated blood cholesterol. Therefore, foods rich in cholesterol but low in saturated fat, such as shrimp, when properly prepared, can be eaten as part of a low-cholesterol, low-saturated fat diet. Therefore, the major emphasis in dietary recommendations is a reduction in fat consumption and particularly saturated fat. See Table 7, page 36, for the cholesterol and saturated fat content of selected foods.

According to the most recent food consumption surveys, Americans currently consume an average of 35% of total calories from fat and 12% of calories from saturated fat. Average daily cholesterol intakes are estimated at below 300 milligrams for women and somewhat above 300 milligrams for men.[30]

TABLE 7

Cholesterol and Saturated Fat Contents of Selected Foods

Type of Food	Milligrams Cholesterol	Grams Saturated Fat
Beef (per 3 oz cooked portion)		
Chuck, Blade Roast - 1/8" fat trim	90	9
Top Round, Steak - 1/8" fat trim	70	3
Poultry (per 3 oz cooked portion)		
Skinless Chicken/Turkey White Meat	55-70	0-0.5
Skinless Chicken/Turkey Dark Meat	65-80	1.5-2.0
Pork (per 3 oz cooked portion)		
Tenderloin Roast - 1/8" fat trim	65	2
Fish (per 3.5 oz portion, raw)		
"Lower" fat varieties (1 g fat/3.5 oz)		
cod, perch, pollock, haddock	42-71	0.1-0.3
"Higher" fat varieties (6-14 g fat/3.5 oz)		
salmon, mackerel, whitefish, herring	55-70	1.0-2.2
Shellfish (1-2 g fat/3.5 oz)		
Lobster	94	0.1
Crab	76	0.1
Shrimp	151	0.3
Squid	231	0.3
Fish Roe (caviar, 1 Tbsp)	105	0.4
Egg Yolk (1 yolk, 17 grams)	94	0.5
Egg White	0	0
Organ Meat (per 3.5 oz portion) raw		
Liver	349	2.0
Kidneys	283	1.5
Sweetbreads (thymus gland)	294	N/A
Whole Milk 3.3% fat (8 fl oz)	31	2.4
Skim Milk (8 fl oz)	4	0
Butter (1 Tbsp)	31	7.6
Cheese (1 oz portion)		
Cheddar	30	6.0
Mozzarella, made from whole milk	25	4.4
Mozzarella, made from part-skim milk	16	2.9

Source: United States Department of Agriculture, Handbook 8.[32 c-j]

Blood cholesterol is cholesterol that is either manufactured in the body or obtained from the food you eat. It is carried in the blood for use by all parts of the body. Scientific studies have shown beyond doubt that high levels of cholesterol in the blood predispose individuals to the development of blockages in the blood vessels of the heart (coronary artery disease).[37,38]

It is important to understand that three dietary factors increase blood cholesterol: (1) eating too much saturated fat; (2) eating too much cholesterol; and (3) eating an excess of calories, resulting in obesity. In the typical American diet, the **saturated fat** content is the strongest contributor to raising blood cholesterol.[39] Excess calories and cholesterol in foods also contribute, but to a lesser extent. Therefore, it is most important to decrease saturated fat to 10% or less of total daily calories, in addition to decreasing dietary cholesterol intake to less than 300 milligrams per day and consuming an appropriate calorie level to attain desirable weight.

Knowing your own cholesterol level is important. The National Cholesterol Education Program Expert Panel sets guidelines for classifying blood cholesterol levels. The Panel advises that a total blood cholesterol level less than 200 mg/dL is desirable for adults over 20 years of age.[35] It has been shown that the risk of developing coronary artery disease steadily increases at cholesterol levels above 218 mg/dL.[40] The average blood cholesterol level for men and women in the United States above the age of 20 is about 206 mg/dL.[41] In men, the risk of death from premature coronary heart disease was observed to be increased at levels above 180 mg/dL.[2]

The effect of dietary change on blood cholesterol varies considerably and is dependent on the amount of dietary fat, the body's ability to absorb fat, and genetic factors. The amount of reduction in blood cholesterol following the dietary recommendations by the National Cholesterol Education Program (i.e., less than 30% total fat, less than 10% saturated fat, less than 300 milligrams cholesterol) ranges from as little as 5% to as much as 30%.[35]

It is important to realize that even small changes in blood cholesterol may reduce risk for heart disease. Scientific studies have shown that for middle-aged men with cholesterol levels exceeding 250 mg/dL, every 1% reduction in blood cholesterol is associated with a 2% reduction in risk for a heart attack. Therefore, a sustained 10-30% reduction of cholesterol may represent a 20-60% reduction in heart attack risk.[42] Furthermore, the benefits of a reduction in dietary saturated fat (i.e., decrease in heart attacks and a decrease in the progression of coronary heart disease) may be additive to the effects associated with a reduction in blood cholesterol.

What are HDL and LDL cholesterol and triglycerides?

You may have heard about the different types of blood cholesterol and their role in determining your risk for coronary artery disease. Because fat and cholesterol do not dissolve in blood, in order for them to be transported in the bloodstream, they must be carried by specialized transport proteins. These transport packages of fat and protein are called lipoproteins. Lipoproteins are classified according to their density.

High-density lipoproteins (HDL): Lipoproteins that appear to carry cholesterol away from the heart and coronary arteries to the liver for reprocessing or removal from the body are called high-density lipoproteins. This process of removing cholesterol from tissues is protective against cholesterol build-up. Persons with higher levels of HDL-cholesterol have a lower incidence of heart disease.[43,44] A level above 60 mg/dL is considered very beneficial and a negative risk factor. Therefore, HDLs have been known as the "good" cholesterol. Conversely, individuals with low levels of HDL-cholesterol (less than 35 mg/dL in men and less than 45 mg/dL in women) are at higher risk for developing coronary heart disease.[35] Even small changes in HDL-cholesterol can have an effect on coronary heart disease risk. For example, for every 1 mg/dL decrease in HDL-cholesterol, the risk for coronary heart disease is increased by 2-3%.[44] Likewise, higher HDL-cholesterol levels appear to afford a degree of protection against coronary heart disease.[43,44]

HDL-cholesterol level is primarily determined by heredity. However, regular exercise, moderate consumption of alcohol, and estrogen replacement therapy in women following menopause can raise HDL-cholesterol. Smoking, a major coronary risk factor, also lowers HDL-cholesterol.[45,46]

Low-density lipoproteins (LDL): Lipoproteins that contain the greatest amount of cholesterol and are responsible for carrying cholesterol to the cells of the body are called low-density lipoproteins. When cholesterol-rich LDL is present in excess, this cholesterol may become deposited in the walls of arteries, contributing to the disease known as atherosclerosis. For this reason, LDL is sometimes called "bad" cholesterol. High levels of LDL-cholesterol are therefore associated with an increased risk of coronary heart disease. A "desirable" level of LDL-cholesterol in adults depends upon the number of coronary heart disease risk factors a person has. In addition to increased levels of LDL-cholesterol, these risk factors include:

- Males 45 years or older
- Females 55 years or older, or who have premature menopause without estrogen replacement therapy
- A family history of premature CHD (definite myocardial infarction or sudden death before 55 years of age in father or other male first-degree relative, or before 65 years of age in mother or other female first-degree relative)
- Current cigarette smoking
- High blood pressure (hypertension defined as blood pressure greater than or equal to 140/90 mm Hg or taking antihypertensive medication)
- diabetes mellitus
- Low HDL-cholesterol (less than 35 mg/dL)

Negative Risk Factor

- High HDL-cholesterol (greater than or equal to 60 mg/dL)

If a person has two or more of these risk factors the goal for LDL-cholesterol levels should be less than 130 mg/dL. If he or she has already been found to have coronary heart disease, LDL-cholesterol levels should be less than 100 mg/dL. For those persons with zero or one risk factor and no coronary heart disease, the goal should be less than 160 mg/dL.[35]

Triglycerides: Triglycerides are fats formed in the intestine following ingestion of dietary fat or in the liver from fats and sugars. Triglycerides are digested in working muscles and are an important source of energy or are deposited in fat stores such as in the abdomen. The normal level of triglyceride is less than 200 mg/dL, and ideally, less than 150 mg/dL.[47] High triglycerides without additional risk factors do not increase the risk of coronary heart disease. However, when associated with other coronary risk factors, such as a low HDL-cholesterol, diabetes mellitus, and hypertension, elevated triglycerides may further increase the risk of heart attacks and atherosclerosis.

The most common reason for finding high blood triglycerides is that a blood sample was taken from an individual who had not properly fasted for 8 to 12 hours. Elevated **fasting** triglycerides can be due to diabetes mellitus, obesity, heredity, excessive dietary fats, sugars, or alcohol, and on occasion, certain medications.[48] High carbohydrate diets may contribute to the increase in blood triglycerides in certain individuals.[49]

How do fats affect cholesterol?

Fats are the major dietary factors that affect cholesterol levels. Some fats will increase blood cholesterol levels, while other fats can decrease cholesterol levels, when substituted in the diet for saturated fats. Dietary fats are a mixture of three major types: saturated, monounsaturated and polyunsaturated. An understanding of this terminology is helpful in becoming familiar with the role of fat in the diet. Saturated, polyunsaturated and monounsaturated are all chemical terms. They refer to the structure and orientation of the molecules of carbon, hydrogen and oxygen.

What is saturated fat?

Saturated fats tend to be solid at room temperature and play a major role in elevating blood cholesterol. They are found predominantly in animal sources but can also be found in some vegetable sources:

SOURCES OF SATURATED FATS

Animal
- Bacon and bacon fat
- Beef tallow
- Chicken fat
- Lamb tallow
- Lard
- Salt Pork

Dairy Products
- Butter
- Cheese
- Cream cheese
- Ice cream
- Sour cream
- Whole and 2% milk

Plant
- Cocoa butter (chocolate)
- Coconut oil
- Palm kernel oil
- Palm oil
- Vegetable shortening or hydrogenated oils made from any of the above

Note: *All foods contain a mixture of fatty acids. The fat in the foods listed in this table consists predominantly of saturated fatty acids.*

What is monounsaturated fat?

Monounsaturated fats tend to be liquid at room temperature. When oils rich in monounsaturated fats, such as canola oil, peanut oil or olive oil, are stored in the refrigerator, they become solid; however, this does not make them saturated. Results from studies that were conducted in the 1950s and 1960s by Keys[50] and Hegsted[51] suggested that oleic acid (a monounsaturated fatty acid) is *neutral* in its effect on blood cholesterol. In 1970 Keys[52] published a major epidemiological study that examined the associations among diet, plasma cholesterol, other risk factors and coronary heart disease (CHD) rates in several different populations in seven countries. This study demonstrated that CHD rates were low in the Mediterranean region where large quantities of olive oil (a rich source of monounsaturated fat) are consumed.[53] More recent clinical research studies[54-56] have shown that monounsaturated fats (oleic acid) are equally effective in lowering LDL-cholesterol as are polyunsaturated fats, when substituted in the diet for saturated fats. In

39

addition, they may not cause HDL-cholesterol levels to decline, as diets high in polyunsaturated fats may do (discussion below).

Significant sources of monounsaturated fats are found in the following vegetable oils, nuts and nut butters.

SOURCES OF MONOUNSATURATED FATS

Vegetable Oils
Avocado oil
Canola oil
High oleic safflower oil
High oleic sunflower oil
Olive oil
Peanut oil

Vegetables/Fruits
Avocados
Olives

Nuts and Nut butters
Acorns
Almonds
Beechnuts
Cashews
Filberts or hazelnuts
Hickory nuts
Macadamia nuts
Peanuts
Pecans

Note: *All foods contain a mixture of fatty acids. The fat in foods listed in this table consists predominantly of monounsaturated fatty acids.*

What is polyunsaturated fat?

Polyunsaturated fats tend to be liquid at room temperature. These oils may become more viscous (thick) or cloudy when refrigerated but will still remain liquid. When replacing saturated fats in the diet, polyunsaturated fats (like monounsaturated fats) may lower LDL-cholesterol.[57] However, there are several potential drawbacks to consuming diets high in polyunsaturated fats. First of all, no large population group has ever consumed large quantities of polyunsaturated fatty acids with proven safety. Secondly, several research studies have shown that diets high in polyunsaturates may also lower the protective HDL-cholesterol levels.[58,59] On the other hand, a recent study showed that HDL-cholesterol is not negatively affected if polyunsaturated fat consumption is kept to the current levels recommended by the National Cholesterol Education Program Step I diet (i.e., 30% or less total fat with 10% or less polyunsaturated fats).[60] Thirdly, it has been speculated that diets high in polyunsaturated fat result in metabolic changes linked to an increased risk for plaque formation in blood vessels. These metabolic changes are attributed to the formation of "oxidized" LDL-cholesterol, which is proposed to be more damaging to the walls of the arteries than LDL-cholesterol that is not oxidatively modified.[61] Finally, a high intake of dietary

polyunsaturated fat is also suspect in increasing the risk for certain types of cancer.[62] Further research to confirm these findings is necessary before firm conclusions can be drawn.

SOURCES OF POLYUNSATURATED FATS

Vegetable Oils
>Corn
>Safflower
>Sesame
>Soybean
>Sunflower

Nuts
>Brazil nuts
>Butternuts
>Pine nuts
>Walnuts

Seeds
>Pumpkin
>Sesame
>Sunflower

Other
>Soft or liquid margarine
>Mayonnaise made from soybean

Note: *All foods contain a mixture of fatty acids. The fat in foods listed in this table consists predominantly of polyunsaturated fatty acids.*

Note
Although cottonseed oil contains 52% polyunsaturated fat, it also contains 26% saturated fat (mostly palmitic acid, which is known to elevate cholesterol). For this reason, it is not listed as a source of recommended polyunsaturated fat. However, cottonseed oil contains predominantly unsaturated fats and is, therefore, an acceptable ingredient in commercially prepared foods.

It is recommended to limit all fats in the diet to less than 30% of daily calories. However, choosing appropriate **types** of fat is just as important as monitoring the **amount** of fat you consume. Table 8, page 42, summarizes the effects of the different fats on blood cholesterol. Use this table to help guide you in your fat selections.

TABLE 8

Sources of Fat and Effect on Blood Cholesterol Levels

Monounsaturated Lowers cholesterol when substituted for Saturated Fats	Polyunsaturated High intakes may lower HDL-Cholesterol	Saturated Elevates LDL-Cholesterol
RECOMMENDATIONS		
Best Choice	Acceptable Choice	Occasional Choice
Vegetable Oils	**Vegetable Oils**	**Animal Fats**
avocado	corn	bacon
canola	safflower	beef fat
high oleic safflower	sesame	chicken fat
high oleic sunflower	soybean	fatty meats
olive	sunflower	lamb fat
peanut	soft margarine	lard
Fruit	mayonnaise	salt pork
avocado		**Dairy Products**
olives	**Nuts**	butter
Nuts	Brazil nuts	cheese
acorns	butternuts	cream
almonds	pine nuts	ice cream
beechnuts	walnuts	whole milk
cashews	**Seeds**	**Nuts**
chestnuts	sesame	coconut
filberts or hazelnuts	sunflower	
hickory nuts	pumpkin	**Tropical Oils**
macadamia nuts		**or Shortenings**
peanuts		coconut
pecans		palm
pistachios		palm kernel
		cocoa butter

Note: *Foods containing fats are a mixture of monounsaturated, polyunsaturated and saturated fatty acids. Foods are listed in the columns according to the type of fatty acid that is most predominant in the food.*

What about hydrogenated oils: Are they good or bad fats?

Hydrogenation is a chemical process that changes liquid vegetable oil (predominantly unsaturated fat) to a more solid shortening (increasing amounts of saturated fat and monounsaturated fat) by adding hydrogen. The commercial food industry uses hydrogenated oils primarily in baked food products, such as breads, crackers, cakes, and cookies. It is necessary to hydrogenate unsaturated oils to a degree in order to produce a desired texture and to increase shelf life. Hydrogenated oils are more stable and resist oxidation, which can cause rancidity and spoilage.

Hydrogenation primarily increases the amount of **monounsaturated** fatty acids and, to a lesser degree, increases the amount of saturated fatty acids (see Table 9). It is important to note that the biggest increase in saturated fat is in the form of stearic acid which has **not** been shown to cause an elevation in blood cholesterol levels in persons who already consume a low cholesterol diet.[63,64] Table 9 illustrates that as soybean oil becomes more hydrogenated, changing from liquid to solid, the most significant change is that monounsaturated fat increases from 23 to 45 grams percent with a subsequent decrease in polyunsaturated fat from 58 to 26 grams percent. Scientists are unsure whether the monounsaturated fatty acids formed by hydrogenation are as beneficial as naturally occurring monounsaturated fatty acids. The reason for this uncertainty is that the process of hydrogenation causes the formation of *trans fatty acids*, which in some recent studies[65] have been suggested to increase LDL-cholesterol and decrease HDL-cholesterol. However, there is no conclusive evidence of this effect. At this point, people concerned about reducing their risk for heart disease are encouraged to lower their saturated fat and total fat intake. *The M-Fit Grocery Shopping Guide* is designed to guide the consumer in selecting food choices that meet this dietary recommendation.

TABLE 9

Effect of Hydrogenation on Fatty Acid Content (grams/100 grams)

Increasing level of hydrogenation ↓	Total Saturated	Stearic	Palmitic	Myristic	Mono-unsaturated	Poly-unsaturated
Soybean oil	14	3.8	10.3	.1	23	58
Soybean oil (hydrogenated)	15	5.0	9.8	.1	43	38
Tub soybean margarine	14	4.7	8.7	.1	37	27
Stick soybean margarine	13	4.9	8.1	.1	38	26
Soybean shortening (soy/cottonseed)	25	10.6	14.1	.4	45	26
Change from oil to shortening	+11	+6.8	+3.8	+.3	+22	-32

The fatty acid values were taken from United States Department of Agriculture, Agriculture Handbook No. 8.[32j]

HOW TO USE THE M-FIT GROCERY SHOPPING GUIDE TO:
CHOOSE A DIET LOW IN FAT,
SATURATED FAT, AND CHOLESTEROL

Choosing the appropriate **type** of fat is just as important as monitoring the **amount** of fat you eat. Although all vegetable fats are cholesterol-free, some still contain significant amounts of saturated fat, which is the key substance that contributes to elevated blood cholesterol. The section on Fats and Oils in *The M-Fit Grocery Shopping Guide,* page 305, lists the types of fats that are recommended in the **"BEST CHOICE,"** and **"ACCEPTABLE CHOICE"** columns, (color-coded "green" and "yellow"). It is recommended that all Fats and Oils be used sparingly because they provide 100% of their calories from fat, and consequently, contribute a significant amount of fat to the diet.

Other foods which can contribute a significant amount of fat to the diet are found in the following sections: Butter and Margarine, page 293; Nut and Seed Butters, page 289; Salad Dressings, page 311; Desserts, page 319; Snack Foods, page 103; Dairy Products, page 197; various Meats, page 207-225; Lunchmeats, page 227; and Meals and Main Dishes, page 255. In all of these food categories, the lower fat options are listed in the **"BEST CHOICE,"** and **"ACCEPTABLE CHOICE"** columns.

Fresh red meats, poultry, game and fish are rated using the USDA's definitions for "Extra Lean," which are in the green **"BEST CHOICE"** column, and "Lean," which are in the yellow **"ACCEPTABLE CHOICE"** column. All other processed and prepared foods are evaluated according to their content of fat and saturated fat. Those products with the least amount of fat are listed in the green **"BEST CHOICE"** columns; those with greater amounts of fat, but still meeting the definition for low-fat are listed in the yellow, **"ACCEPTABLE CHOICE"** columns.

44

CHOOSE A DIET MODERATE IN SUGARS

As discussed on page 28, the term "sugars" is used to describe simple carbohydrates consisting of single or double sugar molecules. They can occur naturally in foods, such as fruits and dairy products, or can be added to foods during processing. Sugars are found in foods in many different forms. They are classified as monosaccharides (glucose, fructose, galactose), and disaccharides (maltose, sucrose, lactose). Foods which contain natural sugars, such as milk (lactose) and fruit (fructose, sucrose), are often good sources of vitamins and minerals. On the other hand, sugars added to processed foods, such as table sugar (sucrose), brown sugar, raw sugar, glucose (dextrose), fructose, maltose, lactose, honey, syrup, molasses, corn syrup, high-fructose corn syrup, and fruit juice concentrate, contribute added calories but few other nutrients.

The *Dietary Guidelines for Americans* recommends that sugars of all types be used only in moderation.[11] While foods with added sugars can serve as a useful source of calories for those individuals who have higher calorie needs, such as active teenagers and athletes, the majority of the adult sedentary population have lower calorie requirements. Limiting the intake of sugar is often useful in reducing calories without reducing nutrient intake.

Most of the added sugars in the typical American diet come from foods such as soft drinks, candy, jams, jellies, syrups and table sugar. Additionally, much of the sugars in the diet also come from prepared foods, such as sweetened bakery products (i.e., cakes and cookies), ice cream, sweetened yogurt, chocolate milk, pre-sweetened cereals, canned or frozen fruit in heavy syrup. Table 10 on page 46 shows the amounts of added sugars in some popular foods. Some of the levels may surprise you!

Both sugars and starches (which the body breaks down into sugars) can contribute to tooth decay. The more often these foods are eaten, and the longer they are exposed to the teeth, the higher the risk of tooth decay. Therefore, excessive snacking of these foods may be more harmful to the teeth than eating them at a meal. Flossing and brushing the teeth regularly with a fluoride toothpaste are important measures in preventing tooth decay. Fluoridation of the public water supply, along with fluoride supplementation for children, has made a tremendous impact on the dental health of this country.

Diets high in sugars have not been shown to cause diabetes.[13] The most common type of diabetes (Type II) occurs in adults who are overweight, but avoiding sugars alone will not correct the problem. Weight loss through a moderately restricted-calorie diet with the addition of exercise is the best way to control this type of diabetes. It is difficult to lose weight and meet your nutrient needs on a diet high in added sugars. This is why keeping sugars to a minimum for those individuals with lower calorie needs is recommended.

TABLE 10

Where are the Added Sugars?

Food Groups	Added Sugars (teaspoons)
Bread, Cereal, Rice, and Pasta	
Bread, 1 slice	0
Muffin, 1 medium	❏ 1
Cookies, 2 medium	❏ 1
Danish pastry, 1 medium	❏ 1
Doughnut, 1 medium	❏❏ 2
Ready-to-eat cereal, sweetened, 1 oz.	(varies)*
Pound cake, no-fat, 1 oz.	❏❏ 2
Angel food cake, 1/12 tube cake	❏❏❏❏❏ 5
Cake, frosted, 1/16 average	❏❏❏❏❏❏ 6
Pie, fruit, 2 crust, 1/6 8" pie	❏❏❏❏❏❏ 6
Fruit	
Fruit, canned in juice, 1/2 cup	0
Fruit, canned in light syrup, 1/2 cup	❏❏ 2
Fruit, canned in heavy syrup, 1/2 cup	❏❏❏❏ 4
Milk, Yogurt, and Cheese	
Milk, plain, 1 cup	0
Chocolate milk, 2 percent, 1 cup	❏❏❏ 3
Lowfat yogurt, plain, 8 oz.	0
Lowfat yogurt, flavored, 8 oz.	❏❏❏❏❏ 5
Lowfat yogurt, fruit, 8 oz.	❏❏❏❏❏❏❏ 7
Ice cream, ice milk, or frozen yogurt, 1/2 cup	❏❏❏ 3
Chocolate shake, 10 fl. oz.	❏❏❏❏❏❏❏❏❏ 9
Other	
Sugar, jam, or jelly, 1 tsp.	❏ 1
Syrup or honey, 1 tbsp.	❏❏❏ 3
Chocolate bar, 1 oz.	❏❏❏ 3
Fruit sorbet, 1/2 cup	❏❏❏ 3
Gelatin dessert, 1/2 cup	❏❏❏❏ 4
Sherbet, 1/2 cup	❏❏❏❏❏ 5
Cola, 12 fl. oz.	❏❏❏❏❏❏❏❏❏ 9
Fruit drink, ade, 12 fl. oz.	❏❏❏❏❏❏❏❏❏❏❏❏ 12

Check product label.   ❏ = 1 teaspoon sugar
Note: 4 grams of sugar = 1 teaspoon

Modified from: The Food Guide Pyramid. U.S. Dept. of Agriculture: 1992. Home and Garden Bulletin #252, pg. 16.

HOW TO USE THE M-FIT GROCERY SHOPPING GUIDE TO:
CHOOSE A DIET MODERATE IN SUGARS

The federal government did not set a "% Daily Value" number on the "Nutrition Facts" panel for sugars. However, the "Nutrition Facts" panel is now required to list the amount of sugars (in grams) present in a serving of the food. The term "sugars" includes both natural sugars in the product (e.g., lactose in milk, fructose in fruit) in addition to sugars added to the product during processing. The reason for the lack of distinction between the two is because there are no analytical methods currently available that can distinguish between naturally-occurring sugars and those added in processing.

Because there is no conclusive scientific evidence that links sugar consumption to disease other than dental carries, the authors of *The M-Fit Grocery Shopping Guide* have elected to include ranking criteria for only those food groups where choices between foods with or without added sugars exist. These food groups are Beverages, page 355, and Fruits, page 179. In both these food categories, the green "BEST CHOICE" ranking is given to the fat-free, *without added sugars,* selections, and the yellow "ACCEPTABLE CHOICE" ranking is given to the low-fat, *with added sugars,* selections. Consumers are therefore informed of the added sugars and are able to make the choice that suits their individual needs.

Other food groups that can provide a substantial amount of sugar to the diet are pre-sweetened cereals and sweetened dessert products. If added sugars are a concern for you or your family, you can evaluate added sugars in foods by reading the ingredient declaration which is part of the "Nutrition Facts" label. Common terms used to describe sugars added to foods include: sugar (sucrose), fructose, maltose, lactose, honey, syrup, corn syrup, high-fructose corn syrup, molasses, and fruit juice concentrate. If one of these sweeteners is listed first or second or if several are listed, the food is likely to be high in added sugars. (Note: Ingredients are listed in order of concentration in the product: largest quantity first, down to the smallest quantity last.)

CHOOSE A DIET
MODERATE IN SALT AND SODIUM

Sodium is an essential mineral needed by the body to regulate blood pressure and body fluids. Sodium is also necessary for the proper functioning of nerves and muscles. Surprisingly, healthy adults under conditions of maximal adaptation and without active sweating only require approximately 115 milligrams of sodium per day. However, in order to account for the wide variations of an individual's patterns of physical activity and climate exposure, the National Academy of Sciences recommends a minimum intake of 500 milligrams of sodium per day.[14] Health authorities also recommend that the general population limit their sodium intake to 2,400 milligrams or less per day. Hence, the Daily Value for sodium used on the food labels is set at 2,400 milligrams per day.

Studies show that most Americans are consuming between 4,000 and 6,000 milligrams of sodium a day,[66] well above the recommended 2,400 milligrams per day level.[14] These values, however, only reflect the amount of sodium naturally found in food or added to food during processing or preparation. They do not include salt added at the table or obtained from non-food sources. Had these sources been taken into account, the average intake would have been even higher.

Currently, approximately one out of every four adults in the United States suffer from high blood pressure (hypertension).[66] Factors that can affect blood pressure include heredity, obesity, and excessive consumption of alcoholic beverages. Research studies have also linked excessive sodium intake with elevated blood pressure in some people.[67] High blood pressure is seen more often in populations where diets are higher in salt than in populations using less salt in their diets. If left untreated, high blood pressure increases an individual's risk of heart attack and stroke.

Perhaps only a small percentage of the American population is truly "salt-sensitive" (meaning their blood pressure goes up with increases in sodium intake).[68,69] Because it is currently difficult to identify who is "salt sensitive," many health professionals believe it is wise for most Americans to consume less salt and sodium.[70]

The major contributor of sodium to the American diet is sodium chloride (table salt). Table salt is 40% sodium and 60% chloride. One teaspoon of salt contains approximately 2,300 milligrams of sodium. Sources of sodium in the typical American diet are:

- ◆ 1/3 occurring naturally in foods,
- ◆ 1/3 added in processed foods, and
- ◆ 1/3 added during cooking or at the table.

To reduce or moderate the use of salt and sodium, follow these tips:

- ◆ Use salt sparingly, if at all, in cooking and at the table.

- ◆ Choose salted snacks, such as chips, crackers, pretzels and nuts less often.

- ◆ Check labels for the amount of sodium in foods and choose those lower in sodium most of the time.

- ◆ Limit your intake of high sodium foods.

Foods that tend to be higher in sodium include many cheeses, processed meats, most frozen dinners and entrees, packaged mixes, seasoning mixes, most canned soups and vegetables, salad dressings and condiments like soy sauce, pickles, olives, catsup and mustard, and foods processed or prepared with monosodium glutamate (MSG).

See page 54 for a description of sodium terminology used in nutrition labeling.

HOW TO USE THE M-FIT GROCERY SHOPPING GUIDE TO:
CHOOSE A DIET
MODERATE IN SALT AND SODIUM

In addition to fat, sodium criteria were used to rank food choices in the following food categories: Vegetables, page 167, Legumes and Meat Alternatives, page 245, and Meals and Main Dishes, page 255. Throughout the book, those food choices meeting the FDA's definition for low sodium (140 milligrams or less per serving) are identified with a ∇ symbol. Additionally, those foods that contain 20% (480 milligrams) or greater of the Daily Value of sodium are identified with a ▲ symbol.

IF YOU DRINK ALCOHOLIC
BEVERAGES, DO SO IN MODERATION

Although alcoholic beverages are excluded from *The M-Fit Grocery Shopping Guide*, a brief discussion of this dietary guideline follows.

According to the Surgeon General's Report on Nutrition and Health excessive alcohol intake is a prominent contributor to 4 of the 10 leading causes of death in the United States—cirrhosis of the liver, motor vehicle and other accidents, suicides, and homicides, in addition to increased risk for oral, esophageal, liver and other types of cancer.[8] Drinking alcoholic beverages is also associated with a higher risk for hypertension and hemorrhagic stroke.[13]

Some studies have suggested that moderate drinking can lower the risk of a heart attack. However, considering the well-established adverse health consequences of excessive alcohol consumption, alcohol is not recommended as a strategy for preventing coronary heart disease.

The *Dietary Guidelines for Americans* **do not** recommend the consumption of alcoholic beverages.[11] However, the guidelines *do* state that if a person elects to drink alcohol, they should do so in moderation; and don't drive. Moderation is defined as no more than 1 drink a day for women and no more than 2 drinks a day for men.

The *Guidelines* also alert the American population to the following conditions in which even moderate drinking is **not** recommended:

- ◆ Women who are pregnant or trying to conceive. Major birth defects have been attributed to heavy drinking by the mother while pregnant. However, evidence that an occasional drink is harmful is not conclusive.

- ◆ Individuals who plan to drive or engage in other activities that require attention or skill. Most people retain some alcohol in the blood up to 2-3 hours after a single drink.

- ◆ Individuals using medications, even those sold over-the-counter. Alcohol may affect the benefits or toxicity of medications. Also, some medications may increase blood alcohol levels or increase the adverse effect of alcohol on the brain.

- ◆ Individuals who cannot keep their drinking at a moderate level. This is a special concern for recovering alcoholics and people whose family members have alcohol problems.

- ◆ Children and adolescents. Use of alcoholic beverages by children and adolescents involves risks to health and other serious problems.

The Bureau of Alcohol, Tobacco and Firearms (BATF) regulates the labeling of most alcoholic beverages. At present, these beverages are not required to provide nutrition information. The FDA regulates the labeling of wine beverages containing less than 7 percent alcohol by volume. These beverages will have the alcohol content (in percentage by volume) stated on the front panel of the label. Some alcoholic beverages such as "Lite" beers and wine coolers may also provide limited nutrient information on their labels for calories, carbohydrate, protein and fat.[16]

Alcohol is second only to fat in calorie density. Alcohol yields 7 calories per gram compared to fat at 9 calories per gram and 4 calories per gram for carbohydrate and protein. Unlike calories supplied from foods rich in protein, carbohydrate and fat, calories supplied from alcohol-containing beverages contain little or no nutrients. Individuals should be particularly careful to limit their intake of nutritionally-deficient alcohol calories, and instead, increase their intake of more nutritionally-dense calories from foods.

LEARN TO USE THE NEW FOOD LABEL
TO SELECT A HEALTHFUL DIET

Healthy eating is a major concern for a growing number of Americans. According to the latest *Trends* report[71] published by the Food Marketing Institute, nutrition is second only to taste as the most important consideration when selecting food. Nutrition outweighs price and product safety, and continues to be a very important factor for three out of four shoppers.

Because Americans typically consume a significant amount of foods that are packaged and processed, learning to read and understand food labels is a critical part of analyzing and improving your diet. Many processed foods contain saturated fat, cholesterol, sugar and sodium. By reading the labels of processed foods, you can make wise food choices that may better suit your health needs.

The new label is designed to help you see how any one food fits into an overall daily diet. It can help you determine the nutritional value of a single food or compare one food with another. You can use it to decide how large a portion to eat or how frequently to eat a particular food. The new label, intended for people age 4 and up, provides important information because what you eat may increase or lower your risk of certain diseases and can help you maintain a desirable weight.

The new labeling regulations require that food manufacturers display a new label format and a list of nutrients on all packaged and processed foods. This new nutrition panel (see Figure 3, page 55) named **"Nutrition Facts"** will help to clear up confusion by standardizing information on all labels.

What's new about the new food label?

The new food label which had its debut in May of 1994, can serve as an important guide to better nutrition. Here's what to look for:

Serving Sizes

All serving sizes on the "Nutrition Facts" panel are standardized and expressed in both common household measures and metric units. Serving sizes on the new food label are based on "reference amounts" established by the FDA and USDA for the purpose of making serving sizes more uniform between similar products. For example, the reference amount established for all snack crackers is 30 grams, whereas the reference amount for all sliced breads is 50 grams. These reference amounts are based on food consumption data and reflect what consumers customarily eat. They are not intended to be recommendations of amounts people should eat. Instead, the reference amounts are designed to help consumers more easily compare the nutrient content of products that are used interchangeably. For example, even though food consumption data show that most Americans drink 1 cup of milk at a sitting, and 3/4 cup of juice at a sitting, the reference amount for serving sizes of food labels was set at 240 milliliters (or 1 cup) for all beverages. This standardization makes it easy for the consumer with a milk allergy, for example, to determine if calcium-fortified orange juice contains about the same amount of calcium as milk.[16] Remember, though, that it is important to compare your actual serving size to the one listed on the package in order to evaluate the number of calories, grams of fat, or other food components that you are actually consuming.

Consumers are sometimes confused because the serving sizes given on the food label may sometimes differ from those of the *Food Guide Pyramid*. The reason for this is that, in addition to

being based on food consumption data, the *Pyramid* serving sizes are also based on two additional considerations—nutrient content and traditional serving sizes used in previous food guides. Therefore, using the example given above, the *Pyramid* serving size for milk is 1 cup, whereas the serving size for juice is 3/4 cup. *Pyramid* serving sizes are not intended to be a prescribed amount to eat but are intended to provide flexibility for people to choose a balanced, nutritionally-adequate diet that suits their taste and lifestyle.[16]

Mandatory Nutrients

The nutrition panel will also display a new set of dietary components. The required nutrients were selected because they reflect today's health concerns. The mandatory components and the order in which they must appear are: total calories, calories from fat, total fat, saturated fat, cholesterol, sodium, total carbohydrate, dietary fiber, sugars, protein, vitamin A, vitamin C, calcium, and iron. The order in which these nutrients must appear address the priority of current dietary recommendations. Other vitamins or minerals may be listed if the manufacturer chooses to do so, or if a product makes a specific nutrient claim.

Daily Value and % Daily Value

The new label contains a new nutritional reference tool called **Daily Value**. These values are set by the government and are based on current nutrition recommendations. Some labels list the Daily Values for 2,000-Calorie and 2,500-Calorie reference diets. This information is printed at the bottom of the "Nutrition Facts" panel in the form of a footnote unless a simplified or shortened form is used.

The U.S. Recommended Daily Allowances (USRDA) values no longer appear on packages. Instead, **% Daily Value** is given for the nutrients (total fat, saturated fat, cholesterol, sodium, total carbohydrate, dietary fiber, vitamin A, vitamin C, calcium, and iron) and gives a general idea of a food's nutrient contributions to a 2,000-calorie reference diet. A daily intake of 2,000 Calories was established as a reference for the food labels because it represents an appropriate amount of calories for weight maintenance for many American women who are relatively inactive and for **very** inactive men. It is also a "round" number that can be easily used in mental calculations to adjust up or down, depending on individual needs (i.e., teenage boys, active men or very active women may require up to 2,800 daily calories, whereas sedentary women and some older adults may require as few as 1,600 daily calories).

You can use the % Daily Value to quickly compare foods or to see if the food fits within your current dietary recommendations. A simple rule of thumb to follow is that if the % Daily Value is 5% or less for a particular nutrient, that food is considered "LOW" in that nutrient. The goal is to choose foods that together give you **no more than** 100% of the Daily Value for fat, saturated fat, cholesterol and sodium and **at least** 100% of the Daily Value for nutrients such as carbohydrate, fiber, calcium, vitamin A, vitamin C, and iron.

Nutrient Content Claims

A **Nutrient Content Claim** (also called a **descriptor**) is a word or phrase used on a food package to describe the level of a nutrient in a serving of food. These claims can only be used if a food meets strict definitions set by the government. The following is a list of some of the more frequently used nutrient claims:

*(Note: The core terms, defined by the government, are in **bold** print).*

- ◆ Calorie **Free** — less than 5 calories
- ◆ **Low** Calorie — 40 calories or less*

- **Reduced** Calorie — at least 25% fewer calories than a regular product
- **Light or Lite** — 1/3 fewer calories or 50% less fat than a regular product (if more than half the calories are from fat, the fat content must be reduced by 50% or more)
- Fat **Free** — less than 1/2 gram fat
- **Low** Fat — 3 grams or less fat*
- **Reduced** Fat — at least 25% less fat than a regular product
- Cholesterol **Free** — less than 2 milligrams cholesterol and 2 grams or less saturated fat*
- **Low** Cholesterol — 20 milligrams or less cholesterol and 2 grams or less saturated fat*
- **Lean** — Meat, poultry, seafood and game meat with less than 10 grams total fat, less than 4 grams saturated fat, and less than 95 milligrams cholesterol per Reference Amount (100 grams). Main dish, meal, and meal-type products with less than 10 grams total fat, less than 4 grams saturated fat, and less than 95 milligrams cholesterol per 100 grams and per labeled serving.
- **Extra Lean** — Meat, poultry, seafood and game meat with less than 5 grams total fat, less than 2 grams saturated fat, and less than 95 milligrams cholesterol per Reference Amount (100 grams). Main dish, meal, and meal-type products with less than 5 grams total fat, less than 2 grams saturated fat, and less than 95 milligrams cholesterol per 100 grams and per labeled serving.

With regard to vitamins and minerals, some helpful terms include:
- **Good Source, Contains, Provides** — product contains 10% to 19% of the Daily Value per serving for the specific vitamin or mineral
- **High, Rich** In, **Excellent Source** Of — product contains 20% or more of the Daily Value per serving for the specific vitamin or mineral
- **More, Fortified, Enriched, Added** — product contains at least 10% more of the Daily Value, compared to the reference food.

For individuals particularly concerned about carbohydrates such as fiber and sugars, some helpful terms to seek out on food labels are:
- **Good Source** of Fiber, **Contains** Fiber, **Provides** Fiber — provides 3 to less than 5 grams of fiber per serving (10% to 19% of the Daily Value for fiber)
- **High** Fiber, **Rich** in Fiber, **Excellent Source** of Fiber — provides 5 grams or more fiber per serving (20% or more of the Daily Value for fiber)

- Sugar **Free** — less than $1/2$ gram sugar per serving
- **Reduced** Sugar, **Less** Sugar — at least 25% less sugar than a regular product.

If you are concerned about sodium, some helpful terms to look for on food packages are:

- **Low** Sodium — 140 milligrams or less sodium*
- **Very Low** Sodium — 35 milligrams or less sodium*
- **Reduced** Sodium — at least 25% less sodium than a regular product
- **Light** in Sodium — 50% less sodium than a regular product.

Note

*The nutrient content claim definitions marked with an asterisk * have to meet additional criteria if the serving size is small; i.e., less than 2 tbs. (30 grams). In that case, the definition must apply to 50 grams (1³/4 oz.) of product as well. For a complete listing of the FDA regulated nutrient content claims and definitions see Appendix C, page 371.*

Health Claims

In addition to the "Nutrition Facts" panel on the side or back of the package, you can check the health claims on the front of the product (see Figure 4). A health claim is an FDA-approved statement that describes the relationship between a nutrient and a disease or health-related condition. A food must meet certain nutrient levels to make a health claim. Only eight health messages are allowed now because they are the only ones that are supported by scientific evidence. These nutrient-disease relationships include:

A DIET: AND	LOWER RISK FOR:
High in calcium	Osteoporosis
High in fiber-containing grain products, fruits and vegetables	Cancer
High in fruits or vegetables	Cancer
High in fiber from fruits, vegetables, and grain products	Coronary Heart Disease
Low in fat	Cancer
Low in saturated fat and cholesterol	Coronary Heart Disease
Low in sodium	High blood pressure
High in folate (in women of child-bearing age)	Neural tube defects in infants

FIGURE 3

The New Food Label at a Glance

The new food label will carry an up-to-date, easier-to-use nutrition information guide, to be required on almost all packaged foods (compared to about 60 percent of products up to now). The guide will serve as a key to help in planning a healthy diet.*

Serving sizes are now more consistent across product lines, are stated in both household and metric measures, and reflect the amounts people actually eat..

The **list of nutrients** covers those most important to the health of today's consumers, most of whom need to worry about getting **too much** of certain nutrients (fat, for example), rather than too few vitamins or minerals, as in the past

The label of larger packages may now tell the number of calories per gram of fat, carbo-hydrate, and protein.

New Title signals that the label contains the newly required information.

Calories from fat are now shown on the label to help consumers meet dietary guidelines that recommend people get no more than 30 percent of the calories in their overall diet from fat.

% Daily Value shows how a food fits into the overall daily diet.

Daily values are also something new. Some are maximums, as with fat (65 grams **or less**); others are minimums, as with carbohydrate (300 grams **or more**). The daily values for a 2,000- and 2,500-calorie diet must be listed on the label of larger packages.

Nutrition Facts

Serving Size 1 cup (228g)
Servings Per Container 2

Amount Per Serving

Calories 260   **Calories from Fat 120**

	% Daily Value*
Total Fat 13g	**20%**
Saturated Fat 5g	**25%**
Cholesterol 30mg	**10%**
Sodium 660mg	**28%**
Total Carbohydrate 31g	**10%**
Dietary Fiber 0g	**0%**
Sugars 5g	
Protein 5g	

Vitamin A 4%	•	Vitamin C 2%	
Calcium 15%	•	Iron 4%	

* Percent Daily Values are based on a 2,000 calorie diet. Your daily values may be higher or lower depending on your calorie needs:

	Calories:	2,000	2,500
Total Fat	Less than	65g	80g
Sat Fat	Less than	20g	25g
Cholesterol	Less than	300mg	300mg
Sodium	Less than	2,400mg	2,400mg
Total Carbohydrate		300g	375g
Dietary Fiber		25g	30g

Calories per gram:
Fat 9 • Carbohydrate 4 • Protein 4

*This label is only a sample. Exact specifications are in the final rules.
Source: Food and Drug Administration, 1994

FIGURE 4

The New Food Label at a Glance

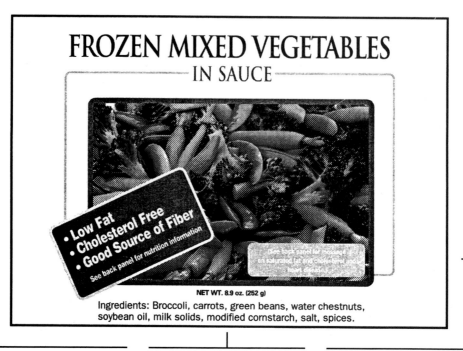

FROZEN MIXED VEGETABLES
IN SAUCE

- Low Fat
- Cholesterol Free
- Good Source of Fiber

See back panel for nutrition information

(See back panel for message on saturated fat and cholesterol and heart disease.)

NET WT. 8.9 oz. (252 g)

Ingredients: Broccoli, carrots, green beans, water chestnuts, soybean oil, milk solids, modified cornstarch, salt, spices.

Claims: While descriptive terms like "low," "good source," and "free" have long been used on food labels, their meaning—and their usefulness in helping consumers plan a healthy diet—have been murky. Now FDA has set specific definitions for these terms, assuring shoppers that they can believe what they read on the package.

Ingredients still will be listed in descending order by weight, and now the list will be required on almost all foods, even standardized ones like mayonnaise and bread.

Health Claims: For the first time, food labels will be allowed to carry information about the link between certain nutrients and specific diseases. For such a "health claim" to be made on a package, FDA must first determine that the diet-disease link is supported by scientific evidence.

Health claim message referred to on the front panel is shown here.

"While many factors affect heart disease, diets low in saturated fat and cholesterol may reduce the risk of this disease."

Source: Adapted from Food and Drug Administration, 1994

STILL CONFUSED ABOUT
THE NEW FOOD LABEL?

Don't worry, help is on the way. *The M-Fit Grocery Shopping Guide* is just what the doctor ordered! Nutrition experts from the University of Michigan Medical Center Preventive Cardiology Program have read and analyzed over 10,000 food product labels. To simplify your job of trying to decide which foods are better choices to reduce risk factors or prevent heart disease, we have grouped food products into three basic categories for healthy eating:

BEST CHOICE

ACCEPTABLE CHOICE

OCCASIONAL CHOICE

The criteria that were developed to evaluate these foods are based on the new FDA food labeling regulations.[10] These criteria have received peer review and have been approved by a panel of national nutrition experts made up of registered dietitians, nutritionists, physicians, and other health professionals.

Finally, here is a publication that you can trust; one that is based on the latest nutrition science; one that is designed to take the guesswork out of selecting healthy foods. *The M-Fit Grocery Shopping Guide* quickly guides you to the healthiest nutritional choices to reduce risk factors or prevent heart disease. There are no numbers to add or percentages to try to remember. *The M-Fit Grocery Shopping Guide* makes it simple to choose foods lower in fat, saturated fat, cholesterol, and sodium, and higher in dietary fiber, which will help you meet the *Dietary Guidelines for Americans*[11] recommended by the U.S. government and many major health organizations.

Best of all, *The M-Fit Grocery Shopping Guide* helps you find the many healthy and delicious products on the supermarket shelves. **The choice is up to you!**

BAKING MIXES
(pancakes, muffins, biscuits)

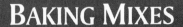

This category contains a large variety of dry baking mixes such as pancakes, muffins, and biscuits. These mixes provide complex carbohydrates to the diet and can be a good source of B-vitamins, iron, and fiber. Baking Mixes vary in the amount of total fat, saturated fat, and cholesterol they contain.

Baking Mixes for products such as pancakes, waffles, muffins, or biscuits are included as part of the "Bread, Cereal, Rice, and Pasta Group" and help make up the base of the *Food Guide Pyramid*. Six to eleven servings each day are recommended from this food group. Serving sizes vary with the type of product; for example, one 4-inch pancake, one medium muffin or biscuit count as one serving each. The FDA has established reference amounts or standardized serving sizes for use on the food label. The reference amount for dry baking mixes is 40 grams (1.4 ounces). This amount is equivalent to 1/4 to 1/3 cup dry mix. (See pages 51 and 52 for an explanation of reference amounts and the difference between serving sizes established by the FDA for food labeling and those recommended by the *Food Guide Pyramid*.)

At first glance, the criteria for this category of foods may seem to be overly restrictive. However, because most of these products require the addition of other ingredients that supply added fat (e.g., oils, milk, and eggs) for preparation, the fat content of these products can be significantly increased. Although many food companies give the nutritional breakdown for both the "As Packaged" and "As Prepared" versions, the "As Prepared" version is voluntary and, therefore, may not be given for all products. Additionally, consumers may, or may not, choose to follow the specified package directions. Consumers are also at liberty to make either higher-fat or lower-fat ingredient substitutions. See Appendix D, page 373, for a listing of ingredient substitutions for lowering fat content. For this reason, the fat content of the "As Packaged" dry mix was used to evaluate these products.

Criteria Key

▲ **Best Choice:**   **Fat Free or Without Added Fats**

Products listed in this category meet the FDA's definition for "Fat Free" (less than ¹/₂ gram fat per serving) in their "As Packaged " form, or are processed without added fats. Many of these food products allow you to add your own ingredients, such as your oil of choice (try reducing the amount called for by half), egg whites, and skim milk. More recipe modification tips are found in Appendix D, page 373.

> *Note: Some products that contain whole grains as their first ingredient will not meet the FDA's "Fat Free" criteria, however, will meet the "without added fats" criteria. The fat content of these products can be as high as 2 grams per serving The fat in this case is naturally-occurring in the whole grain. For this reason, these products are included in the "Best Choice" category.*

▲ **Acceptable Choice:**   **Low Fat**

Products listed in this category meet the FDA's definition for "Low Fat" (3 grams or less fat per serving) in their "As Packaged" form (before preparation).

▲ **Occasional Choice:**   **Contains Greater Than 3 Grams Total Fat**

Products listed in this category **do not** meet the FDA's definition for "Low Fat" in their "As Packaged" form. Since most of these products require the addition of ingredients containing fat (i.e. milk, oil, eggs), these products can provide a significant amount of added fat to the diet. For this reason, they should be used only on occasion.

BRAND	BEST CHOICE	ACCEPTABLE CHOICE	OCCASIONAL CHOICE
	Fat Free OR Without Added Fat	Low Fat	Contains Greater Than 3 Grams Total Fat
Appian Way		Pizza: Regular Crust	

Arrowhead Mills	☆ Biscuit Mix
	★ Bran Muffin Mix
	☆ Cornbread Mix
	★ Griddle Lite Pancake Mix
	☆ Multi-Grain Biscuit Mix
	☆ Multi-Grain Bread Mix
	☆Multi-Grain Corn Bread Mix
	Pancake and Waffle Mix:
	  ★ Buckwheat
	  ☆ Multigrain
	  ★ Oat Bran
	★ Whole Wheat Bread Mix
			Wheat Free Muffin Mix:
			  ★ Oat Bran

Aunt Jemima	Corn Meal Mix:
	  Buttermilk
	  Self Rising White
	Pancake & Waffle Mix:
	  ▲☆ Buckwheat
	  ▲☆ Whole Wheat
	Pancake Mix:
	  ▲ Original
		Original Pancake Batter:
		  ▲ Refrigerate and Pour
		Pancake & Waffle Mix:
		  ▲ Buttermilk Complete
		Pancake Mix:
		  ▲★ Reduced Calorie
		     Buttermilk Complete	

Betty Crocker		Low Fat Muffin Mix:
		  Wild Blueberry
		Muffin Mix:
		  Apple Cinnamon
		  Banana Nut
		  Twice the Blueberries
		  Wild Blueberry
			Coffee Cake & Muffin Mix:
			  Cinnamon Streusel

Bisquick		All Purpose Baking Mix:
		  Reduced Fat
		Shake 'n Pour:
		  ▲ Buttermilk Pancake Mix
			All Purpose Baking Mix:
			  ▲ Original
			Shake 'n Pour:
			  ▲ Blueberry Pancake Mix
			  ▲ Original

Bob's Red Mill	100% Whole Wheat Bread Mix Date-Nut Bran Muffin Mix Spice Apple Bran Muffin Mix Wheat-Free Biscuit & Baking Mix		Cornbread Mix & Cornmeal Muffin Mix Irish Soda Bread Mix Rye Bread Mix

Box Hill	Ready to Bake Home Breads:
	  ∇ White
	  ∇ Whole Wheat		

▲ High Sodium, 480 mg. or greater per serving.
∇ Low Sodium, 140 mg. or less per serving.
☆ Good Source of Fiber, between 2.5 g. and 5 g. per serving.
★ High Fiber, 5 g. or greater per serving.

BRAND	BEST CHOICE	ACCEPTABLE CHOICE	OCCASIONAL CHOICE
	Fat Free OR Without Added Fat	Low Fat	Contains Greater Than 3 Grams Total Fat
Classique Fare		Belgian Waffle Mix	Pancake Mix: Pecan
Daily Bread Company	Quick Loaf: Cinnamon Raisin Garlic & Herbs Hearty Cracked Wheat		
Dromedary Bakery		Bread Machine Mix: All Varieties	
Duncan Hines			Bakery Style Muffin Mix: Blueberry w/Crumb Topping Cinnamon Swirl
Eagle Mill's		Best Loaf Bread Machine Mix Italian White ☆ Whole Wheat	
Fast Shake		▲☆ Real Blueberry Pancake Mix	▲ Buttermilk Pancake Mix
Gold Medal		Blueberry Muffin Mix Golden Corn Muffin Mix Pizza Crust Mix	Apple Cinnamon Muffin Mix Banana Nut Muffin Mix
Hodgson Mill	▲★ Buckwheat Pancake Mix	Bread Mix: ☆ Honey Whole Wheat Wholesome White ▲☆ Buttermilk Pancake Mix ☆ Cornbread and Muffin Mix ▲ Jalapeno Cornbread Mix Muffin Mix: ☆ Bran ▲☆ Whole Wheat	
Jiffy		Pizza Crust Mix	Baking Mix Buttermilk Biscuit Mix Muffin Mix: Apple Cinnamon Banana Nut Blueberry ☆ Bran w/Dates Corn Honey Date Oatmeal

▲ High Sodium, 480 mg. or greater per serving.
☆ Good Source of Fiber, between 2.5 g. and 5 g. per serving.
★ High Fiber, 5 g. or greater per serving.

BRAND	BEST CHOICE	ACCEPTABLE CHOICE	OCCASIONAL CHOICE
	Fat Free OR Without Added Fat	Low Fat	Contains Greater Than 3 Grams Total Fat

Krusteaz	Muffin Mix Fat Free:
	   All Flavors
	Pancake Mix:
	   ▲★Whole Wheat & Honey
		▲ Belgian Waffle Mix
		Honey Cornbread and Muffin Mix
		Muffin Mix:
		   Almond Poppyseed
		Pancake Mix:
		   ▲ Blueberry
		   ▲ Buttermilk
			Biscuit Mix:
			   ▲ Cinnamon Raisin
			Muffin Mix:
			   Oat Bran
			Pancake & Waffle Mix:
			   ▲☆ Harvest Apple Spice

Lund's	Swedish Pancake Mix		
Manischewitz		▲ Potato Pancake Mix	Muffin Mix Passover Gold: Pizza Mix

Maple Grove Farms	Pancake Mix:
	   ▲ Buttermilk & Honey
	   ▲ Honey Buckwheat
		Pancake Mix:
		   ▲☆ Blueberry	

Martha White		Buttermilk Corn Bread Mix
		Deep Pan Pizza Crust Mix
		Muffin Mix:
		   Blueberry
		   Corn
		   Oatmeal Raisin Spice
		Pizza Crust Mix:
		   Crispy Crust
			Bix Mix:
			   ▲ Buttermilk Biscuit Mix
			Flapstax:
			   ▲ Buttermilk Complete
			      Pancake Mix
			Muffin Mix:
			   Banana Nut
			   Blackberry
			   Chocolate Chocolate Chip
			   Lemon Poppyseed
			   Strawberry

Mrs. Butterworth's	▲Old Fashioned Pancake Mix	Buttermilk Complete Pancake Mix:
		   ▲ Lowfat
		▲Complete Pancake & Waffle
		   Mix	

Pillsbury		Bread Machine Mix:
		   Cracked Wheat
		   Crusty White
		Hot Roll Mix:
		   Original
		Hungry Jack:
		   ▲ Buttermilk Complete
		   ▲ Buttermilk Pancake Mix
		Quick Bread Mix:
		   Apple Cinnamon
		   Banana
		   Carrot	

▲ High Sodium, 480 mg. or greater per serving.
☆ Good Source of Fiber, between 2.5 g. and 5 g. per serving.
★ High Fiber, 5 g. or greater per serving.

BRAND	BEST CHOICE	ACCEPTABLE CHOICE	OCCASIONAL CHOICE
	Fat Free OR Without Added Fat	Low Fat	Contains Greater Than 3 Grams Total Fat
Pillsbury (Cont.)		Quick Bread Mix: Cranberry ∇ Date Nut Pumpkin	
Pioneer	▲ Low Fat Biscuit & Baking Mix		
YOUR FAVORITE BAKING MIXES NOT LISTED IN THE *GUIDE*			

▲ High Sodium, 480 mg. or greater per serving.
∇ Low Sodium, 140 mg. or less per serving.

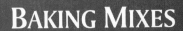

BAKING MIXES
(desserts)

This category contains a variety of dessert-type baking mixes. Although these products are traditionally high in sugar and fat, some products, such as angel food cake and other specially formulated cake mixes, are either fat-free or reduced-fat. Food companies are also including lower-fat recipe instructions for preparation of lower-fat versions of their products.

The *Food Guide Pyramid* considers cakes as part of the "Bread, Cereal, Rice, and Pasta Group." Six to eleven servings each day are recommended from this food group. However, products such as cakes can contain large amounts of fat and sugar, while other foods in this group, such as bread, rice and pasta, and some cereals, are significantly lower in fat and sugar while providing generous amounts of fiber, vitamins, and minerals. The FDA has established reference amounts or standardized serving sizes for use on the food label. The reference amount for cakes ranges from 55 grams (2 ounces) for "light weight" cakes such as angel food, 80 grams (3 ounces) for "medium weight" cakes such as cupcakes or eclairs, to 125 grams (4.5 ounces) for "heavy weight" cakes such as cheesecake. Be sure to read the *Nutrition Facts* label for the serving size information of your choice from this product category. (See pages 51 and 52 for an explanation of reference amounts and the difference between serving sizes established by the FDA for food labeling and those recommended by the *Food Guide Pyramid*.)

At first glance, the criteria for this category of foods may seem to be overly restrictive. However, because most of these products require the addition of other ingredients that supply added fat, (e.g., oils, milk, eggs) for preparation, the fat content of these products can be significantly increased. Although many food companies give the nutritional breakdown for both the "As Packaged" and "As Prepared" versions, the "As Prepared" version is voluntary and, therefore, may not be given for all products. Additionally, consumers may, or may not, choose to follow the specified package directions. Consumers are also at liberty to make either higher-fat or lower-fat ingredient substitutions. (See Appendix D, page 373, for a list of lower-fat substitution suggestions.) For this reason the fat content of the "As Packaged" dry mix was used to evaluate these products.

Criteria Key

▲ Best Choice: Fat Free

Products listed in this category meet the FDA's definition for "Fat Free" (less than ¹/₂ gram fat per serving) in their "As Packaged " form. Many of these food products allow you to add your own ingredients such as your oil of choice (try reducing the amount called for by half), egg whites and skim milk. (See Appendix D, page 373, for a list of lower-fat substitution suggestions.)

▲ Acceptable Choice: Low Fat

Products listed in this category meet the FDA's definition for "Low Fat" (3 grams or less fat per serving) in their "As Packaged" form (before preparation).

▲ Occasional Choice: Contains Greater Than 3 Grams Total Fat

Products listed in this category **do not** meet the FDA's definition for "Low Fat" in their "As Packaged" form. Because most of these products require the addition of ingredients containing fat (e.g., milk, oil, eggs), these products can provide a significant amount of added fat to the diet. For this reason, they should be used only on occasion.

BRAND	BEST CHOICE	ACCEPTABLE CHOICE	OCCASIONAL CHOICE
	Fat Free	Low Fat	Contains Greater Than 3 Grams Total Fat

Betty Crocker	Angel Food Cake Mix:
	  Confetti
	  White
	Fat Free Muffin Mix:
	  Wild Blueberry
	Swirl Angel Food Cake:
	  Chocolate
		Creamy Chilled Desserts:
		  Banana Cream
		Easy Delicious Desserts:
		  Homestyle Carrot Cake
		Fudge Brownie Mix:
		  ∇ Dark Chocolate
		  ∇ Lowfat
		  ∇ Regular
		Muffin Mix:
		  Sunkist Lemon-Poppy Seed
		SuperMoist Cake Mix:
		  Butter Recipe Yellow
		  Yellow
		SuperMoist Light:
		  Devil's Food
		  Yellow
		Supreme Brownie Mix:
		  ∇ Caramel Brownies
		  ∇ Cookies 'n Creme
		  ∇ German Chocolate
		    Brownies
		  ∇ Original
			Creamy Chilled Desserts:
			  Chocolate French Silk
			  Coconut Cream
			  Cookies 'n Creme
			  ∇ Sunkist Lemon Supreme
			∇ Date Bar Mix
			Easy Delicious Desserts:
			  Apple Crisp
			  Chocolate Caramel Crumb
			    Cake
			  Triple Fudge Brownie Cake
			Gingerbread Cake & Cookie
			  Mix
			Golden Pound Cake Mix
			Pineapple Upside Down Cake
			SuperMoist Cake Mix:
			  Butter Pecan
			  Butter Recipe Chocolate
			  Carrot Cake
			  Cherry Chip
			  Chocolate Chip
			  Chocolate Fudge
			  Devil's Food
			  Double Chocolate Swirl
			  French Vanilla
			  German Chocolate
			  Golden Vanilla
			  Lemon
			  Party Cake Swirl
			  Rainbow Chip Party Cake
			  Sour Cream White
			  Strawberry Swirl
			  White
			SuperMoist Light:
			  White
			Supreme Brownie Mix:
			  ∇ Chocolate Chip
			  ∇ Frosted
			  ∇ Hot Fudge
			  ∇ Peanut Butter Candies
			  ∇ Walnut
			  ∇ White Chocolate Swirl
			Supreme Dessert Bar Mix:
			  ∇ Caramel Bars
			  ∇ Chocolate Chunk Bars
			  Reese's Chocolate Peanut
			    Butter Bars

∇ Low Sodium, 140 mg. or less per serving.

BRAND	BEST CHOICE	ACCEPTABLE CHOICE	OCCASIONAL CHOICE
	Fat Free	Low Fat	Contains Greater Than 3 Grams Total Fat

Betty Crocker (Cont.)			Supreme Dessert Bar Mix:
			  ∇ Heath Chocolate Toffee
			  ∇ Easy Layer Bars
			  ∇ Lemon Sunkist Bars
			  ∇ M&M Cookie Bars
			  ∇ Raspberry Bars
			  ∇ Strawberry Swirl
			      Cheesecake

Calhoun Bend Mill	Peach Cobbler Mix		

Duncan Hines	Moist Deluxe Cake Mix:
	  ∇ Angel Food
		Bar Mix:
		  ∇ Double Decker
		  ∇ Milk Chocolate Chunk
		Chocolate Lovers' Brownie Mix:
		  ∇ Chewy Recipe Fudge
		  ∇ Dark Chocolate
		  ∇ Double Fudge
		Cookie Mix:
		  ∇ Golden Sugar
		Moist Deluxe Cake Mix:
		  Yellow Delights
			Bar Mix:
			  ∇ Cinnamon
			Brownie Mix:
			  ∇ Blondies w/Walnuts
			Chocolate Chip Cookie Mix:
			  ∇ Chewy Gooey Cookies
			Chocolate Lovers' Brownie Mix:
			  ∇ Dark Chocolate w/Milk
			      Chocolate Chunks
			  ∇ Milk Chocolate Crunch
			  ∇ Peanut Butter
			  ∇ Walnut
			Duncan Cups Microwave:
			  Brownies w/Chocolate
			      Frosting
			Moist Deluxe Cake Mix:
			  Banana Supreme
			  Butter Recipe Fudge
			  Butter Recipe Golden Caramel
			  Dark Chocolate Fudge
			  Devil's Food
			  French Vanilla
			  Fudge Marble
			  Lemon Supreme
			  Orange Supreme
			  Peach
			  Pineapple Supreme
			  Raspberry
			  Spice
			  Strawberry Supreme
			  White
			  Yellow
			Muffin Mix:
			  Bakery Style Honey Nut
			  Blueberry
			  Chocolate Chip
			  Raspberry
			  ∇ Peanut Butter Cookie Mix

∇ Low Sodium, 140 mg. or less per serving.

BRAND	BEST CHOICE	ACCEPTABLE CHOICE	OCCASIONAL CHOICE
	Fat Free	Low Fat	Contains Greater Than 3 Grams Total Fat
Gold Medal		∇ Chocolate Chip Cookie Mix ∇ Double Chocolate Chunk Cookie Mix ∇ Fudge Brownie Mix	Golden Yellow Cake Mix: Smart Size
Jell-O			No Bake Cheesecake Mix: All Flavors No Bake Dessert: Chocolate Silk Pie Coconut Creme Pie
Jiffy			Brownie Mix: Fudge Cake Mix: ▲ Devil's Food Golden Yellow White Pie Crust Mix
Knorr	Dessert Mix: ∇ Creme Caramel Flan		Dessert Mix: ∇ Dark Chocolate Mousse ∇ Milk Chocolate
Libby's	Pumpkin Pie Mix		.
Manischewitz	∇ Angel Food Cake Mix ∇ Sponge Cake Mix		▲ Chocolate Chocolate Cake Mix Mom's Helper: ∇ Cupcake Mix ∇ Fudgey Gooey Brownie Mix
Martha White		Brownie Mix Chewy Fudge: Family Size ∇ Snack Size	
Nabisco		Honey Maid: ∇ Graham Cracker Crumbs	
Nabisco Royal			Lite Whipped Cheesecake No Bake Pie Mix: Chocolate Mint ▲ Chocolate Peanut Butter Real Cheesecake
Obie's Cookie Jar	Fat Free Cookie Mixes: ∇ Chewy Oatmeal Raisin ∇ French Vanilla w/Almonds	Low Fat Cookie Mixes: ∇ Classic Chocolate Chip ∇ Double Chocolate Fudge	

▲ High Sodium, 480 mg. or greater per serving.
∇ Low Sodium, 140 mg. or less per serving.

BRAND	BEST CHOICE	ACCEPTABLE CHOICE	OCCASIONAL CHOICE
	Fat Free	Low Fat	Contains Greater Than 3 Grams Total Fat

Pillsbury	Cake Mix:
	    Angel Food
		Brownie Mix:
		    ∇ Fudge
		Pillsbury Plus Cake Mix:
		    Butter Recipe
			Bundt Cake Mix:
			    Chocolate Caramel Nut
			    Double Hot Fudge
			    Strawberry Cream Cheese
			Deluxe Bar Mix:
			    ∇ Apple Struesel
			    ∇ Fudge Marble
			    ∇ Lemon Cheesecake
			    ∇ Nutter Butter
			    ∇ Oreo
			Deluxe Brownie Mix:
			    ∇ Cream Cheese Swirl
			    ∇ Hot Fudge
			Lovin' Lites:
			    Yellow Cake Mix
			Pillsbury Plus Cake Mix:
			    Banana
			    Dark Chocolate
			    Devil's Food
			    French Vanilla
			    Funfetti
			    German Chocolate
			    Lemon
			    Sunshine Vanilla
			    White
			    Yellow
			Streusel Swirl:
			    Cinnamon

Salerno		Graham Cracker Crumbs	
Sans Sucre		∇ Cheesecake Mousse Mix	
Sunshine		Graham Cracker Crumbs	

Sweet 'N Low		Cake Mix:
		    ∇ Chocolate
		    ∇ Yellow	

YOUR FAVORITE BAKING MIXES NOT LISTED IN THE *GUIDE*			

∇ Low Sodium, 140 mg. or less per serving.

BREADS

This category contains a large variety of breads such as sliced breads, rolls, and garlic bread. These foods provide complex carbohydrates to the diet and can be a good source of B-vitamins, iron, and fiber. They are also generally low in total fat, saturated fat, and cholesterol.

Bread products are included as part of the "Bread, Cereal, Rice, and Pasta Group" and help make up the base of the *Food Guide Pyramid*. Six to eleven servings each day are recommended from this food group. One slice of bread is considered one serving as is one small dinner roll. It should be noted that many "light" breads report a serving size of two slices on the *Nutrition Facts* label. Although two slices may be equivalent to *one serving* on the food label, consumers need to be aware that this amount is actually considered *two servings* from the *Food Guide Pyramid*. The FDA has established reference amounts or standardized serving sizes for use on the food label. The reference amount for breads is 50 grams (1.8 ounces). The number of bread slices to which this amount is equivalent varies with the type of bread, size of slice, and density of product. Be sure to read the Nutrition Facts label for the serving size information of your bread choice. (See pages 51 and 52 for an explanation of reference amounts and the difference between serving sizes established by the FDA for food labeling and those recommended by the *Food Guide Pyramid*.)

Because Americans consume less than one-half of the fiber recommended by the National Cancer Institute (between 20 and 30 grams per day), fiber was used as part of the criteria to evaluate breads. Breads are a nutritious, low-fat way to provide fiber in daily diets. A greater amount of dietary fiber is found in whole grain products than in their refined alternatives. Criteria were therefore designed to distinguish those products lower in total fat and saturated fat and higher in fiber from their higher-fat, lower-fiber alternatives. Additionally, those breads that meet the definition for "High Fiber" (5 grams or higher per serving) are marked with a ★ symbol. Breads that meet

the definition for "Good Source of Fiber" (between 2.5 grams and 5 grams per serving) are marked with a ☆ symbol.

Sodium content of breads varies between brands and typically ranges from 110 to 175 milligrams per serving. Most breads may, therefore, qualify for the FDA's definition of "Low Sodium" (140 milligrams or less) and will be marked in the book with a ∇ symbol. However, it is important to remember that while individual servings may not seem to contribute large amounts of sodium, the typical American diet consists of several servings from this food category. According to food consumption data, bread is the number one major contributor of sodium in the US diet.[74]

Criteria Key

▲ Best Choice:　　Fat Free or Low Fat, AND Low Saturated Fat, AND Good Source of Fiber

Products listed in this category meet the FDA's definition for "Fat Free" (less than $1/2$ gram fat per serving), or "Low Fat" (3 grams or less fat per serving) and "Low Saturated Fat" (1 gram or less saturated fat per serving). Additionally, products in this category meet the criteria of "Good Source of Fiber" (at least 2.5 grams per serving).

▲ Acceptable Choice:　　Fat Free or Low Fat, AND Low Saturated Fat

These breads are classified as "Acceptable Choice" since they meet the above definitions for "Fat Free" or "Low Fat," and "Low Saturated Fat," but **do not** meet the criteria for "Good Source of Fiber." Consequently these foods do not contribute as much fiber to the overall daily diet.

▲ Occasional Choice:　　Contains Greater Than 3 Grams of Total Fat, OR Greater Than 1 Gram of Saturated Fat

Products listed in this category **do not** meet the FDA's definition for "Low Fat," or "Low Saturated Fat." Generally, bread products that contain greater than 3 grams of total fat or 1 gram of saturated fat should be consumed only on occasion, to make room for the more healthful bread choices.

BRAND	BEST CHOICE	ACCEPTABLE CHOICE	OCCASIONAL CHOICE
	Fat Free or Low Fat AND Low Saturated Fat AND Good Source of Fiber	Fat Free or Low Fat AND Low Saturated Fat	Contains Greater Than 3 Grams Total Fat OR Greater Than 1 Gram of Saturated Fat
American Meal		Premium	

Arnold	Bran'Nola:
	  ∇☆ Nutty Grains
	  ∇☆ Original
	Brick Oven:
	  ☆ 100% Whole Wheat Bread
	  ☆ Wheat Bread
	  ☆ Honey Wheat Berry Bread
	Levy's Old Country Rolls:
	  ☆ Onion
		Bran'Nola:
		  ∇ 7-Grain White Bread
		  Hot Dog Rolls
		Bread:
		  Brick Oven White
		  Country Buttermilk
		  Country Potato
		  ∇ Country Soft Rye
		  Country Soft White
		  Country Wheat
		  Country White
		  ∇ Cranberry
		  Dill Rye
		  Pumpernickel
		  ∇ Raisin Cinnamon
		Dinner Rolls:
		  ∇ Potato
		  ∇ Regular
		Dutch Egg Rolls
		Hot Dog Buns:
		  New England Style
		  Regular
		Hot Dog Rolls:
		  Potato
		Levy's Old Country Rolls:
		  Kaiser
		  Sub
		Levy's Real Jewish Bread:
		  Rye Unseeded
		  Rye w/Caraway
		Pita:
		  Wheat
		  White
		Premium Onion Rolls	

Aunt Ginnie's		Hot Bread:
		  Cinnamon
		  Original	

Aunt Millie's	∇☆ Light Wheat
	Light White Bread:
	  ∇☆ Fat Free
		Fat Free Bread:
		  White Sourdough
		  Potato
		  Wheat, Multi-Grain
		Fat Free Buns:
		  Hamburger Potato
		  Hot Dog Potato	

∇ Low Sodium, 140 mg. or less per serving.
☆ Good Source of Fiber, between 2.5 g. and 5 g. per serving.

BRAND	BEST CHOICE	ACCEPTABLE CHOICE	OCCASIONAL CHOICE
	Fat Free or Low Fat AND Low Saturated Fat AND Good Source of Fiber	Fat Free or Low Fat AND Low Saturated Fat	Contains Greater Than 3 Grams Total Fat OR Greater Than 1 Gram of Saturated Fat

Aunt Millie's (Cont.)		Hamburger Buns
		Homestyle Buttermilk Bread
		Homestyle Cracked Wheat Bread
		Homestyle Oatmeal Bread
		Hot Dog Buns:
		   Restaurant Style
		Hot Rolls:
		   Krusty Enriched Rolls
		Light Italian
		Magnifico Pane Italiano
		Sesame Seed Buns
		∇ Split Top Wheat Bread	

Autumn Grain	∇☆ Light Wheat Bread	∇ Natural Grain Bread	

Baker's Choice		Breadsticks:
		   ∇ Cheese
		   ∇ Garlic
		   ∇ Italian Style
		   ∇ Sesame	

Beefsteak	Bread:
	   ★ Light Soft Rye
		Breads:
		   Hearty Rye, Seeded
		   Hearty Wheat
		   ∇ Robust White
		   Soft Rye, No Seeds
		   Soft Wheat	

Better Way		100% Whole Wheat Bread Natural 7-Grain Bread	

Bread du Jour		Bread Sticks:
		   Original
		   Sourdough
		French Loaves
		Rolls:
		   Bavarian Cracked Wheat
		   Italian
		Soft Rye	

Brownberry	Bran'nola:
	   ∇☆ Hearty Wheat
	   ∇☆ Original
		Bread:
		   ∇ Apple Honey Wheat
		   Natural 12 Grain
		   Natural Caraway Rye
		   Natural Country Wheat
		   Natural Country White	

∇ Low Sodium, 140 mg. or less per serving.
☆ Good Source of Fiber, between 2.5 g. and 5 g. per serving.
★ High Fiber, 5 g. or greater per serving.

74 **Breads**

BRAND	BEST CHOICE	ACCEPTABLE CHOICE	OCCASIONAL CHOICE
	Fat Free or Low Fat AND Low Saturated Fat AND Good Source of Fiber	Fat Free or Low Fat AND Low Saturated Fat	Contains Greater Than 3 Grams Total Fat OR Greater Than 1 Gram of Saturated Fat
Brownberry (Cont.)		Bread: 　Natural Dill Rye 　∇ Natural Health Nut 　∇ Natural Oatmeal 　∇ Natural Orange Raisin 　Natural Pumpernickel Rye 　∇ Raisin Cinnamon 　Natural Thin Sliced Rye 　　Unseeded 　Natural Wheat 　∇ Natural Whole Bran 　∇ Raisin Walnut 　∇ Soft Oatmeal 　∇ Soft Wheat 　∇ Soft White Hot Dog Rolls: 　Sliced 　Wheat Sandwich Buns: 　Wheat 　White	
Butternut	★ Lite Loaf Wheat Bread ★ Lite Loaf White Bread	Dixie Rye Bread Enriched Bread Hearty Rye Bread Honey Wheat Bread Italian Bread	
Chicago Hearth			Enriched Buns
Cole's			Breadsticks: 　Garlic Flavored Garlic Bread: 　Multi-Grain 　Original 　Romano Cheese 　Zesty Italiano Garlic Mini Loaf: 　Butter Flavored
Country Hearth		100% Whole Wheat All Natural: 　Cinnamon Raisin ∇ Deli Rye Honey Wheat Berry Bread Indian Grain Bread ∇ Light Rice Bran and Barley	

∇ Low Sodium, 140 mg. or less per serving.
★ High Fiber, 5 g. or greater per serving.

BRAND	BEST CHOICE	ACCEPTABLE CHOICE	OCCASIONAL CHOICE
	Fat Free or Low Fat AND Low Saturated Fat AND Good Source of Fiber	Fat Free or Low Fat AND Low Saturated Fat	Contains Greater Than 3 Grams Total Fat OR Greater Than 1 Gram of Saturated Fat
Country Hearth (Cont.)		Light Wheat Split Top Wheat w/Oatbran ∇ Stone Ground Wheat	
County Fair		Enriched Buns: All Varieties	

D'Italiano	Real Italian Bread:
	    ☆ Light
		Real Italian Bread:
		    Regular	

Dimpflmeier	☆ Cracked Wheat Bread ☆ Swedish Light Rye Bread	Deli Light Rye Bread Old Fashioned White Bread	
Earthgrains			Garlic Rolls

Father Sam's		▲ Magic Pocketbread
		Pocket Bread:
		    Wheat
		    White	

Garden of Eatin'			Whole Wheat Naan: ☆ All Varieties
Good Hearth		∇ Honey Wheat Berry ∇ Multi-Grain Bread ∇ Oat Bran Bread Stone Ground Wheat Bread	
Great Harvest Bread Co.	☆ Cinnamon Raisin Walnut ☆ Country Molasses ☆ Honey Wheat ☆ Michigan Herb ☆ Nine Grain ☆ Oatberry ☆ Sunflower	White	
Great Lakes		∇ Enriched White Bread	
Great Plains		American Meal Whole Grain Bread	

Holsum		King Size White Enriched
		Sof-Buns:
		    Hamburger
		    Hot Dog	

▲ High Sodium, 480 mg. or greater per serving.
∇ Low Sodium, 140 mg. or less per serving.
☆ Good Source of Fiber, between 2.5 g. and 5 g. per serving.

BRAND	BEST CHOICE	ACCEPTABLE CHOICE	OCCASIONAL CHOICE
	Fat Free or Low Fat AND Low Saturated Fat AND Good Source of Fiber	Fat Free or Low Fat AND Low Saturated Fat	Contains Greater Than 3 Grams Total Fat OR Greater Than 1 Gram of Saturated Fat
Home Pride		Buttertop: Wheat White	
Joseph's	Middle East Style: ∇☆ Whole Wheat Syrian Bread	Middle East Syle: ∇ Enriched Syrian Bread	
Kangaroo	Pocket Bread: ☆ Wheat N Honey	No Pocket Pita: Original Pocket Bread: Onion ∇ White	
King's		∇ Hawaiian Rolls	Hawaiian Bread
Kleen-maid		Enriched Bread Soft Buns: Hamburger Buns Hot Dog	
Koepplinger's	Hamburger Buns: ☆ Lite Wheat Hot Dog Buns: ☆ Lite Wheat Lite Bread: ☆ 100% Whole Wheat ☆ Italian ☆ Oatbran ☆ Wheat	Black Russian Bread Buttersweet: Wheat Bread ∇ White Bread ∇ Buttery Cinnamon Raisin Bread ∇ California Raisin Bread ∇ Cinnamon Wheat and Raisin Bread Early American White Bread Hamburger Buns: Enriched Seeded Enriched White Wheat Hot Dog Buns: Wheat Natural Rye: Seedless Natural Wheat Bread Staff O' Life Health Bread: ∇ Original	
Leon's		Pita Bread Wheat Pita Bread	

∇ Low Sodium, 140 mg. or less per serving.
☆ Good Source of Fiber, between 2.5 g. and 5 g. per serving.

BRAND	BEST CHOICE	ACCEPTABLE CHOICE	OCCASIONAL CHOICE
	Fat Free or Low Fat AND Low Saturated Fat AND Good Source of Fiber	Fat Free or Low Fat AND Low Saturated Fat	Contains Greater Than 3 Grams Total Fat OR Greater Than 1 Gram of Saturated Fat
Less	Hamburger Buns: ☆ Light Wheat Bread: ☆ Light Dark 'N Grainy ☆ Light Oat Bran ☆ Light Wheat ☆ Light White		
Lumber Jack		Bread: ∇ Classic Split Top Country Wheat Enriched White Lumber Camp Style Buns	
Mackinaw Milling Co.		100% Whole Wheat Bread Black Forest Rye Bread ∇ Cinnamon Raisin Bread Deli Rye Honey & Bran Bread Oatmeal Soft Rye Bread Wheat	
Mamma Bella			Garlic Bread
Mrs. Butterworth's		Dinner Rolls: White Enriched White Frozen Bread Dough	
Natural Grains	Lite: ★ Oat Bran ★ Wheat ★ White	12 Grains 7 Whole Grains Bread Oat Bran Oatmeal ∇ Stone Ground Whole Wheat	
Natural Ovens	∇★ 100% Whole Grain Bread ∇☆ Executive Fitness Sunny Millet Bread ∇★ Happiness Bread ∇★ Hunger Filler Bread ∇★ Light Wheat Bread ∇★ Nutty Natural Wheat Bread	∇ English Muffin Bread ∇ Garden Bread ∇ Gourmet Dinner Rolls ∇ Robust German Rye Bread ∇ Soft Sandwich Bread	

∇ Low Sodium, 140 mg. or less per serving.
☆ Good Source of Fiber, between 2.5 g. and 5 g. per serving.
★ High Fiber, 5 g. or greater per serving.

BRAND	BEST CHOICE	ACCEPTABLE CHOICE	OCCASIONAL CHOICE
	Fat Free or Low Fat AND Low Saturated Fat AND Good Source of Fiber	Fat Free or Low Fat AND Low Saturated Fat	Contains Greater Than 3 Grams Total Fat OR Greater Than 1 Gram of Saturated Fat
New York			Garlic Bread

Oven Fresh	☆ Italian Bread
	∇☆ Mom's Choice For Kids
	☆ Reduced Calorie Wheat Bread
		English Muffin Bread
		Golden Wheat:
		   Buttered Split Top
		Romano Italian Bread
		Sloppy Joe Buns
		Soft Hamburger Buns:
		   Seeded
		Soft Hot Dog Buns
		Sub Buns	

Paramount		Non Fat Lavash Bread:
		   ∇ All Varieties
		Pita Bread:
		   ∇ All Varieties	

Parisian		Sourdough Sandwich Rolls	

Pepperidge Farm	French Rolls:
	   ▲☆ Brown and Serve
	Light Style:
	   ★ 7-Grain
	   ★ Oatmeal
	   ★ Vienna
	   ★ Wheat
	☆ Party Rye Bread
	Sandwich Buns:
	   ☆ 7 Grain
	Very Thin:
	   ☆ Wheat
		Cinnamon Swirl:
		   ∇ Cinnamon
		   ∇ Raisin
		Classic Dark Pumpernickel
		   Bread
		Club Rolls
		∇ Cracked Wheat Bread
		Dijon Rye, Seedless Bread
		Dinner Rolls:
		   Country Style
		Frankfurter Rolls:
		   Regular
		French Rolls
		Hamburger Rolls
		Hearty Slices:
		   Country White
		   Crunchy Oat
		   Honey Wheatberry
		   Sesame Wheat
		   Seven Grain
		Jewish Rye Bread:
		   Seedless
		Natural Whole Grain:
		   Nine Grain
		   Whole Wheat
		   ∇ Crunchy Grains
			European Bake Shop Rolls:
			   Twists
			Frankfurter Rolls:
			   Dijon
			Garlic Bread
			Onion Sandwich Buns
			Sandwich Buns:
			   with Sesame Seeds

▲ High Sodium, 480 mg. or greater per serving.
∇ Low Sodium, 140 mg. or less per serving.
☆ Good Source of Fiber, between 2.5 g. and 5 g. per serving.
★ High Fiber, 5 g. or greater per serving.

Breads 79

BRAND	BEST CHOICE	ACCEPTABLE CHOICE	OCCASIONAL CHOICE
	Fat Free or Low Fat AND Low Saturated Fat AND Good Source of Fiber	Fat Free or Low Fat AND Low Saturated Fat	Contains Greater Than 3 Grams Total Fat OR Greater Than 1 Gram of Saturated Fat

Pepperidge Farm (Cont.)		Steak Buns
		∇ Stone Ground 100% Whole Wheat Bread
		Very Thin:
		  White
		Vienna Bread
		Wheat Bread:
		  Old Fashioned
		White Bread:
		  Family
		  ∇ Original
		  Sandwich
		  Toasting	

Perfection Deli		Hoagie Rolls Kaiser Rolls Old World Rye Bread	Super Sub Buns ☆ Wheat Deli Rolls
Pillsbury		Crusty French Loaf Pipin' Hot Loaf: White	
Rich's		Enriched White Bread Dough (frozen)	
Roman Meal		∇ 100% Whole Wheat Bread ∇ Bread	
Rubschlager		Cocktail Pumpernickel Bread Cocktail Rye Bread	
Schafer's		∇ Hillbilly Old Fashioned Bread	

Taystee		Eights Enriched Buns:
		  Hamburger Style
		  Hot Dog Style
		  Sesame Seed
		Golden Split Top:
		  ∇ Wheat	

The Hudson Bay Milling Co.		100% Whole Wheat ∇ Cinnamon Raisin Cottage White ∇ Honey & Bran	

∇ Low Sodium, 140 mg. or less per serving.
☆ Good Source of Fiber, between 2.5 g. and 5 g. per serving.

BRAND	BEST CHOICE	ACCEPTABLE CHOICE	OCCASIONAL CHOICE
	Fat Free or Low Fat AND Low Saturated Fat AND Good Source of Fiber	Fat Free or Low Fat AND Low Saturated Fat	Contains Greater Than 3 Grams Total Fat OR Greater Than 1 Gram of Saturated Fat
The Hudson Bay Milling Co. (Cont.)		Split Top Wheat ∇ White 'N Bran	

Toufayan		Breadsticks:
		  ∇ Garlic
		  ∇ Plain
		  ∇ Sesame
		  Whole Wheat
			Snuggles Hot Dog Buns:
			  White

Wonder	☆ 100% Stoneground Whole Wheat Bread
	Light:
	  ★ Calcium Enriched Bread
	  ★ Sourdough
	  ☆ Wheat
	  ☆ White
		Calcium Enriched Bread
		Enriched Bread:
		  Giant
		  Small
		Family Italian Bread
		Sourdough Bread	

YOUR FAVORITE BREADS NOT LISTED IN THE *GUIDE*			

∇ Low Sodium, 140 mg. or less per serving.
☆ Good Source of Fiber, between 2.5 g. and 5 g. per serving.
★ High Fiber, 5 g. or greater per serving.

BREAD PRODUCTS

This category contains a large variety of prepared bread products such as bagels, muffins, biscuits, English muffins, tortillas, and pizza crusts. These bread products provide complex carbohydrates to the diet and can be a good source of B-vitamins, iron, and fiber. They are also generally low in total fat, saturated fat, and cholesterol. Bread products are included as part of the "Bread, Cereal, Rice, and Pasta Group" and help make up the base of the *Food Guide Pyramid*. Six to eleven servings each day are recommended from this food group. One English muffin is considered two servings, while a large bakery-style bagel may be counted as three to four servings. The FDA has established reference amounts or standardized serving sizes for use on the food label. The reference amount for bread products in this category is approximately 55 grams (2 ounces). The number of pieces to which this amount is equivalent varies with the type of product. Be sure to read the *Nutrition Facts* label for the serving size information of your bread choice. (See pages 51 and 52 for an explanation of reference amounts and the difference between serving sizes established by the FDA for food labeling and those recommended by the *Food Guide Pyramid*.)

The criteria used to evaluate these bread products differ somewhat from those used in the previous bread categories. This is because the bread products listed in this section are bakery-style and are typically made with added fat. For this reason, it seems prudent to recommend that consumers select bread products listed in this category less often than the products listed in the other bread categories.

Although dietary fiber is not part of the evaluation criteria, products that meet the FDA's definition for "Good Source of Fiber" (between 2.5 grams and 5 grams fiber) are marked with a ☆ symbol. Additionally, those products that meet the FDA's definition for "High Fiber" (5 grams or greater) are marked with a ★ symbol.

Criteria Key

▲ **Best Choice:** **Fat Free or Low Fat**

Products listed in this category meet the FDA's definition for "Fat Free" (less than $1/2$ gram fat per serving) or "Low Fat" (3 grams or less fat per serving).

△ **Acceptable Choice:** **Contains Greater Than 3 Grams, but Less Than or Equal to 5 Grams Total Fat**

Products listed in this category **do not** meet the FDA's definition for "Low Fat." They may also contain 5 or less grams of fat per serving. The 5 grams of total fat cut-off was used in order to be consistent with the amount of fat equal to one diabetes diet fat exchange and is also equivalent to 1 teaspoon of added fat.[75] These products contribute a greater amount of fat to the overall daily diet.

▲ **Occasional Choice:** **Contains Greater Than 5 Grams Total Fat**

Those products that contain greater than 5 grams of total fat per serving are listed in this category. These products can contribute a significant amount of fat to the overall daily diet and should be consumed only on occasion.

BRAND	BEST CHOICE	ACCEPTABLE CHOICE	OCCASIONAL CHOICE
	Fat Free or Low Fat	Contains Greater Than 3 Grams But Less Than or Equal to 5 Grams Total Fat	Contains Greater Than 5 Grams Total Fat
Aldons	Original Recipe English Muffins		
All Brands	Bagels English Muffins		Coffee Cakes Croissants Doughnuts Pastries Sweet Rolls

Arnold	Bran'Nola:
	☆ Muffins
	Muffins:
	   Extra Crisp
	   Raisin		

Athens Foods	Fillo Dough		
Auburn Farms	Fat Free Toast 'N Jammers: ☆ All Flavors		

Aunt Jemima	Pancakes:
	▲ Buttermilk
	▲★ Low Fat
	▲ Original
	Waffles:
	▲ Low Fat
		Pancakes:
		▲ Blueberry
			French Toast:
			  Cinnamon Swirl
			  Original
			Waffles:
			  ▲ Blueberry
			  Buttermilk
			  Cinnamon
			  ▲☆ Oatmeal
			  ▲ Original
			  Whole Grain

Aunt Millie's	Fat Free English Muffins:
	☆ All Varieties
			Donut Shoppe:
			  ∇ Old Fashioned Sour Cream
			    Donuts
			  Powder Sugar Donut Treats
			Donut Shoppe Dunking Stix
			Peanutty Dunking Stix

Awrey's Best		Muffins: Blueberry	Assorted Donuts
Azteca	∇ Corn Tortillas Flour Tortillas		∇ Salad Shells
B & M	Brown Bread		

▲ High Sodium, 480 mg. or greater per serving.
∇ Low Sodium, 140 mg. or less per serving.
☆ Good Source of Fiber, between 2.5 g. and 5 g. per serving.
★ High Fiber, 5 g. or greater per serving.

Bread Products (bagels, muffins, pancakes, tortillas) 85

BRAND	BEST CHOICE	ACCEPTABLE CHOICE	OCCASIONAL CHOICE
	Fat Free or Low Fat	Contains Greater Than 3 Grams But Less Than or Equal to 5 Grams Total Fat	Contains Greater Than 5 Grams Total Fat
Bays	English Muffins: ▲ Plain Sourdough		
Boboli	Pizza Crust		
Braun's Bagels	Individually Wrapped Bagels: Cinnamon Raisin Onion Plain Wheat		
Buena Vita	Fat Free Flour Tortillas		
Butternut	Old World Bagels: Cinnamon Raisin Onion Plain		
Chi Chi's			Taco Shells: ∇ White Corn
Cole's	Focaccia: Cheese & Herb Regular		
Country Hearth	English Muffins: Cinnamon Raisin Plain Wheat		
Cracklin' Good		Toaster Pastries	
Dolly Madison Bakery			Blueberry Muffins Cinnamon Rolls Donut Gems: Powdered Sugar
Don Marcos	∇ Corn Tortillas Flour Tortillas		
Downyflake	Crisp & Healthy Waffles: All Varieties	Waffles: ▲ Blueberry ▲ Buttermilk Homestyle	▲ Cinnamon Swirl French Toast
Entenmann's	Fat Free: ∇ Apple Cinnamon Twist		50% Less Fat: Cinnamon Donuts

▲ High Sodium, 480 mg. or greater per serving.
∇ Low Sodium, 140 mg. or less per serving.

BRAND	BEST CHOICE	ACCEPTABLE CHOICE	OCCASIONAL CHOICE
	Fat Free or Low Fat	Contains Greater Than 3 Grams But Less Than or Equal to 5 Grams Total Fat	Contains Greater Than 5 Grams Total Fat
Entenmann's (Cont.)	Fat Free: ∇ Apricot Danish Twist ∇ Blueberry Cheese Rolls ∇ Blueberry Muffins ∇ Cheese Filled Crumb Coffee Cake ∇ Cherry Cheese Coffee Cake ∇ Cinnamon Apple Coffee Cake ∇ Cinnamon Sweet Rolls ∇ Lemon Twist ∇ Pineapple Cheese Coffee Cake ∇ Raspberry Cheese Coffee Cake ∇ Raspberry Twist		50% Less Fat: Donuts, Variety Pack Glazed Donuts Powdered Donuts Apple Puffs Caramel Nut Coffee Cake Cheese Coffee Cake Cheese Filled Crumb Coffee Cake Cheese Topped Sweet Rolls Danish Ring: Pecan Walnut Danish Twist: Lemon Pecan Raspberry Walnut Devil's Food Crumb Donuts Glazed Buttermilk Donuts Glazed Chocolate POPEMS Glazed POPEMS Muffins: Blueberry Rich Frosted Donuts Sour Cream Chip & Nut Loaf
Farm Rich			French Toast Sticks: Cinnamon Swirl
Food For Life	☆ Low Fat Carrot Nut Muffins		
Hostess	Low Fat Muffins: Blueberry		Assorted Donuts Banana Nut Oat Bran Muffins Frosted Donettes Hearty Muffins: Banana Nut Blueberry Lemon Poppyseed Mini Muffins: Banana Walnut Blueberry Chocolate Chip Cinnamon Apple Muffin Loaf: Blueberry Raspberry

∇ Low Sodium, 140 mg. or less per serving.
☆ Good Source of Fiber, between 2.5 g. and 5 g. per serving.

Bread Products (bagels, muffins, pancakes, tortillas) 87

BRAND	BEST CHOICE	ACCEPTABLE CHOICE	OCCASIONAL CHOICE
	Fat Free or Low Fat	Contains Greater Than 3 Grams But Less Than or Equal to 5 Grams Total Fat	Contains Greater Than 5 Grams Total Fat
Hostess (Cont.)			Original Oat Bran Muffins Powdered Donettes
Jimmy Dean			Flapsticks: ▲ Blueberry
Kellogg's	Eggo Waffles: 　Special K Low Fat Pop-Tarts: 　Blueberry 　Cherry 　Strawberry	Pop-Tarts: 　Apple Cinnamon 　Cherry 　Frosted Blueberry 　Frosted Cherry 　Frosted Chocolate Fudge 　Frosted Chocolate Vanilla 　　Creme 　Frosted Strawberry 　Grape 　S'mores	☆ Common Sense Oat Bran 　　Waffles Eggo Minis: 　▲ Blueberry 　▲ Plain Eggo Waffles: 　Blueberry 　Homestyle 　Nut and Honey 　☆ Nutri-Grain 　★ Raisin & Bran Nutri-Grain 　Strawberry Pop-Tarts: 　Blueberry 　Brown Sugar Cinnamon 　Frosted Brown Sugar 　　Cinnamon 　Frosted Raspberry 　Milk Chocolate Graham 　Strawberry
Krusteaz		▲ Blueberry Pancakes ▲☆ Buttermilk Pancakes	▲ Cinnamon Swirl French Toast
La Fronteriza	Flour Tortillas		
Lender's	Bagels: 　Blueberry 　Cinnamon Raisin 　Egg 　Garlic 　Onion 　Plain New York Style Bagels: 　Egg 　Onion 　Raisin Soft Bagels: 　Onion	Soft Bagels: 　Original	

▲ High Sodium, 480 mg. or greater per serving.
☆ Good Source of Fiber, between 2.5 g. and 5 g. per serving.
★ High Fiber, 5 g. or greater per serving.

BRAND	BEST CHOICE	ACCEPTABLE CHOICE	OCCASIONAL CHOICE
	Fat Free or Low Fat	Contains Greater Than 3 Grams But Less Than or Equal to 5 Grams Total Fat	Contains Greater Than 5 Grams Total Fat
Little Debbie			Coffee Cake: Apple Streusel Donut Sticks
Lupita	▽ White Corn Tortillas ▽ Yellow Corn Tortillas		
Mama Mary's		▽ Pizza Crust	
Millspring	Bagels: All Flavors		

Mission	▽ Corn Tortillas
	Flour Tortillas:
	   Fajita Style
		Flour Tortillas:
		   Soft Taco Size	

Mrs. Butterworth's			Cinnamon Sweet Rolls: ▲ Ready to Eat
Nabisco		Toastettes: All Flavors	

Natural Ovens	Bagels:
	   ★ Brainy
	   ★ Whole Grain
		Muffins:
		   ▽ Blueberry-Oat
			Muffins:
			   ▽ 24-Karrot Gems

Newlyweds	English Muffins		
New York Flatbreads	Low Fat Flatbreads: ▽ All Flavors		

Olivieri	Italian Pizza Shell:
	   The Flourentine
	   The Original		

Pepperidge Farm	English Muffins:
	   Cinnamon Raisin
	   Plain
		Butter Crescents	

Pillsbury	All Ready Pizza Crust
	Biscuits:
	   ▲ Buttermilk
	   ▲ Country
	Soft Breadsticks
		Big Country Biscuits:
		   Butter Tastin'
		   Buttermilk
		   Southern Style
		   ▲ Butterflake Dinner Rolls
		Cinnamon Rolls
			Caramel Rolls w/Nuts
			Cinnamon Raisin Rolls
			Cornbread Twists
			Crescent Dinner Rolls:
			   Original
			Crescent Rolls:
			   ▲ Cheese

▲ High Sodium, 480 mg. or greater per serving.
▽ Low Sodium, 140 mg. or less per serving.
★ High Fiber, 5 g. or greater per serving.

BRAND	BEST CHOICE	ACCEPTABLE CHOICE	OCCASIONAL CHOICE
.	Fat Free or Low Fat	Contains Greater Than 3 Grams But Less Than or Equal to 5 Grams Total Fat	Contains Greater Than 5 Grams Total Fat
Pillsbury (Cont.)		Tender Layer Biscuits: ▲ Buttermilk	Grands!: ▲ Butter Tastin' ▲ Buttermilk ▲ Flaky Biscuits Hungry Jack: ▲ Butter Tastin' Flaky Biscuits ▲ Buttermilk Flaky ▲ Flaky Biscuits Orange Sweet Rolls: with Icing Toaster Strudel: All Flavors
Quaker	Toasted Oatmeal Waffles		
Rhodes	Pizza Dough and Italian Bread ☆ Raisin Bread Dough ☆ Whole Wheat Texas Rolls		
Rich's	Enriched Homestyle Roll Dough		
Sara Lee	Premium Bagels: ▲ Blueberry ▲ Egg Premium Toaster Size Bagels: Cinnamon Raisin Onion Plain		Coffee Cake: Butter Streusel Crumb Pecan
Sun Maid	English Muffins: Raisin		
The Hudson Bay Milling Co.	☆ English Muffins		
The University of Michigan	M-Fit Muffin: ☆ Blueberry Apple ☆ Cranberry Orange ☆ Pumpkin Raisin ☆ Raisin Apple Bran		
Thomas'	Bagels: ☆ Cinnamon Raisin Egg Onion		

▲ High Sodium, 480 mg. or greater per serving.
☆ Good Source of Fiber, between 2.5 g. and 5 g. per serving.

90 **Bread Products (bagels, muffins, pancakes, tortillas)**

BRAND	BEST CHOICE	ACCEPTABLE CHOICE	OCCASIONAL CHOICE
	Fat Free or Low Fat	Contains Greater Than 3 Grams But Less Than or Equal to 5 Grams Total Fat	Contains Greater Than 5 Grams Total Fat
Thomas' (Cont.)	English Muffins: ☆ Honey Wheat Oat Bran Original Raisin Sourdough		
Toast'em		Toaster Fruit Pastries: All Varieties	
Uncle B's	Bakery Bagels: Cinnamon Raisin Honey Wheat		
Weight Watchers	Low Fat Muffins: Apple Cinnamon Blueberry Carrot Chocolate Chip Cranberry Orange Lemon Poppy	Breakfast On-The-Go!: ☆ Blueberry Muffins Glazed Cinnamon Rolls	
Wonder	English Muffins: Raisin Rounds Soft Wraps		
YOUR FAVORITE BREAD PRODUCTS NOT LISTED IN THE *GUIDE*			

☆ Good Source of Fiber, between 2.5 g. and 5 g. per serving.

CEREALS

This category contains a large variety of cereals—from ready-to-eat dry varieties to hot cereals. Cereals provide complex carbohydrates to the diet and can be a good source of many vitamins and minerals and fiber. They are also generally low in total fat, saturated fat, and cholesterol.

Some cereals are also high in simple sugar, such as added sucrose, honey, brown sugar, corn syrup, and other sweeteners. The *Dietary Guidelines for Americans*[11] recommends that foods high in sugar be consumed in moderation by most healthy people and sparingly by people who need to limit their caloric intake. Dietary sugar also may contribute to the development of dental caries.[13] Those persons concerned with limiting their intake of sugar should check the *Nutrition Facts* label. "Sugar" is listed as part of "Total Carbohydrate" and includes all sugars added during processing or packing, including ingredients that contain sugars (e.g., fruit juices, applesauce, dried fruit).

Cereals are included as part of the "Bread, Cereal, Rice, and Pasta Group" and help make up the base of the *Food Guide Pyramid*. Six to eleven servings are recommended each day from this food group. Serving size for cereals is one ounce ready-to-eat, or 1/2 cup cooked. The FDA has established reference amounts or standardized serving sizes for use on the food label. The reference amount for cereals ranges from 15 grams (1/2 ounce) to 55 grams (2 ounces), which is generally equivalent to 1/4 cup to 1 1/3 cups, depending on the type of cereal (e.g., granola, puffed, biscuit-type). Be sure to read the *Nutrition Facts* label for the serving size information of your cereal choice. (See pages 51 and 52 for an explanation of reference amounts and the difference between serving sizes established by the FDA for food labeling and those recommended by the *Food Guide Pyramid*.)

Because Americans consume less than one-half of the fiber recommended by the National Cancer Institute (between 20 and 30 grams per day), fiber was used as part of the criteria to evaluate cereals. Cereals are a good, low-fat way to provide

fiber in daily diets. A greater amount of dietary fiber is found in the whole grain products than in their refined alternatives. Criteria were therefore designed to distinguish those products lower in total fat, saturated fat, and higher in fiber from their higher-fat, lower-fiber alternatives. Additionally, those cereals that meet the definition for "High Fiber" (5 grams or higher per serving) are marked with a ★ symbol.

Criteria Key

▲ **Best Choice:**   **Fat Free or Low Fat, AND Low Saturated Fat, AND Good Source of Fiber**

Products listed in this category meet the FDA's definition for "Fat Free" (less than 1/2 gram fat per serving) or "Low Fat" (3 grams or less fat per serving), and "Low Saturated Fat" (1 gram or less saturated fat per serving), and "Good Source of Fiber" (between 2.5 grams and 5 grams fiber).

▲ **Acceptable Choice:**   **Fat Free or Low Fat, AND Low Saturated Fat**

These cereals are classified as "Acceptable Choice" since they meet the above definition for "Fat Free," "Low Fat," and "Low Saturated Fat," but **do no**t meet the definition for "Good Source of Fiber." Consequently, these cereals do not contribute as much fiber to the overall daily diet.

▲ **Occasional Choice:**   **Contains Greater Than 3 Grams of Total Fat, or Greater Than 1 Gram Saturated Fat**

Cereals that do not meet the FDA's definition for "Low Fat" or "Low Saturated Fat" are listed in this category.

BRAND	BEST CHOICE	ACCEPTABLE CHOICE	OCCASIONAL CHOICE
	Fat Free or Low Fat AND Low Saturated Fat AND Good Source of Fiber	Fat Free or Low Fat AND Low Saturated Fat	Contains Greater Than 3 Grams Total Fat OR Greater Than 1 Gram Saturated Fat
Alpen		Lowfat Swiss Style Cereal: ∇ No Added Sugar Swiss Style Cereal: ∇ Original	
American Prairie	Hot Cereal: ∇★ 5 Grain ∇☆ Creamy Rye & Rice		
Arrowhead Mills	∇☆ Amaranth Flakes Bits O Barley: ∇★ Barley Grits ∇☆ Kamut ∇★ Maple Corns Cereal ∇☆ Multi-Grain Flakes ∇☆ Nature O's ∇☆ Nature Whole Grain O's ∇☆ Oat Bran Flakes ∇★ Seven Grain ∇☆ Spelt Flakes	∇ Bear Mush ∇ Puffed Corn ∇ Puffed Millet ∇ Puffed Rice ∇ Puffed Wheat ∇ Raw Wheat Germ ∇ Rice and Shine	
Barbara's	Frosted Funnies: ∇☆ Frosted Corn Flakes ★ High 5 ☆ Multigrain Shredded Spoonfuls ∇★ Shredded Wheat	Startoons: ∇ Frosted Cocoa Crunch ∇ Frosted Honey Crunch	
Bob's Red Mill	∇☆ 5 Grain Rolled Hot Cereal ∇☆ 10 Grain Hot Cereal ∇★ Grande Whole Grains Cereal/Pilaf ∇☆ Oat Bran Hot Cereal ∇☆ Rolled Oats	Brown Rice Farina: ∇ Creamy Rice Hot Cereal ∇ Cracked Wheat Hot Cereal ∇ Old Country Style Muesli ∇ Rolled Wheat ∇ Scottish Oatmeal	
Breadshop's	Granola: ∇☆ Blueberry 'n Cream ∇☆ Raspberry 'n Cream ∇☆ Strawberry 'n Cream	∇ Cinnamon Grins ∇ Health Nuggets ∇ Krinklie Grains ∇ Puffs 'n Honey ∇ Shapes'n Honey	Granola: ∇☆ Crunchy Oat Bran ∇ Super Natural
Elam's	∇★ Miller's Bran		
Erewhon	∇☆ Apple Cinnamon Instant Oatmeal	∇ Apple Stroodles ∇ Aztec Cereal	Granola: ∇☆ Date Nut

∇ Low Sodium, 140 mg. or less per serving.
☆ Good Source of Fiber, between 2.5 g. and 5 g. per serving.
★ High Fiber, 5 g. or greater per serving.

BRAND	BEST CHOICE	ACCEPTABLE CHOICE	OCCASIONAL CHOICE
	Fat Free or Low Fat AND Low Saturated Fat AND Good Source of Fiber	Fat Free or Low Fat AND Low Saturated Fat	Contains Greater Than 3 Grams Total Fat OR Greater Than 1 Gram Saturated Fat
Erewhon (Cont.)	∇☆ Apple Raisin Instant Oatmeal ∇☆ Barley Plus ∇★ Fruit 'N Wheat Cereal ∇☆ Instant Oatmeal w/ Added Oat Bran ∇☆ Kamut Flakes ∇☆ Maple Spice Instant Oatmeal ∇★ Oat Bran w/Toasted Wheat Germ ∇★ Raisin Bran ∇★ Raisin Grahams ∇☆ Spelt Flakes ∇★ Wheat Flakes	∇ Banana-O's ∇ Brown Rice Cream ∇ Corn Flakes Crispy Brown Rice: 　∇ No Salt Added 　Original ∇ Galaxy Grahams ∇ Honey Crisp Corn ∇ Poppets	Granola: 　∇☆ Honey Almond 　∇☆ Maple 　∇★ Number 9 w/Bran 　∇☆ Spiced Apple 　∇☆ Sunflower Crunch
Familia	∇★ Light Granola Swiss Muesli: 　∇★ No Added Sugar 　∇★ Original		∇☆ Crunchy Swiss Muesli
General Mills	☆ Basic 4 Cheerios: 　☆ Original ☆ Crispy Wheats 'n Raisins ∇★ Fiber One ☆ Multi Grain Cheerios Nature Valley: 　☆ Low Fat Fruit Granola ☆ Oatmeal Crisp w/Apples Ripple Crisp: 　★ Honey Bran ☆ Sun Crunchers ★ Total Raisin Bran Wheaties: 　☆ Whole Grain ☆ Whole Grain Total	Body Buddies Booberry Cereal ∇ Bunuelitos Cheerios: 　Apple Cinnamon 　Honey Nut Cocoa Puffs Count Chocula Country Corn Flakes Frankenberry Golden Grahams Hidden Treasures Kaboom Kix: 　Berry Berry 　Regular Lucky Charms Oatmeal Raisin Crisp Ripple Crisp: 　Honey Corn S'Mores Grahams ∇ Sprinkle Spangles Total Corn Flakes Triples ∇ Trix	Cinnamon Toast Crunch ☆ Clusters ☆ Oatmeal Crisp w/Almonds ★ Raisin Nut Bran

∇ Low Sodium, 140 mg. or less per serving.
☆ Good Source of Fiber, between 2.5 g. and 5 g. per serving.
★ High Fiber, 5 g. or greater per serving.

BRAND	BEST CHOICE Fat Free or Low Fat AND Low Saturated Fat AND Good Source of Fiber	ACCEPTABLE CHOICE Fat Free or Low Fat AND Low Saturated Fat	OCCASIONAL CHOICE Contains Greater Than 3 Grams Total Fat OR Greater Than 1 Gram Saturated Fat

General Mills (Cont.)		Wheaties:
		  Dunk-A-Balls
		  Honey Gold	

Golden Temple	∇★ Cinnamon Apple Raisin
	    Cereal
			Crisp 'n Crunchy Granola:
			  ∇☆ Reduced Fat
			  ∇☆ Super Nutty Granola
			  ∇☆ Wild Blueberry Granola

Grainfields	∇☆ Raisin Bran	∇ Corn Flakes ∇ Crispy Rice Multi Grain Flakes: ∇ w/Rice Bran	

Health Valley	10 Bran Cereal:
	  ∇☆ Almond Flavor O's
	  ∇☆ Apple and Cinnamon O's
	  ∇☆ High Fiber O's
	100% Natural Bran Cereal:
	  ∇★ Apples and Cinnamon
	  ∇★ Raisins
	∇☆ 100% Organic Raisin
	    Bran Flakes
	∇☆ Amaranth Flakes
	∇☆ Banana Amaranth
	∇☆ Blue Corn Flakes
	Fat Free Granola:
	  ∇★ All Flavors
	∇☆ Fiber 7 Flakes
	∇☆ Healthy Fiber Flakes
	Oat Bran Flakes:
	  ∇☆ Almonds, Dates
	  ∇☆ Regular
	  ∇☆ w/Raisins
	∇☆ Oat Bran O's
	∇★ Raisin Bran Cereal
	∇☆ Sprouts 7 Cereal
		Fruit Lites:
		  ∇ Brown Rice
		  ∇ Golden Corn
		∇ Honey Crisp Corn Cereal
			Real Oat Bran Cereal:
			  ∇★ Almond Crunch

Healthy Choice	☆ Multi-Grain Flakes ☆ Multi-Grain Flakes w/Raisins ∇★ Multi-Grain Squares		

Heartland	Granola:
	  ∇☆ Low Fat
			Granola:
			  ∇☆ Raisin
			  ☆ Regular

∇ Low Sodium, 140 mg. or less per serving.
☆ Good Source of Fiber, between 2.5 g. and 5 g. per serving.
★ High Fiber, 5 g. or greater per serving.

BRAND	BEST CHOICE	ACCEPTABLE CHOICE	OCCASIONAL CHOICE
	Fat Free or Low Fat AND Low Saturated Fat AND Good Source of Fiber	Fat Free or Low Fat AND Low Saturated Fat	Contains Greater Than 3 Grams Total Fat OR Greater Than 1 Gram Saturated Fat
Hodgson Mill	∇★ Cracked Wheat Cereal ∇★ Oat Bran ∇★ Wheat Bran ∇☆ Wheat Germ		
Kashi	Breakfast Pilaf: 　∇★ 7 Whole Grain and 　　Sesame	∇ Medley ∇ Puffed 7 Grains and Sesame	
Kellogg's	★ All Bran ★ All Bran w/Extra Fiber ☆ Apple Raisin Crisp ★ Bran Buds ☆ Common Sense Oat Bran ★ Complete Bran Flakes ☆ Frosted Bran Frosted Mini Wheats: 　∇★ Bite Size 　∇★ Original Size Just Right: 　☆ Crunchy Nuggets 　☆ Fruit and Nuts Low Fat Granola: 　∇☆ w/Raisins Mueslix: 　☆ Crispy Blend, Raisin, 　　Date and Almond NutriGrain: 　☆ Almond Raisin 　★ Golden Wheat & Raisins 　☆ Wheat ★ Raisin Bran Squares: 　∇★ Apple Cinnamon 　∇★ Blueberry 　∇★ Raisin 　∇★ Strawberry	Apple Cinnamon Rice Krispies ∇ Apple Jacks Cinnamon Mini Buns Cocoa Krispies Corn Flakes ∇ Corn Pops Crispix Double Dip Crunch Frosted Froot Loops Frosted Flakes Frosted Krispies Low Fat Granola: 　∇ Regular Nut & Honey Crunch Pop-Tart Crunch: 　Brown Sugar Cinnamon 　∇ Frosted Strawberry Product 19 Rice Krispies Rice Krispies Treats ∇ Smacks Special K Temptations: 　French Vanilla Almond 　Honey Roasted Pecan	★ Cracklin' Oat Bran Mueslix: 　★ Apple and Almond Crunch
Kölln	∇★ Oat Bran Crunch ∇☆ Oat Bran Crunch with Fruit	∇ Crispy Oats	
Kretschmer	★ Toasted Wheat Bran Wheat Germ: 　∇☆ Regular	Wheat Germ: 　∇ Honey Crunch	

∇ Low Sodium, 140 mg. or less per serving.

☆ Good Source of Fiber, between 2.5 g. and 5 g. per serving.

★ High Fiber, 5 g. or greater per serving.

BRAND	BEST CHOICE	ACCEPTABLE CHOICE	OCCASIONAL CHOICE
	Fat Free or Low Fat AND Low Saturated Fat AND Good Source of Fiber	Fat Free or Low Fat AND Low Saturated Fat	Contains Greater Than 3 Grams Total Fat OR Greater Than 1 Gram Saturated Fat
Lifestream	∇★ 8 Grain Flakes ∇☆ Berry Granola ∇☆ Fruit & Nut Muesli ∇☆ Multigrain Honey Puffs		
Little Crow		∇ Coco Wheats	

Malt-O-Meal		Cocoa-Roos
		Crispy Rice
		∇ Golden Sugar Puffs
		∇ Maple & Brown Sugar
		∇ Puffed Rice
		Puffed Wheat:
		    ∇ No Added Salt or Sugar
		∇ Quick Malt-O-Meal
		Toasty O's:
		    Apple Cinnamon
		    Honey Nut
		    Regular
		∇ Tootie Fruities	

Manischewitz	★ Raisin Bran	∇ Fruity's Cereal ∇ Honey Stars Cereal	
Martha White		∇ Quick Cooking Grits ∇ Yellow Grits	
Maypo	Instant Oatmeal: ∇☆ Maple Flavor		

Michaelene's	Gourmet Granola:
	    ∇☆ Lowfat Apple-
	      Raspberry Honey Crunch
	    ∇☆ Lowfat Apple-Spice &
	      Everything Nice
		Gourmet Granola:
		    ∇ Fat Chance, Honey!	

Mother's	Hot Cereal: ∇☆ Rolled Whole Wheat ∇☆ Instant Oatmeal ∇★ Oat Bran Hot Cereal ∇☆ Rolled Oats		
Nabisco	∇★ 100% Bran ∇★ Frosted Wheat Bites	∇ Cream of Rice Instant Cream of Wheat: Fruit Variety Pack	

∇ Low Sodium, 140 mg. or less per serving.
☆ Good Source of Fiber, between 2.5 g. and 5 g. per serving.
★ High Fiber, 5 g. or greater per serving.

BRAND	BEST CHOICE	ACCEPTABLE CHOICE	OCCASIONAL CHOICE
	Fat Free or Low Fat AND Low Saturated Fat AND Good Source of Fiber	Fat Free or Low Fat AND Low Saturated Fat	Contains Greater Than 3 Grams Total Fat OR Greater Than 1 Gram Saturated Fat
Nabisco (Cont.)	Fruit Wheats: 　∇☆ Blueberry 　∇☆ Raspberry ∇☆ Shredded Wheat ∇★ Spoon Size Shredded 　　Wheat	Instant Cream of Wheat: 　Original 　∇ Regular Mix 'n Eat Cream of Wheat: 　Apple Granola Crunch 　Apple 'n Cinnamon 　Variety Pack ∇ Quick Cream of Wheat Team Flakes	
Nature's Path	∇☆ Corn Flakes ∇★ Heritage Muesli ∇☆ Millet Rice Oatbran 　　Flakes ∇☆ Multigrain and Raisins 　　Cereal		
New Morning		∇ Fruit-E-O's	
Pacific Grain		∇ Nutty Rice Nutty Rice Cereal: 　∇ w/Raisins & Almonds	
Pillsbury		Farina: 　∇ Original	
Post	★ Bran Flakes Bran'nola: 　★ Original 　★ w/Raisins Fruit and Fibre: 　★ Dates, Raisins, Walnuts 　★ Peaches, Raisins and 　　Almonds ∇☆ Grape-Nut Flakes ☆ Grape-Nuts ★ Natural Bran Flakes ★ Raisin Bran	Alphabits Cocoa Pebbles Crispy Critters Fruity Pebbles ∇ Golden Crisp Honey Bunches of Oats: 　Almonds 　Honey Roasted Honeycomb Marshmallow Alphabits Toasties Corn Flakes	☆ Banana Nut Crunch Blueberry Morning ☆ C. W. Post Great Grains: 　☆ Crunchy Pecan 　☆ Raisin, Date, Pecan
Pritikin	Hearty Hot Cereal: 　∇☆ Apple Raisin Spice 　∇☆ Multi Grain		

∇ Low Sodium, 140 mg. or less per serving.
☆ Good Source of Fiber, between 2.5 g. and 5 g. per serving.
★ High Fiber, 5 g. or greater per serving.

BRAND	BEST CHOICE	ACCEPTABLE CHOICE	OCCASIONAL CHOICE
	Fat Free or Low Fat AND Low Saturated Fat AND Good Source of Fiber	Fat Free or Low Fat AND Low Saturated Fat	Contains Greater Than 3 Grams Total Fat OR Greater Than 1 Gram Saturated Fat
Quaker	100% Natural Low Fat: 　∇☆ Crispy Whole Grain w/ Raisins ★ Cinnamon Oat Squares ★ Crunchy Corn Bran Instant Oatmeal: 　∇☆ Apple & Cinnamon 　☆ Cinnamon & Spice 　☆ Maple & Brown Sugar 　☆ Raisin & Spice 　☆ Raisin, Date, Walnut 　∇☆ Regular Kids Choice Oatmeal: 　☆ Variety Package Life Cereal: 　☆ Cinnamon ∇★ Multi Grain Oatmeal Oat Bran: 　∇★ Hot Cereal 　★ Regular ☆ Oat Squares ∇☆ Old Fashioned Quaker Oats ∇☆ Quick Quaker Oats ∇★ Shredded Wheat	Cap'n Crunch: 　Crunch Berries 　Deep Sea Crunch 　Original 　Peanut Butter Honey Graham Oh's Instant Grits Instant Oatmeal: 　Bananas & Cream 　∇ Blueberries & Cream 　Cinnamon Toast 　Fruit & Cream Variety 　Peaches & Cream 　Strawberries & Cream King Vitaman Life Cereal: 　Regular Marshmallow Safari ∇ Old Fashioned Grits Popeye: 　∇ Cocoa Blasts 　Fruit Curls 　∇ Jeepers Cereal Oat'mmms 　∇ Sweet Puffs ∇ Puffed Rice ∇ Puffed Wheat ∇ Quick Grits Sweet Crunch Toasted Oatmeal: 　∇ Honey Nut	100% Natural: 　∇☆ Oats & Honey 　∇☆ Oats, Honey & Raisins Sun Country Granola: 　∇☆ w/Almonds 　∇☆ w/Raisin and Dates Toasted Oatmeal: 　Original
Ralston	★ Multi Bran Chex Peach Muesli: 　☆ w/Pecans Raspberry Muesli: 　☆ w/Almonds ☆ Strawberry Muesli Wheat Chex: 　★ 100% Whole Grain	∇ Chocolate Chip Cookie Crisp Corn Chex Double Chex Graham Chex Graham Chex and Crispy Mini Grahams Rice Chex Sun Flakes: 　Multi-Grain Cereal	Banana Muesli: 　☆ w/Walnuts ∇☆ Blueberry Muesli w/ Pecans ☆ Honey Almond Delight
Sovex	Good Shepherd: 　∇★ Wheat Bran Granola ∇★ Oat Bran Hot Cereal		

∇ Low Sodium, 140 mg. or less per serving.
☆ Good Source of Fiber, between 2.5 g. and 5 g. per serving.
★ High Fiber, 5 g. or greater per serving.

Cereals 101

BRAND	BEST CHOICE	ACCEPTABLE CHOICE	OCCASIONAL CHOICE
	Fat Free or Low Fat AND Low Saturated Fat AND Good Source of Fiber	Fat Free or Low Fat AND Low Saturated Fat	Contains Greater Than 3 Grams Total Fat OR Greater Than 1 Gram Saturated Fat
Sunbelt	∇☆ Five Grain Muesli		∇☆ Banana Nut Granola ∇☆ Fruit & Nut Granola
Sunshine	∇★ Bite Size Shredded Wheat ∇★ Shredded Wheat		
Sweethome Farm	∇☆ Low-Fat Granola w/ Raisins	Muesli: ∇ Lowfat w/Apples & Almonds	100% Natural Cereal: ∇☆ Honey Oat Clusters w/ Almonds ∇☆ Honey Oat Clusters w/ Raisins
T. Abraham's		Crispy-O's Cereal: ∇ Cocoa ∇ Fruit Flavored ∇ Regular	
Weetabix	∇☆ Weetabix Whole Wheat Cereal		
Wheatena	Hi Fiber Wheat Cereal: ∇★ Original		
YOUR FAVORITE CEREALS NOT LISTED IN THE *GUIDE*			

∇ Low Sodium, 140 mg. or less per serving.
☆ Good Source of Fiber, between 2.5 g. and 5 g. per serving.
★ High Fiber, 5 g. or greater per serving.

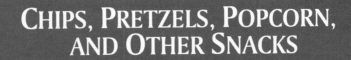

CHIPS, PRETZELS, POPCORN, AND OTHER SNACKS

This category contains a wide range of snack products. Snack-type foods may provide complex carbohydrates, B-vitamins, iron, and fiber to the diet; however, if not chosen carefully, these foods can also can be significant contributors of fat, sodium, and excess calories. Fortunately, a larger variety of products such as potato chips and tortilla chips are now available in reduced-fat and fat-free varieties. Pretzels and rice or popcorn cakes have always been low-fat options and are available in a variety of flavors. Plain, air-popped popcorn is also low in fat and provides added fiber to the diet.

Snack foods in this product category are produced from foods (e.g., potatoes, corn, rice, fruit) that are part of different groups of the *Food Guide Pyramid*. However, snack foods as a whole are not considered part of any particular *Pyramid* group and, therefore, serving recommendations are not given.

The FDA has established reference amounts or standardized serving sizes for use on the food label. The reference amount for snack foods such as those in this category is 30 grams (one ounce). The number of pieces to which this amount is equivalent varies with the type of product. Be sure to read the *Nutrition Facts* label for the serving size information of your snack choice.

Food choices from this category range from those that are higher in total fat and saturated fat to those that are fat free or low in fat. Criteria were therefore designed to distinguish those products lower in total fat and saturated fat from their higher-fat alternatives. Many of these products also contribute a significant amount of sodium. Those products that contain 480 milligrams sodium or more per serving (20% of the Daily Value), are considered high in sodium and are marked with a ▲ symbol.

Criteria Key

▲ **Best Choice:**   **Fat Free or Low Fat, AND Low Saturated Fat**

Products listed in this category meet the FDA's definition for "Fat Free" (less than $1/2$ gram fat per serving), or "Low Fat" (3 grams or less fat per serving) and "Low Saturated Fat" (1 gram or less saturated fat per serving).

▲ **Acceptable Choice:**   **Contains Greater Than 3 Grams, but Less Than or Equal to 5 Grams Total Fat, AND Low Saturated Fat**

Products listed in this category **do not** meet the FDA's definition for "Low Fat," but **do** meet the criteria for "Low Saturated Fat." The 5 grams of total fat cut-off was used in order to be consistent with the amount of fat equal to one diabetes diet fat exchange and is also equivalent to 1 teaspoon of added fat.[75] Although these products contribute a greater amount of fat to the overall daily diet, they are acceptable if consumed in moderation.

▲ **Occasional Choice:**   **Contains Greater Than 5 Grams Total Fat, or Greater Than 1 Gram Saturated Fat**

Products listed in this category **do not** meet the FDA's definition for either "Low Fat," or "Low Saturated Fat." These products can contribute a significant amount of fat to the overall daily diet and should be consumed only on occasion.

BRAND	BEST CHOICE	ACCEPTABLE CHOICE	OCCASIONAL CHOICE
	Fat Free or Low Fat AND Low Saturated Fat	Contains Greater Than 3 Grams but Less Than or Equal To 5 Grams Total Fat AND Low Saturated Fat	Contains Greater Than 5 Grams Total Fat OR Greater Than 1 Gram Saturated Fat
Act II	96% Fat Free Microwave Popcorn: ▲☆ Butter	Light Microwave Popcorn ★ Butter	Flavor Lover's Microwave Popcorn: ☆ Cheese ∇★ Cinnamon Toffee Glaze
All Brands	∇☆ Popcorn Kernels		
American Grains	Popsters: Herb & Garlic ★ Original		
Anderson	Bavarian Dutch Style Pretzels Bavarian Pretzels: ∇ Baldies, No Salt Added ▲ Sourdough Hard Pretzels		
Auburn Farms	98% Fat Free Spud Bakes: ∇ Cheddar Cheese ∇ Mesquite Barbeque Original ∇ Sour Cream & Onion ∇ Fat Free Butterscotch Corn ∇ Fat Free Caramel Corn Fat Free Only Chips: Cajun Cheddar ∇ Mesquite Barbecue ∇ Original ∇ Sour Cream & Onion		
Barbara's	Honeysweet Pretzels: ∇☆ Organic Whole Wheat		Blue Corn Chips: ∇ Regular ∇ Unsalted ∇ Natural Cheese Puffs Pinta Chips ∇ Sweet Potato Chips
Bearitos	∇ Lite Cheddar Puffs Microwave Popcorn: ∇★ No Salt, No Oil Popcorn: ∇ No Salt, No Oil		Crunchitos: Mexicali Cheddar Tangy Cheddar Popcorn: Jalapeno Jack White Cheddar

▲ High Sodium, 480 mg. or greater per serving.
∇ Low Sodium, 140 mg. or less per serving.
☆ Good Source of Fiber, between 2.5 g. and 5 g. per serving.
★ High Fiber, 5 g. or greater per serving.

BRAND	BEST CHOICE	ACCEPTABLE CHOICE	OCCASIONAL CHOICE
	Fat Free or Low Fat AND Low Saturated Fat	Contains Greater Than 3 Grams but Less Than or Equal To 5 Grams Total Fat AND Low Saturated Fat	Contains Greater Than 5 Grams Total Fat OR Greater Than 1 Gram Saturated Fat

Bearitos (Cont.)			Popcorn Lite:
			  50% Less Oil
			Tortilla Chips:
			  ∇ Organic Blue Corn
			  ∇ Organic White Corn
			  ∇ Organic Yellow Corn

Better Made			Potato Chips:
			  Barbeque
			  ∇ Salt & Vinegar
			  ∇ Sour Cream & Onion
			  ∇ Waves

Betty Crocker	Light Bugles:
	  BBQ
	  Cheddar Cheese
	  Original
	Bugs Bunny Fruit Snacks:
	  ∇ Assorted Fruit
	By Request Microwave Popcorn:
	  ☆ Butter
	  ☆ Natural
	Fruit By The Foot:
	  ∇ All Flavors
	Fruit Roll-Ups:
	  ∇ All Flavors
	Fruit Snacks:
	  ∇ All Flavors
	Gushers:
	  ∇ All Flavors
	String Thing:
	  ∇ All Flavors
		Pop Chips:
		  Butter
		  Original
			Bugles:
			  Nacho Cheese
			  Original
			  Ranch
			  Sour Cream & Onion
			FundaMiddles:
			  ∇ ChocoMania
			Pop-Secret:
			  ☆ Cheddar Cheese
			Pop-Secret Light:
			  ☆ Butter
			  ☆ Butter Snack Size Bags
			  ☆ Buttery Burst
			  ☆ Natural Flavor
			Pop-Secret Original:
			  ☆ Butter
			  ☆ Butter Snack Size Bags
			  ☆ Natural Flavor

Black Jewell	∇☆ Popcorn Kernels		Microwave Popcorn:
			  ∇☆ Butter
			  ∇☆ Natural Flavor

Borden			Potato Chips:
			  ∇ Calypso Sweet & Sour
			    Caribbean

Brock	Fruit Snackers: ∇ All Flavors		
Bruno & Luigi's	Pasta Chips: ∇ All Flavors		

∇ Low Sodium, 140 mg. or less per serving.
☆ Good Source of Fiber, between 2.5 g. and 5 g. per serving.

BRAND	BEST CHOICE	ACCEPTABLE CHOICE	OCCASIONAL CHOICE
	Fat Free or Low Fat AND Low Saturated Fat	Contains Greater Than 3 Grams but Less Than or Equal To 5 Grams Total Fat AND Low Saturated Fat	Contains Greater Than 5 Grams Total Fat OR Greater Than 1 Gram Saturated Fat
Burns & Ricker	Fat Free Bagel Crisps: All Flavors	Mini Bagel Crisps: Garlic Original Bagel Crisps: ∇ Plain Low Sodium Pita Crisps: Sesame Garlic	Original Bagel Crisps: Sesame Pita Crisps: Poppy Seed & Wild Onion
Butterfield			∇ Shoestring Potato Sticks
Cabana			Pork Rinds: All Flavors Tostados: ∇ Lightly Salted
Cain's			Potato Chips: Bar-B-Q Marcelle Dip Style Thin Potato Chips
Camacho's			∇ Nacho Corn Chips
Cape Cod			Popcorn: White Cheddar Cheese Potato Chips: ∇ No Salt Added ∇ Regular ∇ Sea Salt & Vinegar
Casa Ricardo		Tortilla Thins 40% Less Fat: ∇ All Flavors	Tortilla Chips: Nacho Cheese
Cheese Shoppe	Pretzels: Bite Size		Nacho Chips: ∇ Unsalted Tortilla Chips: ∇ Traditional
Chi Chi's			Tortilla Chips: ∇ No Salt ∇ Plain
Chico San	Popcorn Cakes: ∇ Carousel Caramel ∇ Double Feature Butter ∇ Whoppin' White Cheddar		
Chifles			∇ Plantain Chips

∇ Low Sodium, 140 mg. or less per serving.

Chips, Pretzels, Popcorn, Snacks 107

BRAND	BEST CHOICE	ACCEPTABLE CHOICE	OCCASIONAL CHOICE
	Fat Free or Low Fat AND Low Saturated Fat	Contains Greater Than 3 Grams but Less Than or Equal To 5 Grams Total Fat AND Low Saturated Fat	Contains Greater Than 5 Grams Total Fat OR Greater Than 1 Gram Saturated Fat
Childers	∇ Fat Free Potato Chips		

Combos		Combos:
		  Cheddar Cheese
		  Mustard Pretzel
		  Nacho Cheese Pretzels
		  Pizzeria Pretzel
			Combos:
			  Cheddar Cheese Crackers
			  Pepperoni Pizza

Cornnuts		Toasted Corn:
		  Barbecue
		  Nacho Cheese
		  Original	

Cousin Willie's		Microwave Popcorn:
		  ☆ Light Butter
			Microwave Popcorn:
			  ∇☆ Butter
			☆ Original Popcorn

Cracker Jack	Fat Free Cracker Jack:
	  ∇ Butter Toffee
	  ∇ Original
	∇ Original Cracker Jack
			Nutty Deluxe:
			  Butter Toffee

Crunch 'n Munch	∇ Caramel Popcorn w/Peanuts	Buttery Toffee Popcorn w/ Peanuts Maple Flavored Popcorn w/ Walnuts	

Del Monte			Fruit Snacks:
			  ∇ Sierra Trail Mix
			Yogurt Raisins:
			  ∇ Original
			  ∇ Strawberry

Eagle	Bavarian Hard Pretzels:
	  Sourdough
	Pretzel Sticks:
	  No Fat
	  Mini Bites
	  Thin Twists
			∇ El Grande Restaurant Style Rounds
			Nacho Thins
			Potato Chips:
			  Idaho Russet, Dark and Crunchy
			Ranch Thins
			Ripples:
			  Mesquite BBQ
			  Natural
			  Sour Cream and Onion

∇ Low Sodium, 140 mg. or less per serving.
☆ Good Source of Fiber, between 2.5 g. and 5 g. per serving.

BRAND	BEST CHOICE	ACCEPTABLE CHOICE	OCCASIONAL CHOICE
	Fat Free or Low Fat AND Low Saturated Fat	Contains Greater Than 3 Grams but Less Than or Equal To 5 Grams Total Fat AND Low Saturated Fat	Contains Greater Than 5 Grams Total Fat OR Greater Than 1 Gram Saturated Fat

Eagle (Cont.)			Snack Mix
			Thins:
			   ∇ Crispy Cooked Potato
			     Chips
			   Mesquite BBQ Potato Chips
			   Potato Chips
			   Sour Cream & Onion

El Rio			Tortilla Chips: ∇ White Corn

Estee	Caramel Popcorn:
	   ∇ No Sugar Added
	Pretzels:
	   ∇ Unsalted		

Farley's	Fat Free Fruit Snacks:
	   ∇ All Flavors
	Fruit Funnies:
	   ∇ Trolls In Trouble - All
	     Flavors
	Fruit Rolls:
	   ∇ All Varieties
	Fruit Snacks:
	   ∇ All Flavors		

Fiddle Faddle	Fat Free Caramel Popcorn		Caramel Corn w/Peanuts
Flavor Tree			☆ Hot N' Spicy Mix Party Mix ☆ Sesame Chips Sour Cream & Onion Sesame Sticks

Frito Lay	Baked Lays:
	   Original
	Baked Tostitos:
	   ∇ Regular
	   ∇ Unsalted
	Rold Gold Pretzels:
	   Bavarian
	   Fat Free Thins
	   Rods
	   Sticks
			Chee-tos:
			   Crunchy
			   Curls
			   Paws
			   Puffs
			Chester's:
			   Butter, Caramel & Cheese
			   ☆ Cheddar Cheese Popcorn
			Doritos:
			   Cooler Ranch

∇ Low Sodium, 140 mg. or less per serving.
☆ Good Source of Fiber, between 2.5 g. and 5 g. per serving.

BRAND	BEST CHOICE	ACCEPTABLE CHOICE	OCCASIONAL CHOICE
	Fat Free or Low Fat AND Low Saturated Fat	Contains Greater Than 3 Grams but Less Than or Equal To 5 Grams Total Fat AND Low Saturated Fat	Contains Greater Than 5 Grams Total Fat OR Greater Than 1 Gram Saturated Fat

Frito Lay (Cont.)	Rold Gold Pretzels:
	▲ Thins
	Tiny Twists
			Doritos:
			  Nacho Cheesier
			  Taco Supreme Tortilla Chips
			  Taco Tortilla Chips
			  Zesty Cheese
			Fritos:
			  Bar-B-Q
			  Chili Cheese
			  King Size
			  Original
			  ∇ Scoops
			  Wild n' Mild Ranch
			Funyons
			Lays Potato Chips:
			  Bar-B-Q
			  KC Masterpiece
			  ∇ Regular
			  Sour Cream and Onion
			  Tangy Ranch
			Munchos:
			  Potato Crisps
			Ruffles Potato Chips:
			  Cheddar & Sour Cream
			  ∇ Mesquite Grille BBQ
			  ∇ Original
			  Ranch
			  ∇ Reduced Fat
			Santitas:
			  ∇ Tortilla Chips - 100% White Corn
			Sun Chips:
			  ∇ French Onion
			  Harvest Cheddar
			  Original
			Taco Bell:
			  ∇ Tortilla Chips
			Taco Bell White Corn Chips:
			  ∇ Restaurant Style
			Tortilla Thins:
			  ∇ Original
			  Salsa 'N Cheese
			Tostitos:
			  ∇ 100% White Corn Crispy Tortilla Chips

▲ High Sodium, 480 mg. or greater per serving.
∇ Low Sodium, 140 mg. or less per serving.

BRAND	BEST CHOICE	ACCEPTABLE CHOICE	OCCASIONAL CHOICE
	Fat Free or Low Fat AND Low Saturated Fat	Contains Greater Than 3 Grams but Less Than or Equal To 5 Grams Total Fat AND Low Saturated Fat	Contains Greater Than 5 Grams Total Fat OR Greater Than 1 Gram Saturated Fat

Frito Lay (Cont.)			Tostitos:
			  ∇ Bite Size
			  ∇ Restaurant Style
			Wavy Lays:
			  Au-Gratin
			  ∇ Original

Garden of Eatin	California Bakes:
	  ∇ All Flavors
		ToTopos Cantina Chips:
		  ∇ Chili & Lime
		  ∇ Salted
			Blue Chips:
			  ∇ No Salt Added
			  ∇ Salted
			Chili Chips:
			  ∇ Black Bean
			Corn Chips:
			  ∇ Mini
			  ∇ Red Hot Blues
			  ∇ Sesame Blues
			  ∇ Sunny Blues
			∇ Corntilla Chips
			Tortilla Chips:
			  ∇ Black Bean

Gardetto's		Pretzel Mix:
		  Mustard Flavor
			Snak-ens:
			  Original

General Mills		Cheerios Snack Mix:
		  Cheddar Cheese
		  Original	

Grandma Shearer's			Potato Chips:
			  ▲ Bar-B-Q
			  ∇ Country Cooked
			  ∇ Kettle Style
			Tortilla Chips:
			  ∇ Ripples
			  ∇ Restaurant Style

Greenfield	Air Popped Popcorn: ∇ Caramel		
Guiltless Gourmet	Baked Tortilla Chips: Nacho		

▲ High Sodium, 480 mg. or greater per serving.
∇ Low Sodium, 140 mg. or less per serving.

Chips, Pretzels, Popcorn, Snacks 111

BRAND	BEST CHOICE	ACCEPTABLE CHOICE	OCCASIONAL CHOICE
	Fat Free or Low Fat AND Low Saturated Fat	Contains Greater Than 3 Grams but Less Than or Equal To 5 Grams Total Fat AND Low Saturated Fat	Contains Greater Than 5 Grams Total Fat OR Greater Than 1 Gram Saturated Fat
Guiltless Gourmet (Cont.)	Baked Tortilla Chips: ∇☆ No Salt Added ☆ Salted ∇ White Corn		
Hain	Fat Free Mini Popcorn Rice Cakes: ∇ Butter ∇ Caramel Fat Free Mini Rice Cakes: ∇ Apple-Cinnamon ∇ Honey Nut ∇ Teriyaki Mini Popcorn Rice Cakes: ∇ Lightly Salted ∇ Mild Cheddar ∇ White Cheddar Mini Rice Cakes: ∇ Cheese ∇ Plain	Mini Rice Cakes: Ranch	
Harry's	Sourdough Pretzels: Regular ∇ Unsalted Whole Wheat Honeys: ∇ Pretzels w/Sesame Seeds		
HBO			Microwave Popcorn: ☆ Butter Flavor ☆ Movie Butter Flavor
Health Valley	Fat Free Caramel Corn Puffs: ∇ All Flavors Fat Free Cheese Puffs: All Flavors Fat Free Corn Puffs: ∇ All Flavors		
Jays			100% White Corn Crispy Rounds: ∇ Tortilla Chips 100% White Corn Restaurant Style: ∇ Tortilla Chips Hot Stuff Potato Chips

∇ Low Sodium, 140 mg. or less per serving.
☆ Good Source of Fiber, between 2.5 g. and 5 g. per serving.

BRAND	BEST CHOICE	ACCEPTABLE CHOICE	OCCASIONAL CHOICE
	Fat Free or Low Fat AND Low Saturated Fat	Contains Greater Than 3 Grams but Less Than or Equal To 5 Grams Total Fat AND Low Saturated Fat	Contains Greater Than 5 Grams Total Fat OR Greater Than 1 Gram Saturated Fat
Jays (Cont.)			O-Ke-Doke Popcorn: Buttery Cheese White White Cheddar Potato Chips: ▽ No Salt Added Tortilla Chips: Nacho Cheese
Jiffy Pop	Glazed Popcorn Clusters: ▽ Caramel		Popcorn: ☆ Butter Flavor
Keebler	Pretzels: ▲ Butter Braids ▲ Butter Knots ▲ Traditional Bavarian ▲ Traditional Knots		Chacho's: Cheesy Quesadilla ▽ Cinnamon Crispana Restaurant Style Original Salsa Verde O'Boisies: Cheddar Original Sour Cream and Onion Pizzarias: Cheese Pizza Pizza Supreme Zesty Pepperoni Ripplin's: Barbecue Original Ranch Tato Wilds Criss Cross: Barbecue Original Tato Wilds Tato Skins: Cheese n' Bacon Original Baked Potato Sour Cream n' Onion
Kettle Krisp		▽ Toffee Caramel Popcorn w/Peanuts	
Krunchers			Potato Chips: Jalapeño Mesquite Original

▲ High Sodium, 480 mg. or greater per serving.
▽ Low Sodium, 140 mg. or less per serving.
☆ Good Source of Fiber, between 2.5 g. and 5 g. per serving.

Chips, Pretzels, Popcorn, Snacks 113

BRAND	BEST CHOICE	ACCEPTABLE CHOICE	OCCASIONAL CHOICE
	Fat Free or Low Fat AND Low Saturated Fat	Contains Greater Than 3 Grams but Less Than or Equal To 5 Grams Total Fat AND Low Saturated Fat	Contains Greater Than 5 Grams Total Fat OR Greater Than 1 Gram Saturated Fat

Louise's	Fat Free Potato Chips:
	  Maui Onion
	  Mesquite BBQ
	  Original
	  ∇ Original No Salt
	  Vinegar & Salt
	Low Fat Popcorn:
	  ☆ Buttered
	  Caramel
	  ∇☆ Lightly Salted
	Low Fat Potato Chips:
	  Original
	Low Fat Tortilla Chips:
	  Nacho Cheese
	  Ranch
	  White Corn		

Manischewitz	Bagel Shaped Pretzels:
	  All Flavors
	Passover Gold:
	  Matzo Crackers
		Bagel Chips:
		  Cinnamon Spice & Raisin	

McCleary's	Elite Quality:
	  ∇ Caramel Corn
			Elite Quality Tortilla Chips:
			  ∇ Blue Corn
			  Deli Style
			  ∇ No Salt Deli Style
			  ∇ Restaurant Style

Michael Season's	Organic Pretzels:
	  Lightly Salted Mini Twists
	  ∇ Unsalted Mini Twists
	Party Mix
	Potato Bakes:
	  All Flavors
	Pretzels:
	  Lightly Salted Dutch
	  Lightly Salted Mini Twists
	  Lightly Salted Twists
	  ∇ Unsalted Twists
	Shape Ups:
	  ∇ Original
	  ∇ Salsa
		Corn Tostados:
		  ∇ Bite Size, Lightly Salted
			40% Less Fat Potato Chips:
			  Honey Barbecue
			  ∇ Lightly Salted
			  ∇ Unsalted
			  ∇ Yogurt & Green Onion
			White Corn Tortilla Chips:
			  ∇ Lightly Salted

∇ Low Sodium, 140 mg. or less per serving.
☆ Good Source of Fiber, between 2.5 g. and 5 g. per serving.

114   **Chips, Pretzels, Popcorn, Snacks**

BRAND	BEST CHOICE	ACCEPTABLE CHOICE	OCCASIONAL CHOICE
	Fat Free or Low Fat AND Low Saturated Fat	Contains Greater Than 3 Grams but Less Than or Equal To 5 Grams Total Fat AND Low Saturated Fat	Contains Greater Than 5 Grams Total Fat OR Greater Than 1 Gram Saturated Fat
Mother's	Minis Rice Cakes: ∇ All Flavors Popped Corn Cakes: ∇ Butter, Sodium Free ∇ Natural Butter Flavor ∇ White Cheddar Rice Cakes: ∇ Multi-Grain, Unsalted ∇ Plain, Sodium Free ∇ Sesame ∇ Sesame, Sodium Free		
Mr. Phipps	Pretzel Chips: ▲ Fat Free Lower Sodium ▲ Original	Tater Crisps: Bar-B-Que Original Sour Cream & Onion Tortilla Crisps: Nacho Cheese ∇ Original	
Nabisco	Mister Salty Pretzels: Fat Free, All Varieties ▲ Regular, All Varieties Mr. Salty: ▲ Fat Free Pretzel Chips ▲ Pretzel Chips		Ritz Snack Mix: Traditional
Nature's Favorite		Apple Chips: ∇★ Caramel ∇★ Crispy Cinnamon ∇★ Crispy Original ∇★ Crispy Tart	
New York		Bagel Chips: Cajun ∇ Cinnamon Raisin Sesame	Bagel Chips: Garlic ∇ Original/Low Sodium Bite Size Bagel Chips: Hot 'n Spicy
Newman's Own	Microwave Popcorn: ∇☆ Butter Flavor Light ∇☆ Light ∇★ Popcorn		Microwave Popcorn: ☆ All Natural Flavor ☆ Butter ∇☆ No Salt

▲ High Sodium, 480 mg. or greater per serving.
∇ Low Sodium, 140 mg. or less per serving.
☆ Good Source of Fiber, between 2.5 g. and 5 g. per serving.
★ High Fiber, 5 g. or greater per serving.

Chips, Pretzels, Popcorn, Snacks 115

BRAND	BEST CHOICE	ACCEPTABLE CHOICE	OCCASIONAL CHOICE
	Fat Free or Low Fat AND Low Saturated Fat	Contains Greater Than 3 Grams but Less Than or Equal To 5 Grams Total Fat AND Low Saturated Fat	Contains Greater Than 5 Grams Total Fat OR Greater Than 1 Gram Saturated Fat

Newman's Own (Cont.)	Pretzels:
	  Salted Rounds
	  Salted Sticks
	  ∇ Unsalted Rounds		

North Castle			Jarlsberg Cheese Crisps:
			  Cheese
			  ∇ Cheese Pizza

Orville Redenbacher	Gourmet Popcorn:
	  ∇ Original-Lower Fat Recipe
	Smart-Pop:
	  ★ Butter
		Microwave Popcorn:
		  ★ Butter Light
		  ★ Natural Light
		Redden Budders:
		  ★ Movie Theatre Butter
		  Light
			Gourmet Popping Corn:
			  ∇☆ White
			Microwave Popcorn:
			  ☆ Butter Flavor
			  ∇★ Butter Flavor, Unsalted
			  ∇ Caramel Flavored
			  ☆ Cheddar Cheese
			  ★ Natural
			  ★ Snack-Size Butter
			Redden Budders:
			  ☆ Movie Theater Butter
			  ☆ Zesty Butter

Pacific Grain	No Fries: ∇ All Flavors		

Pacific Snax		Popcorn Shaped Rice:
		  ∇ Honey Mustard
		  ∇ Lightly Salted
		  Santa Fe Cheddar
			Popcorn Shaped Rice:
			  ∇ White Cheddar

Pepperidge Farm			Goldfish:
			  ☆ Tortilla Crisps
			Goldfish Party Mix:
			  w/Honey Roasted Peanuts
			Snack Sticks:
			  Sesame
			  Pumpernickel
			  Three Cheese

Planters			Cheez Balls Cheez Curls
Pow-Wow			Puffs: Cheese

∇ Low Sodium, 140 mg. or less per serving.
☆ Good Source of Fiber, between 2.5 g. and 5 g. per serving.
★ High Fiber, 5 g. or greater per serving.

BRAND	BEST CHOICE	ACCEPTABLE CHOICE	OCCASIONAL CHOICE
	Fat Free or Low Fat AND Low Saturated Fat	Contains Greater Than 3 Grams but Less Than or Equal To 5 Grams Total Fat AND Low Saturated Fat	Contains Greater Than 5 Grams Total Fat OR Greater Than 1 Gram Saturated Fat
Prime Time			Microwave Popcorn: Butter

Pringles			Potato Crisps:
			  BBQ
			  Cheez Ums
			  Original
			  ∇ Ranch
			  ∇ Sour Cream 'n Onion
			Ridges:
			  Original
			Right Crisps:
			  ∇ Original
			  ∇ Ranch
			  ∇ Sour Cream 'n Onion

Pritikin	Rice Cakes: ∇ All Varieties		

Quaker	Corn Cakes:
	  ∇ All Varieties
	Rice Cakes:
	  ∇ All Flavors		

Quinlan	Pretzels: All Shapes		

R W Frookie	∇ Fat Free Frisps
	Frisps:
	  ∇ Apple Cinnamon
	  ∇ Honey Crunch		

Ralston		Chex Mix:
		  Barbeque
		  Golden Cheddar Cheese
		  Traditional
		  Zesty Ranch	

Roman Meal	Corn Cakes:
	  ∇ All Varieties
	Rice Cakes:
	  ∇ All Varieties		

Sargento			MooTown Snackers:
			  Cheese & Pretzels
			  Cheese & Sticks

∇ Low Sodium, 140 mg. or less per serving.

BRAND	BEST CHOICE	ACCEPTABLE CHOICE	OCCASIONAL CHOICE
	Fat Free or Low Fat AND Low Saturated Fat	Contains Greater Than 3 Grams but Less Than or Equal To 5 Grams Total Fat AND Low Saturated Fat	Contains Greater Than 5 Grams Total Fat OR Greater Than 1 Gram Saturated Fat
Seyfert's	Pretzel Rods: Butter		Cheese Twistees
Skinny			Corn Chips: Barbeque Nacho Cheese ∇ No Salt ∇ Original Lightly Salted ∇ Sour Cream & Onion
Smart Choice	Fruit Snacks: ∇ Space and Pirates		
Smart Temptations	No Oil Tortilla Chips: ∇ No Salt ∇ Regular		
Smartfood			Popcorn: White Cheddar Cheese
Snack Appeal	95% Fat Free Snacks: All Varieties Fat Free Pretzels: All Varieties		
Snack Time			Potato Chips: Bar-B-Q Cain's
Snyder's of Hanover	Hard Pretzels: ▲ Sourdough ∇ Unsalted Sourdough ∇ Honey Wheat Pretzels w/Sesame Seeds Old Fashioned Dipping Sticks Olde Tyme Pretzels: Regular ∇ Unsalted Pretzel Minis: ▲ Regular ∇ Unsalted Pretzels: Logs ▲ Nibblers Oat Bran	Sourdough Pretzel Pieces: Buttermilk Ranch Honey Mustard & Onion	Potato Chips: Grilled Steak & Onion Kosher Dill ∇ No Salt ∇ Regular ∇ Ripple Chips Salt & Vinegar Sausage Pizza Sour Cream & Onion Pretzel Pieces: Cheddar Cheese Snack Mix Sourdough Pretzel Pieces: Cheddar Cheese Creamy Caramel Pepperoni Pizza

▲ High Sodium, 480 mg. or greater per serving.
∇ Low Sodium, 140 mg. or less per serving.

BRAND	BEST CHOICE	ACCEPTABLE CHOICE	OCCASIONAL CHOICE
	Fat Free or Low Fat AND Low Saturated Fat	Contains Greater Than 3 Grams but Less Than or Equal To 5 Grams Total Fat AND Low Saturated Fat	Contains Greater Than 5 Grams Total Fat OR Greater Than 1 Gram Saturated Fat

Snyder's of Hanover (Cont.)	Pretzels:
	  Rods
	  Stix
	  ▲ Ultra-Thin		

Sunkist	Fruit Rolls: ∇ All Flavors		

Sunshine		Cheez-it:
		  Party Mix
		Old San Francisco Style Pretzel Pieces:
		  All Flavors	

Tastee			Apple Chips: ∇ All Flavors

Terra			Terra Chips:
			  ∇☆ Regular
			  ∇☆ Spiced Taro

The Allens			∇ Shoestring Potato Sticks

The Fat Free Gourmet	Baked Potato Corns:
	  Nacho
	Baked Tortilla Chips:
	  Nacho
	  Natural
	  Salsa
	Sourdough Pretzels:
	  ▲ Salted
	  ∇ Unsalted		

TreeTop	∇ Crispy Apple Chips		
Ultra Slim Fast	Cheese Curls		
Utz	Hard Pretzels: Sourdough		
Vic's			∇ Gourmet Cheese Popcorn ☆ Gourmet White Popcorn

▲ High Sodium, 480 mg. or greater per serving.
∇ Low Sodium, 140 mg. or less per serving.
☆ Good Source of Fiber, between 2.5 g. and 5 g. per serving.

BRAND	BEST CHOICE	ACCEPTABLE CHOICE	OCCASIONAL CHOICE
	Fat Free or Low Fat AND Low Saturated Fat	Contains Greater Than 3 Grams but Less Than or Equal To 5 Grams Total Fat AND Low Saturated Fat	Contains Greater Than 5 Grams Total Fat OR Greater Than 1 Gram Saturated Fat

Weight Watchers	∇☆ Apple Chips
	Crunchy Snacks:
	    ∇ Barbeque Flavored Curls
	Fruit Snack:
	    ∇ All Flavors
	∇★ Microwave Popcorn
	Smart Snackers:
	    ∇☆ Butter Flavor Popcorn
	    ∇ Cheese Curls
	    Ranch Curls
		Smart Snackers:
		    ∇ White Cheddar Cheese	

Westbrae Natural	Rice Cakes: ∇ All Flavors		

White Kernel			Popcorn:
			    ☆ Buttery
			    Reduced Sodium

Wise	Lowfat Pretzel Stixs:
	    ▲ Butter
			Cottage Fries:
			    ∇ No Salt Added
			Potato Chips:
			    Barbecue
			    Cheddar & Sour Cream
			    ∇ Lightly Salted
			    Onion and Garlic
			    Original
			    Ridged
			    Salt & Vinegar

FROZEN			

SuperPretzel	Baked Soft Pretzels
	    ∇ Unsalted
	Soft Pretzel Bites:
	    ∇ Unsalted
	Softstix:
	    Cheese Filled Soft Pretzel
	        Sticks		

YOUR FAVORITE SNACK FOODS NOT LISTED IN THE GUIDE			

▲ High Sodium, 480 mg. or greater per serving.
∇ Low Sodium, 140 mg. or less per serving.
☆ Good Source of Fiber, between 2.5 g. and 5 g. per serving.
★ High Fiber, 5 g. or greater per serving.

120   **Chips, Pretzels, Popcorn, Snacks**

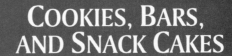

COOKIES, BARS, AND SNACK CAKES

This product category contains a large variety of cookies and cookie-type bars. These snack foods can add variety to the diet, but if quantities are not controlled, they can also contribute excessive calories. Many companies are now producing reduced-fat or fat-free versions of their regular cookies, bars, and snack cakes. However, when choosing low-fat or fat-free cookies or bars, it is important to remember that although they may be fat-free, they are unlikely to be calorie-free. Another important point of which to be aware is that the product claim of "Fat Free" or "Low Fat" applies only to the standard serving size identified on the package label. The serving size for some cookies can be as small as one cookie. If you eat several cookies at one sitting, you can conceivably be eating a substantial amount of fat. Make sure to read the *Nutrition Facts* label for the serving size, calories, and fat content of that specific product.

The *Food Guide Pyramid* considers cookies as part of the "Bread, Cereal, Rice, and Pasta Group." Six to eleven servings are recommended each day from this food group. Two medium cookies count as a serving from this food group. However, products such as cookies can contain liberal amounts of fat and sugar, while other foods in this group, such as bread, rice and pasta, and some cereals, are significantly lower in fat and sugar while providing generous amounts of vitamins, minerals, and fiber. The FDA has established reference amounts or standardized serving sizes for use on the food label. The reference amount for cookies ranges from 30 grams (one ounce) for most cookies to 40 grams (1.4 ounces) for most granola and breakfast-type bars. Be sure to read the *Nutrition Facts* label for the serving size information of your cookie choice. (See pages 51 and 52 for an explanation of reference amounts and the difference between serving sizes established by the FDA for food labeling and those recommended by the *Food Guide Pyramid*.)

Criteria Key

▲ **Best Choice:**   **Fat Free or Low Fat AND Low Saturated Fat**

Products listed in this category meet the FDA's definition for "Fat Free" (less than $1/2$ gram fat per serving) or "Low Fat" (3 grams or less fat per serving) and "Low Saturated Fat" (1 gram or less saturated fat per serving).

▲ **Acceptable Choice:**   **Contains Greater Than 3 Grams but Less Than or Equal to 5 Grams Total Fat, AND Low Saturated Fat**

Products listed in this category **do not** meet the FDA's definition for "Low Fat," but **do** meet the definition for "Low Saturated Fat." These products are, therefore, higher in total fat than those listed in the "Best Choice" category but are low in saturated fat. The 5 grams of total fat cut-off was used in order to be consistent with the amount of fat equal to one diabetes diet fat exchange and is also equivalent to 1 teaspoon of added fat.[75]

▲ **Occasional Choice:**   **Contains Greater Than 5 Grams Total Fat or Greater Than 1 Gram Saturated Fat**

Products listed in this category do not meet the FDA's definition for either "Low Fat" or "Low Saturated Fat." These products contain greater than 5 grams of total fat or greater than 1 gram saturated fat per serving. These products can contribute a significant amount of fat to the overall daily diet and should be consumed only on occasion.

BRAND	BEST CHOICE	ACCEPTABLE CHOICE	OCCASIONAL CHOICE
	Fat Free or Low Fat AND Low Saturated Fat	Contains Greater Than 3 Grams but Less Than or Equal to 5 Grams Total Fat AND Low Saturated Fat	Contains Greater Than 5 Grams Total Fat OR Greater Than 1 Gram Saturated Fat
A Whale of a Snack	Fat Free Bars: 　All Flavors		
All Star Foods	∇ Low Fat Oatmeal Cookie Miracle Meal: 　∇★ Meal In One Cookie	∇ Brownie Cookie	
Archway	∇ Apple Filled Oatmeal Fat Free Cookies: 　∇ Chocolate 　∇ Lemon Nuggets 　∇ Sugar ∇ Fat Free Apple Bar ∇ Fat Free Fig Bar ∇ Fat Free Fruit Bar ∇ Fat Free Granola Bar Fat Free Oatmeal Raisin Bar Fat Free Oatmeal Raspberry Bar ∇ Oatmeal Cookies Old Fashioned Molasses 　Cookies	∇ Apple 'n Raisin Carrot Cake Cookies Dark Molasses Cookies ∇ Date Filled Oatmeal ∇ Frosty Lemon Cookie ∇ Gingersnaps ∇ Oatmeal Raisin ∇ Raspberry Filled Cookies ∇ Ruth's Golden Oatmeal ∇ Soft Sugar Drop Cookies Sugar Cookies ∇ Windmill Cookies	∇ Cherry Filled Cookies ∇ Chocolate Chip and Toffee 　Cookies ∇Chocolate Chip Drop Cookie ∇ Chocolate Chip Ice Box 　Cookies ∇ Lemon Snaps ∇ Oatmeal Pecan ∇ Peanut Butter Cookie ∇ Pecan Ice Box ∇ Rocky Road Gourmet Cookies ∇ Strawberry Filled Cookies
Auburn Farms	Fat Free Brownies: 　∇ All Flavors Fat Free Jammers: 　∇ All Flavors		
Aunt Fanny's			Fried Pies: 　▲ All Flavors
Awrey's Best		∇ Date Nut Pastry ∇ Date Oatmeal Pastry	
Bahlsen		∇ Deloba	∇ Apple Crumblies Choco Leibniz: 　∇ Milk Chocolate 　∇ Dark Chocolate ∇ Choco Star ∇ Dark Chocolate Waffeletten ∇ Delice ∇ Hannover-Waffeln ∇ Leibniz Butter Cookies ∇ Milk Chocolate Waffeletten

▲ High Sodium, 480 mg. or greater per serving.
∇ Low Sodium, 140 mg. or less per serving.
★ High Fiber, 5 g. or greater per serving.

BRAND	BEST CHOICE	ACCEPTABLE CHOICE	OCCASIONAL CHOICE
	Fat Free or Low Fat AND Low Saturated Fat	Contains Greater Than 3 Grams but Less Than or Equal to 5 Grams Total Fat AND Low Saturated Fat	Contains Greater Than 5 Grams Total Fat OR Greater Than 1 Gram Saturated Fat
Bakery Wagon	Fat Free Chewy Fruit Cookies: ∇ All Flavors Mini Iced Molasses		∇ Ginger Snaps
Barbara's	∇ Fat Free Double Chocolate Mini Cookies Nature's Choice Cereal Bars: ∇ All Flavors Nature's Choice Grrr-nola Treats: ∇ Chocolate Chip		Small Indulgence: ∇ Butter Pecan Bites ∇ Chocolate Chip Crisps ∇ Coffee Cake Crunch ∇ Lemon Almond Delights
Betty Crocker	Pop-Secret Popcorn Bars: ∇ All Flavors		Dunkaroos: ∇ Cinnamon Graham Cookies w/Vanilla Frosting ∇ Graham Cookies w/ Chocolate Frosting
Bursting With Fruit	Fat Free Fruity Chewy Cookies: ∇ Peach Apricot		
Carnation			Breakfast Bars: ∇ Chewy Chocolate Chip ∇ Chewy Peanut Butter w/Chocolate Chips ∇ Chocolate Chunk Granola ∇ Honey and Oats Granola
Carr's			Home Wheat: ∇ Chocolate Topped Graham Cookies
Chadwick Farms		∇ Vanilla Wafers	
Colonial		∇ Maple Leaf Sandwich Cremes	
Dare			∇ Harvest From the Rainforest Cookies
Delicious	Vanilla Wafers	Musselman's: Applesauce Oatmeal Cookie Power Rangers Dinozord Sandwich Cookies: ∇ All Flavors	∇ Butterfinger Cookies Chiquita: ∇ BananaRamas Heath: ∇ English Toffee Cookies

∇ Low Sodium, 140 mg. or less per serving.

124 **Cookies, Bars, and Snack Cakes**

BRAND	BEST CHOICE	ACCEPTABLE CHOICE	OCCASIONAL CHOICE
	Fat Free or Low Fat AND Low Saturated Fat	Contains Greater Than 3 Grams but Less Than or Equal to 5 Grams Total Fat AND Low Saturated Fat	Contains Greater Than 5 Grams Total Fat OR Greater Than 1 Gram Saturated Fat
Delicious (Cont.)		∇ Raisinets Oatmeal Cookies	Land-O-Lakes: ∇ Frosted Butter Cookies Skippy: ∇ Peanut Butter Cookies
Dolly Madison Bakery			Cupcakes: Creme Filled Devil's Food
Dutch Twins		∇ Fudge Sticks	∇ Assorted Creme Wafers ∇ Party Stix Yes! Yes!: ∇ Fudge Caramel & Toasted Coconut
Earth Bar	∇ Ocean Berry Bar	∇ Desert Delight Bar ∇ Mountain Majesty Bar	∇ Rainforest Frost Bar ∇ Tropical Splendor Bar
Entenmann's	Fat Free: ∇ Chocolate Brownie Cookies ∇ Fudge Brownie ∇ Oatmeal Chocolate Chip Cookies ∇ Oatmeal Raisin Cookies	50% Less Fat: ∇ Chocolate Chip Cookies	∇ Butter Cookies ∇ Chocolate Chip Cookies ∇ English Toffee Cookies
Estee	Fig Bars Low Fat: ∇☆ All Flavors	∇ Oatmeal Raisin Cookies Sandwich Cookies: ∇ Vanilla	∇ Chocolate Chip Cookies ∇ Coconut Cookies Creme Wafers: ∇ Chocolate ∇ Lemon ∇ Peanut Butter ∇ Triple Decker Creme Wafers Sugar Free: ∇ Vanilla/Strawberry ∇ Fudge Cookies ∇ Lemon Cookies Sandwich Cookies: ∇ Chocolate ∇ Original ∇ Peanut Butter ∇ Vanilla Cookies
Famous Amos	Fat Free Fruit Bar Cookies: ∇ All Flavors	Cookies: ∇ Oatmeal Raisin Cinnamon	Cookies: ∇ Chocolate Chip ∇ Chocolate Sandwich ∇ Chocolate Chip & Pecans ∇ Oatmeal Macaroon Sandwich ∇ Peanut Butter Sandwich

∇ Low Sodium, 140 mg. or less per serving.
☆ Good Source of Fiber, between 2.5 g. and 5 g. per serving.

Cookies, Bars, and Snack Cakes 125

BRAND	BEST CHOICE	ACCEPTABLE CHOICE	OCCASIONAL CHOICE
	Fat Free or Low Fat AND Low Saturated Fat	Contains Greater Than 3 Grams but Less Than or Equal to 5 Grams Total Fat AND Low Saturated Fat	Contains Greater Than 5 Grams Total Fat OR Greater Than 1 Gram Saturated Fat

Fi-Bar	Berry Best:
	  ∇☆ Cranberry & Wildberry
	  ∇☆ Raspberry
	  ∇☆ Strawberry
	Fruit & Nuts:
	  ∇☆ Strawberry Oatmeal & Almond
	One Gram Granola Bars:
	  ∇ All Flavors
		Fruit & Nuts:
		  ∇☆ Apple, Oatmeal, & Spice
		  ∇☆ Banana Nut
			Chewy & Nutty:
			  ∇ Cocoa Almond Crunch
			  ∇ Cocoa Peanut Butter Crunch
			  ∇ Vanilla Almond Crunch
			  ∇ Vanilla Peanut Butter Crunch
			Nectar Granola Bars:
			  ∇ Milk Chocolate Peanut Butter Crunch

Fifty 50			∇ Assorted Cream Filled Wafers ∇ Chocolate Chip Cookies ∇ Hearty Oatmeal Cookies ∇ Peanut Butter Cookies
Fireside	∇ Fig Bars		
General Henry	Fruit Bars: ∇ All Flavors		
Goteborgs			∇ Dinosaurs Chocolate Cookies

Greenfield	Healthy Foods:
	  ∇ Blonde Brownie
	  ∇ Fat Free Brownie		

Guiltless Low-Fat	Cookies:
	  ∇ Chocolate Chip
	  ∇ Double Chocolate
	  ∇ Oatmeal Apple Spice
	  ∇ Oatmeal Raisin
	  ∇ Peanut Butter		

Health Valley	100% Natural Bars:
	  ∇ Apple Bakes
	100% Natural Fruit Bars:
	  ∇ Date Bakes
	  ∇ Raisin Bakes
	Breakfast Bar:
	  ∇☆ Strawberry Apple
	Fat Free Bakes:
	  ∇☆ All Flavors
	Fat Free Breakfast Bars:
	  ∇☆ All Flavors		

∇ Low Sodium, 140 mg. or less per serving.
☆ Good Source of Fiber, between 2.5 g. and 5 g. per serving.

BRAND	BEST CHOICE	ACCEPTABLE CHOICE	OCCASIONAL CHOICE
	Fat Free or Low Fat AND Low Saturated Fat	Contains Greater Than 3 Grams but Less Than or Equal to 5 Grams Total Fat AND Low Saturated Fat	Contains Greater Than 5 Grams Total Fat OR Greater Than 1 Gram Saturated Fat
Health Valley (Cont.)	Fat Free Brownie Bars: ∇☆ All Flavors Fat Free Chocolate Cookies with Fruit Centers: ∇☆ All Flavors Fat Free Fruit Bars: ∇☆ All Flavors Fat Free Fruit Centers: ∇ All Flavors Fat Free Fruit Chunks Cookies: ∇☆ All Flavors Fat Free Granola Bars: ∇☆ All Flavors Fat Free Healthy Tarts: ∇ All Flavors Fat Free Jumbo Cookies: ∇☆ All Flavors Fat Free Mini Fruit Center Cookies: ∇ All Flavors ∇ Fruit and Nut Bars Healthy Chips: ∇☆ Original Healthy Tarts: ∇☆ All Flavors Jumbo Fruit Cookies: ∇☆ Fat Free All Flavors Oat Bran Jumbo Fruit Bars: ∇ All Flavors		
Hostess	Lights: ∇ Low Fat Brownies ∇ Low Fat Crumb Cakes Low Fat Cup Cakes Low Fat Twinkies		Brownie Bites: ∇ Regular ∇ Walnut Choco-licious ▲ Cup Cakes Fruit Pies: All Flavors Ho Hos King Dons Sno Balls Suzy Q's Twinkies

▲ High Sodium, 480 mg. or greater per serving.
∇ Low Sodium, 140 mg. or less per serving.
☆ Good Source of Fiber, between 2.5 g. and 5 g. per serving.

BRAND	BEST CHOICE	ACCEPTABLE CHOICE	OCCASIONAL CHOICE
	Fat Free or Low Fat AND Low Saturated Fat	Contains Greater Than 3 Grams but Less Than or Equal to 5 Grams Total Fat AND Low Saturated Fat	Contains Greater Than 5 Grams Total Fat OR Greater Than 1 Gram Saturated Fat
Keebler	Chips Deluxe: ∇ Reduced Fat Elfin Delights Fat Free: ∇ Devil's Food Cookies ∇ Devil's Food Cookies w/ Vanilla Middles Elfin Delights Reduced Fat: ∇ Caramel Apple Oatmeal Cookies Pecan Sandies: ∇ Reduced Fat Raisin Ruckus: ∇ Chocolate Covered Raisins ∇ Plump Raisins Soft Batch: ∇ Oatmeal Raisin	Elfin Delights Reduced Fat: ∇ Chocolate Sandwich Cookie w/Fudge Creme Chocolate Sandwich Cookie w/Vanilla Creme ∇ Creme Sandwich Cookies ∇ French Vanilla Creme Cookies Original Cookie Classics: ∇ Chocolate Fudge ∇ Pitter Patter Soft Batch: ∇ Chocolate Chip ∇ Walnut Chocolate Chip Vanilla Wafers: ∇ Reduced Fat	Chips Deluxe: ∇ Bakery Crisp ∇ Bite Size ∇ Chocolate Lovers ∇ Original ∇ Pecan ∇ Rainbow ∇ Coconut Chocolate Drop Cookies ∇ Deluxe Grahams E.L. Fudge: ∇ Butter Cookie w/Fudge Creme ∇ Fudge Cookies w/Fudge Creme ∇ Fudge N'Caramel ∇ Fudge Sticks ∇ Fudge Stripes ∇ Golden Vanilla Wafers ∇ Grasshopper ∇ Iced Animal Cookies Mini Middles: ∇ Chocolate Chip ∇ Shortbread ∇ P.B. Fudgebutters Pecan Sandies: ∇ Bite Size ∇ Pecan Sandies & Praline Creme Rainbow Chips Deluxe: ∇ Bite Size ∇ Sweetspots ∇ Toffee Sandies ∇ Toffee Toppers
Kellogg's	Low Fat Granola Bars: ∇ All Flavors NutriGrain Cereal Bars: ∇ All Flavors	Pop-Tarts Minis: Frosted Chocolate Frosted Strawberry	Rice Krispies: ∇ Chewy Granola Bars
Kudos	Low Fat Bars: ∇ Blueberry ∇ Strawberry Whole Grain Bars: ∇ Chocolate Chunk ∇ Honey Nut ∇ Oatmeal Raisin		Reduced Fat Bars: ∇ All Flavors Whole Grain Bars: ∇ Milk Chocolate-Chocolate Chip ∇ Nutty Fudge ∇ Peanut Butter

∇ Low Sodium, 140 mg. or less per serving.

BRAND	BEST CHOICE Fat Free or Low Fat AND Low Saturated Fat	ACCEPTABLE CHOICE Contains Greater Than 3 Grams but Less Than or Equal to 5 Grams Total Fat AND Low Saturated Fat	OCCASIONAL CHOICE Contains Greater Than 5 Grams Total Fat OR Greater Than 1 Gram Saturated Fat
Lance			Van O Lunch: ∇ Cookies
Little Debbie	Brownie Lights Fat Free Figaroos ∇ Fat Free Strawberry Fruit Cookies ∇ Ginger Cookies Lowfat Angel Cakes: ∇ Raspberry Oatmeal Lights Snacks	∇ Figaroos ∇ Lemon Creme Wafers ∇ Marshmallow Supremes ∇ Pecan Spinwheels ∇ Raisin Creme Pies	∇ Animal Cookies ∇ Apple Delights Banana Twins Cakes ∇ Caramel Cookie Bars Chocolate Chips Cakes ∇ Christmas Tree Cakes Coconut Cakes Devil Creme Cakes Devil Squares Fudge Brownies w/English Walnuts ∇ Fudge Crispy Golden Cremes Cakes ∇ Mint Creme Wafers ∇ Nutty Bar Oatmeal Cream Pies Spice Cakes ∇ Star Crunch Strawberry Shortcake Rolls Swiss Cake Rolls Tiger Cakes Zebra Cakes
Lotte			Koala Yummies: Peanut Butter ∇ Regular
Lu		Milk Lunch: New England Biscuits	∇ Dipped Chocolatiers Le Petit Beurre ∇ Lu Chocolatiers Wafers Marie Lu Cookies ∇ Pim's Orange ∇ Pim's Raspberry The Little Schoolboy: ∇ Dark Chocolate ∇ Milk Chocolate Truffle Lu
Mama's	Fig Bars	∇ Peanut Butter Cremes	∇ 2-in-1 Cremes Butter Thins Coconut Bars ∇ Duplex Cremes Dutch Windmill Cookies Fudge Cremes ∇ Lemon Cremes

∇ Low Sodium, 140 mg. or less per serving.

Cookies, Bars, and Snack Cakes 129

BRAND	BEST CHOICE	ACCEPTABLE CHOICE	OCCASIONAL CHOICE
	Fat Free or Low Fat AND Low Saturated Fat	Contains Greater Than 3 Grams but Less Than or Equal to 5 Grams Total Fat AND Low Saturated Fat	Contains Greater Than 5 Grams Total Fat OR Greater Than 1 Gram Saturated Fat
Mama's (Cont.)			▽ Striped Delights ▽ Vanilla Wafers
Manischewitz			▽ Chocolate Chunk Macaroons w/Cherry Bits ▽☆ Rocky Road Macaroons
Mother's	▽ Whole Wheat Fig Bars		

Mrs. Alisons		Cookies:
		  ▽ Almond Windmill
		  ▽ Shortbread
			Cookies:
			  ▽ Chocolate Chip
			  ▽ Iced Oatmeal
			  ▽ Jelly Tops
			  ▽ Macaroons
			  ▽ Oatmeal

Murray	Low Fat Cookies:
	  Ginger Snaps
	  Iced Chocolate
	  Iced Lemon
	  Iced Oatmeal		

Nabisco	Family Favorites:
	  ▽ Iced Oatmeal
	  ▽ Oatmeal Cookies
	Fat Free Newtons:
	  ▽ All Flavors
	▽ Fig Newtons
	Ginger Snaps
	SnackWell's:
	  Chocolate Sandwich Cookies
	  ▽ Cinnamon Graham Snacks
	  ▽ Creme Sandwich Cookies
	  ▽ Devil's Food Cookie Cakes
	  ▽ Double Fudge Cookie Cakes
	  ▽ Fat Free Cereal Bars
	  ▽ Oatmeal Raisin Cookies
		Bugs Bunny Graham Cookies
		Bugs Bunny Graham Snacks:
		  ▽ Chocolate
		  ▽ Cinnamon
		▽ Cameo Creme Sandwich
		Granola Bars:
		  Chips Ahoy!
		  Nutter Butter
		  Oreo
		Mystic Mint:
		  ▽ Sandwich Cookies
		▽ Nilla Wafers
		Oreo:
		  Reduced Fat
		Pecan Passion:
		  ▽ Pecan Shortbread Cookies
		Teddy Grahams:
		  Chocolate
		  Cinnamon
		  Honey
			Biscos:
			  ▽ Sugar Wafers
			Chips Ahoy!:
			  ▽ Chewy
			  ▽ Chunky
			  ▽ Mini
			  ▽ Original
			  Reduced Fat
			  ▽ Sprinkled
			  ▽ Striped
			▽ Chocolate Covered Ritz
			Cookie Break:
			  ▽ Vanilla Flavored Creme Sandwich
			Family Favorites:
			  ▽ Fudge Covered Grahams
			  ▽ Fudge Striped Shortbread
			  ▽ Vanilla Sandwich Cookies
			Famous Chocolate Wafers
			▽ Fudge Covered Oreo
			▽ Imported Danish Cookies
			▽ Lorna Doone
			▽ Marshmallow Twirls
			▽ Nutter Butter Bites

▽ Low Sodium, 140 mg. or less per serving.
☆ Good Source of Fiber, between 2.5 g. and 5 g. per serving.

BRAND	BEST CHOICE	ACCEPTABLE CHOICE	OCCASIONAL CHOICE
	Fat Free or Low Fat AND Low Saturated Fat	Contains Greater Than 3 Grams but Less Than or Equal to 5 Grams Total Fat AND Low Saturated Fat	Contains Greater Than 5 Grams Total Fat OR Greater Than 1 Gram Saturated Fat

Nabisco (Cont.)			Nutter Butter Cookies:
			    ∇ Original
			    ∇ Peanut Creme Patties
			Oreo:
			    Double Stuff
			    Original
			    ∇ White Fudge Covered
			∇ Pecan Supremes
			SnackWell's:
			    Chocolate Chip Cookies
			    ∇ Sprinkled Chips Ahoy
			T. G. Bearwich:
			    ∇ Chocolate w/Vanilla Creme
			    ∇ Cinnamon w/Vanilla Creme

Nature Valley	Low Fat Chewy Granola Bars:
	    ∇ All Flavors
			Granola Bars:
			    All Flavors

Nature's Choice	Granola Bars:
	    ∇ Carob Chip
	    ∇☆ Cinnamon and Raisin
	    ∇ Oats and Honey
	    ∇ Peanut Butter
	Real Fruit Bars:
	    ∇ Apricot
	    ∇ Cherry
	    ∇ Grape
	    ∇ Raspberry		

Nestle			Sweet Success Snack Bars: ∇☆ All Flavors

Original Lady Cookies		100% Natural:
		    ∇ Chocolate Chunk
		    ∇ Date Pecan
		    ∇ Oatmeal Raisin
			100% Natural:
			    ∇ Peanut Butter

Peek Freans	Reduced Fat:
	    Chocolate Creme
	    ∇ Creme Sandwich
		∇ Arrowroot Biscuits
		∇ Ginger Crisp Biscuits
			∇ Assorted Creme
			∇ Coffee Creme
			∇ Fruit Creme Biscuits
			∇ Nice Biscuits

∇ Low Sodium, 140 mg. or less per serving.
☆ Good Source of Fiber, between 2.5 g. and 5 g. per serving.

BRAND	BEST CHOICE	ACCEPTABLE CHOICE	OCCASIONAL CHOICE
	Fat Free or Low Fat AND Low Saturated Fat	Contains Greater Than 3 Grams but Less Than or Equal to 5 Grams Total Fat AND Low Saturated Fat	Contains Greater Than 5 Grams Total Fat OR Greater Than 1 Gram Saturated Fat
Peek Freans (Cont.)			∇ Petit Beurre Biscuits Rich Tea Biscuits ∇ Shortcake Biscuits Sweetmeal Biscuits
Pepperidge Farm	Fruitful Cookies: 　∇ Cherry Cobbler 　∇ Peach Tart 　∇ Raspberry Tart	∇ Ginger Man Cookies Santa Fe: 　∇ Oatmeal Raisin	Beacon Hill: 　∇ Chocolate Chocolate 　　Walnut ∇ Bordeaux Cookies ∇ Brussels Cookies ∇ Brussels Mint Cookies ∇ Cafe Favorites Cookie 　　Collection Charleston Milk Chocolate: 　∇ Toffee Pecan Cookies Chesapeake: 　∇ Chocolate Chunk Pecan ∇ Chessman Butter Cookies ∇ Chocolate Chip ∇ Dessert Favorites ∇ Double Chocolate Milano Fruitful Cookies: 　∇ Apricot Raspberry Cup 　∇ Strawberry Cup ∇ Geneva Cookies Goldfish Cookies: 　∇ Real Chocolate 　∇ Real Vanilla ∇ Hazelnut Milano ∇ Ice Cream Favorites ∇ Lido Cookies ∇ Milano Cookies ∇ Milk Chocolate Bordeaux ∇ Milk Chocolate Milano ∇ Mint Milano Nantucket: 　∇ Chocolate Chunk ∇ Orange Milano Cookies ∇ Party Favorites ∇ Pecan Shortbread Cookies Sausalito: 　∇ Milk Chocolate 　　Macadamia ∇ Shortbread Cookies

∇ Low Sodium, 140 mg. or less per serving.

BRAND	BEST CHOICE	ACCEPTABLE CHOICE	OCCASIONAL CHOICE
	Fat Free or Low Fat AND Low Saturated Fat	Contains Greater Than 3 Grams but Less Than or Equal to 5 Grams Total Fat AND Low Saturated Fat	Contains Greater Than 5 Grams Total Fat OR Greater Than 1 Gram Saturated Fat
Pepperidge Farm (Cont.)			Soft Baked Cookies: ∇ Caramel Pecan ∇ Chewy Brownie Walnut ∇ Chocolate Chunk ∇ Milk Chocolate Macadamia ∇ Sugar Cookies ∇ Tahoe White Chunk Macadamia
Power Bar	Power Bar: ∇☆ Apple-Cinnamon ∇☆ Malt-Nut ∇☆ Wild Berry		
Quaker	Chewy Low Fat Granola Bars: ∇ All Varieties	Chewy Granola Bars: ∇ Caramel Apple ∇ Trail Mix	Chewy Granola Bars: ∇ S'Mores
R W Frookie	Fat Free Brownies: All Flavors Fruitins: ∇ Fat Free Fig ∇ Fat Free Raspberry ∇ Fig ∇ Oatmeal Raisin	∇ 7-Grain Oatmeal ∇ Apple Cinnamon Oat Bran ∇ Chocolate Chip Fortune Cookies: ∇ All Flavors Frookwich: ∇ All Flavors ∇ Ginger Spice ∇ Mandarin Orange Chocolate Chip ∇ Mint Chocolate Chip Power Grahams: ∇ Cinnamon Cookies	Dream Creams: ∇ Strawberry ∇ Vanilla
Rippin' Good	∇ Fat Free Mini Bits Fig Bars		Cookie Stix: ∇ All Flavors ∇ Fudge Fluffs Cookies ∇ Mint Creme Cookie Patties
Royal	∇ Apple Cakes	∇ Devil's Food Cakes ∇ Raisin Cakes	∇ Brownie Rounds ∇ Chocolate Chip Cookies ∇ Granola Cookies ∇ Oatmeal Cookies
Salerno	∇ Dinosaur Grrrahams	∇ Almond Windmill Cookies ∇ Animal Crackers	∇ Alyce's Mint Creme Cookies

∇ Low Sodium, 140 mg. or less per serving.
☆ Good Source of Fiber, between 2.5 g. and 5 g. per serving.

Cookies, Bars, and Snack Cakes 133

BRAND	BEST CHOICE	ACCEPTABLE CHOICE	OCCASIONAL CHOICE
	Fat Free or Low Fat AND Low Saturated Fat	Contains Greater Than 3 Grams but Less Than or Equal to 5 Grams Total Fat AND Low Saturated Fat	Contains Greater Than 5 Grams Total Fat OR Greater Than 1 Gram Saturated Fat
Salerno (Cont.)		∇ Ginger Snaps Mini Dinosaur Grrrahams: 　∇ Cinnamon 　∇ Original ∇ Vanilla Wafers	∇ Assorted Sugar Wafers ∇ Bonnie Shortbread Cookies Butter Cookie Cremes: 　∇ Angel Creme 　∇ Chocolate Creme ∇ Butter Cookies ∇ Caramel Patties Chips Supreme Cinnamon Grahams ∇ L'il Chips ∇ Mini Butter Cookies Mini Butter Cremes: 　∇ Angel Creme 　∇ Chocolate Creme Reduced Fat Butter Cookies ∇ Royal Grahams Cookies ∇ Royal Stripes ∇ Sierra Peanut Butter Patties
Sargento			MooTown Snackers-Cookies & Creme: 　∇ Honey Graham & Vanilla Creme 　∇ Vanilla Sticks & Chocolate Creme
Stella D'oro	∇ Almond Toast ∇ Anisette Sponge Anisette Toast ∇ Breakfast Treats Fat Free Fruit Delight Cookies: 　∇ All Flavors ∇ Fat Free Fruit Slices	∇ Anginetti Golden Bars: 　∇ Low Sodium	∇ Angel Wings ∇ Biscottini Cashews ∇ Chinese Dessert Cookies ∇ Lady Stella Assortment ∇ Margherite ∇ Margherite Combination ∇ Roman Egg Biscuits ∇ Swiss Fudge Cookies
Sun Maid		∇ Raisin Oatmeal Cookies	
Sunshine	Golden Fruit: 　∇ Apple Biscuits 　∇ Cranberry Biscuits 　∇ Raisin Biscuits	∇ Animal Crackers ∇ Grahamy Bears OH! Berry: 　∇ Fudge Dipped Cookies	∇ Assorted Sugar Wafers ∇ Butter Flavored Cookies ∇ Chip-a-Roos

∇ Low Sodium, 140 mg. or less per serving.

BRAND	BEST CHOICE	ACCEPTABLE CHOICE	OCCASIONAL CHOICE
	Fat Free or Low Fat AND Low Saturated Fat	Contains Greater Than 3 Grams but Less Than or Equal to 5 Grams Total Fat AND Low Saturated Fat	Contains Greater Than 5 Grams Total Fat OR Greater Than 1 Gram Saturated Fat
Sunshine (Cont.)	OH! Berry: ∇ Fat Free Strawberry Wafers	OH! Berry: Reduced Fat Reduced Fat: ∇ Hydrox ∇ Vienna Wafers	Classics: ∇ Chocolate Chip ∇ Chocolate Chip Shortbread w/Pecans ∇ Chocolate Chip w/ Walnuts ∇ Chocolate Chocolate Chip w/Walnuts Country Style Oatmeal Cookies ∇ Fudge Dipped Graham Crackers ∇ Fudge Mint Patties ∇ Fudge Striped Shortbread ∇ Hydrox ∇ Lemon Coolers Cookies ∇ Peanut Butter Sugar Wafers ∇ Vanilla Wafers ∇ Vienna Fingers
Sweetzels	∇ Ginger Snaps		
Tastykake			Butterscotch Krimpets Creamies: ∇ All Flavors Kandy Kakes: All Flavors Tasty Too: Lemon Krimpets
Tiger's Milk	Light Bar: ∇☆ Cocoa Yogurt Fudge Tiger Crunchie Tiger Sport Bar: ∇ Chocolate ∇ Coffee		Nutrition Bar: ∇ Protein Flavor
Twix			∇ Caramel Cookie Bars ∇ Cookies-n-Creme Cookie Bars ∇ Fudge & Crunchy Cookie Bars ∇ Peanut Butter Cookie Bars
Ultra Slim Fast	∇ Chocolate Sandwich Cookies		Bars: ∇ Chewy Caramel Crunch

∇ Low Sodium, 140 mg. or less per serving.
☆ Good Source of Fiber, between 2.5 g. and 5 g. per serving.

BRAND	BEST CHOICE	ACCEPTABLE CHOICE	OCCASIONAL CHOICE
	Fat Free or Low Fat AND Low Saturated Fat	Contains Greater Than 3 Grams but Less Than or Equal to 5 Grams Total Fat AND Low Saturated Fat	Contains Greater Than 5 Grams Total Fat OR Greater Than 1 Gram Saturated Fat
Ultra Slim Fast (Cont.)	Fat Free Breakfast Bars: All Flavors ∇ Fig Cookies		Bars: ∇☆ Chocolate Chip Crunch ∇☆ Cocoa Almond Crunch ∇☆ Mint Chocolate Crunch ∇ Peanut Caramel Crunch
Vista		Double Fudge Cremes	
Voortman	∇ Oatmeal Apple	∇ Dutch Fudge Cookies ∇ Gingerboys ∇ Oatmeal Chip ∇ Windmill Cookies	∇ Almond Krunch ∇ Almonettes ∇ Chocolate Chips ∇ Peanut Delight ∇ Shortbread Cookies Wafers: ∇ All Flavors
Walkers			∇ Almond Shortbread ∇ Chocolate Chip Shortbread ∇ Chocolate Shortbread Rings ∇ Hazelnut Shortbread ∇ Shortbread Fingers ∇ Shortbread Petticoat Tails ∇ Shortbread Rounds
Weight Watchers	Smart Snackers: ∇ Fig ∇ Oatmeal Raisin Cookies ∇ Raspberry Filled ∇ Vanilla Sandwich Cookies	Smart Snackers: Chocolate Sandwich Cookies	Smart Snackers: ∇ Chocolate Chip Cookies
Westbrae Natural			Chocolate Chip Classics: ∇ Crisp Chocolate Chip ∇ Crisp Chocolate Chip Walnut ∇ Soft Chocolate Chip Coconut ∇ Soft Chocolate Chip Pecan ∇ Soft Chocolate Chocolate Chip Cookie Jar Classics: ∇ Dutch Apple Cinnamon ∇ Honey Almond ∇ Oatmeal Raisin

∇ Low Sodium, 140 mg. or less per serving.
☆ Good Source of Fiber, between 2.5 g. and 5 g. per serving.

BRAND	BEST CHOICE	ACCEPTABLE CHOICE	OCCASIONAL CHOICE
	Fat Free or Low Fat AND Low Saturated Fat	Contains Greater Than 3 Grams but Less Than or Equal to 5 Grams Total Fat AND Low Saturated Fat	Contains Greater Than 5 Grams Total Fat OR Greater Than 1 Gram Saturated Fat
Westbrae Natural (Cont.)			Cookie Jar Classics: ∇ Peanut Butter Nut ∇ Raspberry Vanilla
Wholesome Accents	Lowfat Cookies: All Varieties		
World Classics		∇ Lemon Creme Cookies	∇ Milk Chocolate Chip & Macadamia Nut Cookies ∇ Oatmeal Raisin Cookies ∇ Peanut Butter Chip & Nut Cookies
REFRIGERATED & FROZEN COOKIE DOUGH			
Nestle			Cookie Dough: ∇ Chocolate Chocolate Chip ∇ Oatmeal w/Raisinettes ∇ Sugar Cookie w/Bits of Butterfinger
Pillsbury	Teddy Bears: ∇ Brown Sugar Cookie w/ Chocolate	Cookie Dough: ∇ Skippy Peanut Butter ∇ Reduced Fat Chocolate Chip Cookie Dough	Cookie Dough: ∇ Chocolate Chip ∇ Oatmeal Chocolate Chip ∇ Sugar ∇ w/M&M's ∇ Fudge Brownie Dough
YOUR FAVORITE COOKIES, BARS, AND SNACK CAKES NOT LISTED IN THE *GUIDE*			

∇ Low Sodium, 140 mg. or less per serving.

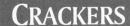

This category contains a large variety of crackers. Crackers may provide complex carbohydrates, B-vitamins, iron, and fiber to the diet. However, if not chosen carefully, these foods can also be significant contributors of fat, sodium, and excess calories. Many "snack" crackers now come in reduced-fat or fat-free varieties. Low-fat cracker choices include many brands of saltines, rye crackers, crisp breads, melba toast, and bread sticks.

Crackers are included as part of the "Bread, Cereal, Rice, and Pasta Group" and help make up the base of the *Food Guide Pyramid*. Six to eleven servings each day are recommended from this food group. Five to six small crackers are considered a serving. The FDA has established reference amounts or standardized serving sizes for use on the food label. The reference amount for crackers varies, depending on the type of cracker. For crackers that are not typically consumed as a snack, such as melba toast, or hard bread sticks, the reference amount per serving is 15 grams (1/2 ounce). On the other hand, products that are typically consumed as snacks, such as saltines or graham crackers, have a serving size of 30 grams (1 ounce). Be sure to read the *Nutrition Facts* label for the serving size information of your cracker choice. (See pages 51 and 52 for an explanation of reference amounts and the difference between serving sizes established by the FDA for food labeling and those recommended by the *Food Guide Pyramid*.)

Food choices from this category range from those that are higher in total fat, saturated fat, and sodium to those that are fat free or low in fat. The criteria were therefore designed to distinguish those crackers lower in total fat and saturated fat from their higher-fat alternatives. Those products that contain 480 milligrams sodium or more per serving (20% of the Daily Value) are considered high in sodium and are marked with a ▲ symbol.

Criteria Key

▲ **Best Choice:**   **Fat Free or Low Fat AND Low Saturated Fat**

Products listed in this category meet the FDA's definition for "Fat Free" (less than 1/2 gram fat per serving), or "Low Fat," (3 grams or less fat per serving), and "Low Saturated Fat" (1 gram or less saturated fat per serving). These crackers are the preferred choices because they are lower in fat content.

▲ **Acceptable Choice:**   **Contains Greater Than 3 Grams, but Less Than or Equal to 5 Grams Total Fat, AND Low Saturated Fat**

Products listed in this category **do not** meet the FDA's definition for "Low Fat." These crackers contain 5 or less grams of fat per serving. The 5 grams of total fat cut-off was used in order to be consistent with the amount of fat equal to one diabetes diet fat exchange and is also equivalent to 1 teaspoon of added fat.[75] These products contribute a greater amount of fat to the overall daily diet.

▲ **Occasional Choice:**   **Contains Greater Than 5 grams Total Fat, or Greater Than 1 Gram Saturated Fat**

Products listed in this category **do not** meet the FDA's definition for either "Low Fat," or "Low Saturated Fat." These products can contribute a significant amount of fat to the overall daily diet and should be consumed only on occasion.

BRAND	BEST CHOICE	ACCEPTABLE CHOICE	OCCASIONAL CHOICE
	Fat Free or Low Fat AND Low Saturated Fat	Contains Greater Than 3 Grams but Less Than or Equal to 5 Grams Total Fat AND Low Saturated Fat	Contains Greater Than 5 Grams Total Fat OR Greater Than 1 Gram Saturated Fat
Ak-Mak	☆ 100% Stone Ground Crackers		

Auburn Farms	Fat Free 7-Grainers:
	  Onion
	  Original
	  Rye
	  ∇ Veggie		

Austin			Cheese on Cheese Crackers Toasty Peanut Butter on Crackers Whole Wheat Crackers w/ Cheddar Cheese

Barbara's	Wheatines:
	  ∇ Cracked Pepper
	  ∇ Sesame		

Blue Diamond	Nut-Crackers:
	  ∇ Hazelnut
		Nut-Crackers:
		  ∇ Almond	

Bremner	Wafers:
	  Low Sodium
	  Regular		

Campbell's	∇ Soup & Oyster Crackers		

Carr's	∇ Assorted Biscuits for Cheese
	∇ Croissant Crackers
	Table Water Crackers:
	  ∇ Regular
	  ∇ w/Cracked Pepper
	  ∇ w/Sesame Seeds
		∇ Poppy & Sesame Crackers
		∇ Wheatmeal Biscuits
		∇ Whole Wheat Crackers
			∇ Cheddar Crackers

Dare			Breton:
			  ∇ Low Sodium
			  ∇ Sesame
			  ∇ Thin Wheat Cracker w/ Wheat Germ
			Caberet Crackers
			Vivant:
			  ∇ Vegetable Crackers

∇ Low Sodium, 140 mg. or less per serving.
☆ Good Source of Fiber, between 2.5 g. and 5 g. per serving.

BRAND	BEST CHOICE	ACCEPTABLE CHOICE	OCCASIONAL CHOICE
	Fat Free or Low Fat AND Low Saturated Fat	Contains Greater Than 3 Grams but Less Than or Equal to 5 Grams Total Fat AND Low Saturated Fat	Contains Greater Than 5 Grams Total Fat OR Greater Than 1 Gram Saturated Fat

Devonsheer	Fat Free Melba Rounds:
	  ∇ All Flavors
	Low Fat Melba Rounds:
	  ∇ All Flavors		

Finn Crisp	∇☆ Dark w/Caraway		

Frito Lay			Doritos:
			  ▲ Nacho Cheese Sandwich
			  Crackers

Hain	Fat Free Crackers:
	  Herb
	  ∇ Onion
	  ∇ Vegetable
	  ∇ Whole Wheat
	∇ Honey Grahams		

Health Valley	Fat Free Crackers:
	  ∇ All Flavors
	Fat Free Graham Crackers:
	  ∇☆ All Flavors		

Jacobsen's	Snack Toast:
	  ∇ Cinnamon
	  ∇ Cinnamon Raisin
	  ∇ Original		

Jardine's	∇ Cracked Pepper Crackers ∇ Garlic & Herb Crackers ∇ Sun Dried Tomato Crackers		

KA-ME	Rice Crunch Crackers:
	  Cheese
	  ∇ Onion
	  ∇ Sesame		

Kavli	Whole Grain Crispbread:
	  ∇ Crispy Thin
	  ∇☆ Hearty Thick		

▲ High Sodium, 480 mg. or greater per serving.
∇ Low Sodium, 140 mg. or less per serving.
☆ Good Source of Fiber, between 2.5 g. and 5 g. per serving.

142   **Crackers**

BRAND	BEST CHOICE	ACCEPTABLE CHOICE	OCCASIONAL CHOICE
	Fat Free or Low Fat AND Low Saturated Fat	Contains Greater Than 3 Grams but Less Than or Equal to 5 Grams Total Fat AND Low Saturated Fat	Contains Greater Than 5 Grams Total Fat OR Greater Than 1 Gram Saturated Fat

Keebler	Club Partners:
	  ∇ Garlic Bread
	  Original
	  ∇ Reduced Sodium
	  Touch of Cheddar
	Elfin Delights Low Fat:
	  ∇ Animal Crackers
	∇ Export Soda Crackers
	Graham Selects:
	  Lowfat Cinnamon Crisp
	  Lowfat Honey
	  ∇ Original
	Toasteds 50% Reduced Fat:
	  Wheat
	Townhouse:
	  50% Reduced Fat
	Zesta:
	  ∇ 50% Reduced Sodium
	  ∇ Fat Free
	  Original
		Graham Selects:
		  Apple Cinnamon
		  Cinnamon Crisp
		Munch 'ems:
		  Ranch
		  Seasoned Original
		Munch 'ems Less Fat:
		  Chili Cheese
		  Salsa
		Townhouse:
		  ∇ 50% Reduced Sodium
		  Classic Crackers
		Wheatables:
		  50% Reduced Fat
			Cracker Paks:
			  Cheese and Peanut Butter
			  Club & Cheddar
			  Graham & Chocolate Creme
			  Toast & Peanut Butter
			Graham Selects:
			  ∇ Chocolate
			  ∇ Honey
			Munch 'ems:
			  Cheddar
			  Sour Cream and Onion
			Toasteds:
			  Buttercrisp
			  Onion
			  Rye
			  Sesame
			  Wheat
			Townhouse:
			  Wheat
			Wheatables:
			  All Flavors

Kraft			Handi Snacks:
			  Cheez' n Breadsticks
			  Cheez' n Crackers
			  Cheez' n Pretzels
			  Peanut Butter' n Crackers
			  ∇ Peanut Butter' n Graham
			    Sticks

Lance	∇ Wheat Twins		Captain's Wafers:
			  with Chives
			Cheese on Wheat
			∇ Malt Crackers
			Rye Cheese Crackers
			Toastchee Crackers
			Toasty Peanut Butter
			  Crackers

Lifestream	Stoneground Wheat Crackers:
	  ☆ Garden Vegetable
	  ∇ Sesame Seed
	  ∇ Wheat & Onion		

∇ Low Sodium, 140 mg. or less per serving.
☆ Good Source of Fiber, between 2.5 g. and 5 g. per serving.

Brand	Best Choice	Acceptable Choice	Occasional Choice
	Fat Free or Low Fat AND Low Saturated Fat	Contains Greater Than 3 Grams but Less Than or Equal to 5 Grams Total Fat AND Low Saturated Fat	Contains Greater Than 5 Grams Total Fat OR Greater Than 1 Gram Saturated Fat
Little Debbie			Cheese Crackers w/Peanut Butter Toasty Crackers w/Peanut Butter Wheat Crackers w/Cheddar Cheese
Mama's	∇ Oyster Crackers		

Manischewitz	Matzo:
	  Egg and Onion
	  Savory Garlic
	  ∇ Thin Salted
	  ∇ Unsalted
	  ∇☆ Whole Wheat
			Premium Gold Matzo:
			  Lightly Salted Tops
			  Regular
			  Snack Bits
			  ∇ Unsalted Tops
			Tam Tam Crackers

Master Old Country	☆ Hardtack Crisp Rye Crackers		
Mi-Del	∇ 100% Whole Wheat Honey Grahams		
Murray	∇ Honey Grahams	∇ Cinnamon Grahams	

Nabisco	Grahams
	Honey Maid Grahams:
	  Chocolate
	  Cinnamon
	  Honey
	  ∇ Oatmeal Crunch
	Premium:
	  Soup and Oyster Crackers
	Premium Crackers:
	  ∇ Fat Free
	  ∇ Low Sodium
	  Original
	  ∇ Unsalted Tops
	Ritz Crackers:
	  ∇ Reduced Fat
	SnackWell's:
	  Cheese Crackers
	  Classic Golden Crackers
	  Cracked Pepper Crackers
	  French Onion Crackers
	  Wheat Crackers
	  Zesty Cheese Crackers
		Barnum's Animal Crackers
		Cheese Nips:
		  Reduced Fat
		Garden Crisps:
		  Vegetable
		Harvest Crisps:
		  5-Grain
		Ritz Crackers:
		  ∇ Low Sodium
		  ∇ Regular
		Sociables Savory Crackers
		Triscuit:
		  ☆ Deli-Style Rye
		  ∇☆ Garden Herb
		  ∇☆ Low Sodium
		  ☆ Original
		∇ Waverly
		Wheat Thins:
		  Multi-Grain
		  Reduced Fat
		Wheatsworth:
		  Stone Ground
			Better Cheddar:
			  ∇ Low Salt
			  Reduced Fat
			  Regular
			Cheese Nips:
			  Original
			Cheese Tid-Bits
			Chicken in a Biskit
			Doo Dads Snack Mix:
			  Original Recipe
			Nabs:
			  Cheese Cracker w/Real Peanut Butter
			  Toast Cracker w/Real Peanut Butter
			Oat Thins:
			  Toasted Snack Crackers
			Ritz Bits:
			  Regular

∇ Low Sodium, 140 mg. or less per serving.

☆ Good Source of Fiber, between 2.5 g. and 5 g. per serving.

BRAND	BEST CHOICE	ACCEPTABLE CHOICE	OCCASIONAL CHOICE
	Fat Free or Low Fat AND Low Saturated Fat	Contains Greater Than 3 Grams but Less Than or Equal to 5 Grams Total Fat AND Low Saturated Fat	Contains Greater Than 5 Grams Total Fat OR Greater Than 1 Gram Saturated Fat
Nabisco (Cont.)	Triscuit: ☆ Reduced Fat		Ritz Bits Sandwiches: ∇ Peanut Butter Real Cheese Ritz Cracker Sandwiches: with Peanut Butter with Real Cheese Snack Crackers: Bacon Snorkels Fun Crackers: Cheddar Swiss Cheese Snack Crackers Twigs: Sesame & Cheese Snack Sticks Vegetable Thins Wheat Thins: ∇ Low Sodium Original
O.T.C.	Soup, Chowder & Oyster Crackers Wine Crackers: ∇ Original		
Old London	Melba Snacks: ∇ Bacon ∇ Garlic ∇ Mexicali Corn ∇ Onion Rye ∇ Sesame ∇ White ∇ Whole Grain Melba Toast: ∇ Onion ∇ Rye ∇ Sesame ∇ Wheat ∇ White ∇ Whole Grain		
Pepperidge Farm	∇ Butter Thins	∇ Hearty Wheat Crackers	

∇ Low Sodium, 140 mg. or less per serving.
☆ Good Source of Fiber, between 2.5 g. and 5 g. per serving.

BRAND	BEST CHOICE	ACCEPTABLE CHOICE	OCCASIONAL CHOICE
	Fat Free or Low Fat AND Low Saturated Fat	Contains Greater Than 3 Grams but Less Than or Equal to 5 Grams Total Fat AND Low Saturated Fat	Contains Greater Than 5 Grams Total Fat OR Greater Than 1 Gram Saturated Fat

Pepperidge Farm (Cont.)	Goldfish:
	  Pretzel
	  ∇ Three Cracker Assortment
			Goldfish:
			  Cheddar Cheese
			  Original
			  Parmesan
			  Pizza
			  ∇ Reduced Sodium Cheddar Cheese
			Nutty Deluxe

R W Frookie	Fat Free Crackers:
	  ∇ Cracked Pepper
	  Garlic & Herb
	  ∇ Water
	  ∇ Whole Wheat
	Frook Wheats Snacker Crackers:
	  ∇ Onion Poppy		

Red Oval Farms	Entertainer:
	  ∇ Sesame Crackers
	Some of Each:
	  ∇ Assorted Crackers
	Stoned Wheat Thins:
	  Mini
	  ∇ Regular		

Ry-Krisp	∇☆ Natural Ry-Krisp Crackers		

Ryvita	Whole Grain Crisp Bread:
	  ∇☆ Tasty Dark Rye
	  ∇☆ Tasty Light Rye
	  ∇☆ Flavorful Fiber		

Salerno	∇ Fat Free Oyster Crackers
	Saltine Crackers:
	  ∇ Fat Free
	Sea Crisp Crackers:
	  ∇ Unsalted Tops
		Graham Crackers:
		  Milk & Honey
			Mini Golden Rounds:
			  Mild Cheddar
			  Regular
			Salsa Crisps

Sunshine	Krispy:
	  Cracked Pepper
	  ∇ Fat Free
	  Mild Cheddar
	  Original
		Cheez-it:
		  Reduced Fat
		Hi Ho Deluxe:
		  Reduced Fat
		  ∇ Honey Grahams
			Cheez-it:
			  Hot & Spicy Snack Crackers
			  ∇ Low Sodium
			  Regular
			  White Cheddar

∇ Low Sodium, 140 mg. or less per serving.
☆ Good Source of Fiber, between 2.5 g. and 5 g. per serving.

BRAND	BEST CHOICE	ACCEPTABLE CHOICE	OCCASIONAL CHOICE
	Fat Free or Low Fat AND Low Saturated Fat	Contains Greater Than 3 Grams but Less Than or Equal to 5 Grams Total Fat AND Low Saturated Fat	Contains Greater Than 5 Grams Total Fat OR Greater Than 1 Gram Saturated Fat

Sunshine (Cont.)	Krispy:
	    Soup & Oyster
	    ∇ Unsalted Tops
	    ∇ Whole Wheat
			Cinnamon Grahams
			Hi Ho:
			    Butter Flavor
			    Cracked Pepper
			    Multi Grain
			Hi Ho Deluxe:
			    Regular
			    Whole Wheat

Tender Toasts	∇ Garlic ∇ Sesame ∇ Wheat		
Venus	Fat Free Crackers: All Varieties		
Vista	Soup & Oyster Crackers		

Wasa	Crispbread:
	    ∇☆ Fiber Plus
	    ∇ Fruit 'N Nut
	    ∇ Golden Rye
	    ∇ Lite Rye
	    ∇☆ Sesame Rye
	    ∇ Sesame Wheat		

YOUR FAVORITE CRACKERS NOT LISTED IN THE *GUIDE*			

∇ Low Sodium, 140 mg. or less per serving.
☆ Good Source of Fiber, between 2.5 g. and 5 g. per serving.

PASTA, POTATOES, STUFFING, AND GRAINS

This category contains a wide range of products and is subdivided into four different sections: Pasta and Pasta Mixes, Stuffing Mixes and Croutons, Grain and Grain Mixes, and Potato and Potato Mixes. These foods provide complex carbohydrates to the diet and can be a good source of B-vitamins. Pasta, potatoes, and rice can be combined with smaller amounts of lean meat, fish, or poultry for a tasty main dish that can be low in fat and calories.

Depending on the type of product, foods in these categories are included either as part of the "Bread, Cereal, Rice, and Pasta Group" or the "Vegetable Group" (e.g., potato dishes are considered part of the "Vegetable Group," pasta dishes are considered part of the "Bread, Cereal, Rice, and Pasta Group"). The recommended serving sizes will vary depending on their food group classification. Six to eleven half-cup servings are recommended for those products in the "Bread, Cereal, Rice and Pasta Group," whereas three to five half-cup servings are recommended for those products in the "Vegetable Group." The FDA has established reference amounts or standardized serving sizes for use on the food label. The reference amount for foods in this category varies depending on type of product. These reference amounts range from 45 grams (1½ ounces) to 100 grams (3½ ounces) of dry product, and 140 grams (5 ounces) of prepared product. Be sure to read the *Nutrition Facts* label for the serving size information of your product choice. (See pages 51 and 52 for an explanation of reference amounts and the difference between serving sizes established by the FDA for food labeling and those recommended by the *Food Guide Pyramid*.)

This food category contains a variety of products ranging from those that have little or no fat to those made with creamy sauces. Because most of these products require the addition of other ingredients that supply added fat (e.g., milk, butter, margarine) for preparation, the fat content of these products can be significantly increased. Although many food companies give the nutritional breakdown for both the "As Packaged" and "As Prepared" versions, the "As Prepared" version

is voluntary and, therefore, may not be given for all products. Additionally, consumers may, or may not, choose to follow the specified package directions. Consumers are also at liberty to make either higher-fat or lower-fat ingredient substitutions. For this reason, the fat content of the "As Packaged" dry mix was used to evaluate these products. See Appendix D, page 373, for a listing of ingredient substitutions for lowering fat content.

Criteria were therefore designed to distinguish those products lower in total fat and saturated fat from their higher-fat alternatives. Some prepared products can also contain a substantial amount of sodium. Those products that contain 480 milligrams sodium or more per serving (20% of the Daily Value) are considered high in sodium and are marked with a ▲ symbol. *Tip: For those products that include seasoning packets, the sodium content of the finished product can be significantly lowered by adding only 1/3 to 1/2 of the packet.*

Criteria Key

▲ **Best Choice:**   **Fat Free or Low Fat AND Low Saturated Fat**

Products listed in this category meet the FDA's definition for "Fat Free" (less than 1/2 gram fat per serving), or "Low Fat" (3 grams or less fat per serving), and "Low Saturated Fat" (1 gram or less per serving).

▲ **Acceptable Choice:**   **Contains Greater Than 3 Grams but Less Than or Equal to 5 Grams Total Fat OR Contains Less Than or Equal to 5 Grams Total Fat and Greater Than 1 Gram Saturated Fat**

Products listed in this category **do not** meet the FDA's definition for "Low Fat." They may also contain 5 or less grams of fat per serving. The 5 grams of total fat cut-off was used in order to be consistent with the amount of fat equal to one diabetes diet fat exchange and is also equivalent to 1 teaspoon of added fat.[75] These products contribute a greater amount of fat or saturated fat to the overall daily diet.

▲ **Occasional Choice:**   **Contains Greater Than 5 Grams Total Fat**

Those products that contain greater than 5 grams of total fat per serving are listed in this category. These products can contribute a significant amount of fat to the overall daily diet and should be consumed only on occasion.

BRAND	BEST CHOICE	ACCEPTABLE CHOICE	OCCASIONAL CHOICE
	Fat Free or Low Fat AND Low Saturated Fat	Contains Greater Than 3 Grams But Less Than or Equal To 5 Grams Total Fat OR Contains Less Than or Equal to 5 Grams Total Fat and Greater Than 1 Gram Saturated Fat	Contains Greater Than 5 Grams Total Fat

GRAIN AND GRAIN MIXES

BRAND	BEST CHOICE	ACCEPTABLE CHOICE	OCCASIONAL CHOICE
A Taste of THAI	∇ Soft Jasmine Rice		
All Brands	∇☆ Barley ∇ Buckwheat Groats (Kasha) ∇ Bulgar Wheat ∇ Corn Grits ∇ Instant Rice ∇☆ Long Grain Brown Rice ∇ Medium Grain Brown Rice ∇ Millet ∇☆ Oats ∇ Rye ∇ Short Grain Brown Rice ∇ White Rice ∇ Wild Rice		
Bascam's	∇ Barley		

Betty Crocker	Dinner Sensations:
	  ▲ Beef Teriyaki
	  Sweet & Sour Chicken
	Hamburger Helper:
	  ▲ Mushroom and Wild Rice		

Birdseye			▲ French Style Rice
Casbah	Lentil Pilaf Mix Nutted Pilaf Mix Rice Pilaf Mix Spanish Pilaf Mix		
Fantastic Foods	Tabouli Salad Mix		
Green Giant		Rice Originals: ▲☆ White 'n Wild w/French Style Green Beans	
Kane	∇ Bean Threads		
Knorr	Basmati Rice Pilaf: Tomato & Herbs		

▲ High Sodium, 480 mg. or greater per serving.
∇ Low Sodium, 140 mg. or less per serving.
☆ Good Source of Fiber, between 2.5 g. and 5 g. per serving.

Pasta, Potatoes, Stuffings and Grains 151

BRAND	BEST CHOICE	ACCEPTABLE CHOICE	OCCASIONAL CHOICE
	Fat Free or Low Fat AND Low Saturated Fat	Contains Greater Than 3 Grams But Less Than or Equal To 5 Grams Total Fat OR Contains Less Than or Equal to 5 Grams Total Fat and Greater Than 1 Gram Saturated Fat	Contains Greater Than 5 Grams Total Fat

Knorr (Cont.)	Harvest Pilaf:
	  Rice Medley & Carrots
	Jasmine Rice Pilaf:
	  ∇ Lemon & Herbs		

La Preferida	∇ Extra Long Grain Enriched Rice		
Lawry's	Chicken 'n Rice: Fajitas Flavor ▲ Nacho Rice ▲★ Santa Fe Rice		

Lipton	Rice and Sauce:
	  ▲☆ Cajun Style
	  ▲ Cheddar Broccoli Chicken
	  ▲ Chicken Broccoli
	  ▲ Mushroom
	  ▲ Original Long Grain and Wild Rice
	  ▲ Rice Medley
	  ▲ Spanish
		Golden Saute:
		  ▲ Chicken
		  ▲ Chicken & Broccoli
		  ▲ Oriental
		  ▲ Savory Herb Pilaf w/ Garlic
		  ▲ Spanish Fiesta
		Rice and Sauce:
		  ▲ Alfredo Broccoli
			Rice and Sauce:
			  ▲ Creamy Chicken

Lundberg	One Step Entree:
	  ★ Chili
	  ★ Curry
	  ▲★ Garlic Basil		

Luzianne	▲ Etouffee Dinner ▲ Gumbo Dinner ▲ Jambalaya Dinner ▲ Shrimp Creole Dinner		
Mahatma	∇ Extra Long Grain Enriched Rice ▲★ Red Beans w/Rice ▲ Saffron Yellow Rice ▲ Wild Rice w/Seasonings		

▲ High Sodium, 480 mg. or greater per serving.
∇ Low Sodium, 140 mg. or less per serving.
☆ Good Source of Fiber, between 2.5 g. and 5 g. per serving.
★ High Fiber, 5 g. or greater per serving.

BRAND	BEST CHOICE	ACCEPTABLE CHOICE	OCCASIONAL CHOICE
	Fat Free or Low Fat AND Low Saturated Fat	Contains Greater Than 3 Grams But Less Than or Equal To 5 Grams Total Fat OR Contains Less Than or Equal to 5 Grams Total Fat and Greater Than 1 Gram Saturated Fat	Contains Greater Than 5 Grams Total Fat
Marrakesh Express	Cous Cous: ▽ Lentil Curry ▽ Wild Mushroom		
Minute	Boil-in-Bag: ▽ Long Grain Rice ▽ Instant Whole Grain Brown Rice ▽ Minute Original Rice ▽ Premium Long Grain Rice		
Near East	▲ Curry Rice Mix ▲ Long Grain and Wild Rice Pilaf Mix: ☆ Barley ▲★ Garden Vegetable Bean & Rice ▲★ Lentil ▲☆ Red Beans & Rice ▲ Regular ▲★ Tomato Herb Bean & Rice ▲☆ Wheat ▲ Spanish Rice Mix ☆ Taboule Wheat Salad Mix		
Nishiki	Sushi Rice: ▽ Medium Grain		
Quaker	▽ Quick Barley		
Rice-A-Roni	⅓ Less Salt: ▲ Beef ▲ Chicken ▲ Fried Rice ▲ Beef ▲ Chicken ▲ Chicken & Broccoli ▲ Fried Rice ▲ Long Grain and Wild Rice ▲ Rice Pilaf	⅓ Less Salt: ▲ Broccoli Au Gratin ▲ White Cheddar & Herbs	▲ Broccoli Au Gratin Savory Classics: ▲ Broccoli au Gratin

▲ High Sodium, 480 mg. or greater per serving.
▽ Low Sodium, 140 mg. or less per serving.
☆ Good Source of Fiber, between 2.5 g. and 5 g. per serving.
★ High Fiber, 5 g. or greater per serving.

BRAND	BEST CHOICE	ACCEPTABLE CHOICE	OCCASIONAL CHOICE
	Fat Free or Low Fat AND Low Saturated Fat	Contains Greater Than 3 Grams But Less Than or Equal To 5 Grams Total Fat OR Contains Less Than or Equal to 5 Grams Total Fat and Greater Than 1 Gram Saturated Fat	Contains Greater Than 5 Grams Total Fat
Rice-A-Roni (Cont.)	Savory Classics: ▲ Almond Chicken and Wild Rice ▲ Oriental Stir Fry ▲ Spanish Rice		
Riceland	∇ Extra Long Grain Enriched Rice		
RiceSelect	∇ Texmati Brown Rice ∇ Texmati Rice		
Sapporo			Ichiban: ▲★ All Flavors
Success	∇ Brown Rice ∇ Natural Long Grain Rice		
Uncle Ben's	Brown & Wild Rice: Mushroom ∇ Brown Rice Converted Rice: ∇ Boil-in-Bag ∇ Original Long Grain ∇ Instant Brown Rice ∇ Instant Rice Long Grain & Wild Rice: Chicken Stock Sauce w/ Vegetables ▲ Fast Cooking Recipe ▲ Garden Vegetable ▲ Original Recipe Specialty Blends: ∇ Rice Trio ∇ Wild Blend	Country Inn Recipes: ▲ Broccoli & White Cheddar ▲ Broccoli Rice Au Gratin ▲ Creamy Mushroom & Wild Rice ▲ Green Bean Almondine ▲ Herbed Rice au Gratin	Country Inn Recipes: ▲ Chicken & Broccoli ▲ Chicken & Vegetables Country Inn Rice: ▲ Homestyle Chicken & Vegetable
Valsugana	∇★ Instant Polenta		
Van Camp's	▲ Spanish Rice		
Vigo	Mexican Style Rice Dinner: ▲ Chicken		

▲ High Sodium, 480 mg. or greater per serving.
∇ Low Sodium, 140 mg. or less per serving.
★ High Fiber, 5 g. or greater per serving.

154   **Pasta, Potatoes, Stuffings and Grains**

BRAND	BEST CHOICE	ACCEPTABLE CHOICE	OCCASIONAL CHOICE
	Fat Free or Low Fat AND Low Saturated Fat	Contains Greater Than 3 Grams But Less Than or Equal To 5 Grams Total Fat OR Contains Less Than or Equal to 5 Grams Total Fat and Greater Than 1 Gram Saturated Fat	Contains Greater Than 5 Grams Total Fat
Watermaid	∇ Enriched Rice		
Wolff's	Kasha, Roasted Buckwheat: ∇ All Flavors		
PASTA AND PASTA MIXES			
Al Dente	Pasta: ∇ All Varieties Pasta & Sauce: Garlic Herb Spring Pesto	Pasta & Sauce: Alfredo Sauce	
All Brands	∇ Couscous ∇ Egg Noodles ∇ Lasagna ∇ Linguini ∇ Macaroni ∇ Mostaccioli ∇ Rigatoni ∇ Shells ∇ Spaghetti ∇ Torroncini ∇ Vermicelli Whole Wheat: ∇★ Lasagna ∇★ Macaroni ∇★ Spaghetti ∇ Ziti		
American Beauty	Pasta: ∇ All Varieties		
Ancient Harvest	∇☆ Quinoa Pasta		
Annie's		Cheddar Shells	
Antoine's	∇ Fettucini ∇ Fettucini w/Herbs		

∇ Low Sodium, 140 mg. or less per serving.

☆ Good Source of Fiber, between 2.5 g. and 5 g. per serving.

★ High Fiber, 5 g. or greater per serving.

Pasta, Potatoes, Stuffings and Grains 155

BRAND	BEST CHOICE	ACCEPTABLE CHOICE	OCCASIONAL CHOICE
	Fat Free or Low Fat AND Low Saturated Fat	Contains Greater Than 3 Grams But Less Than or Equal To 5 Grams Total Fat OR Contains Less Than or Equal to 5 Grams Total Fat and Greater Than 1 Gram Saturated Fat	Contains Greater Than 5 Grams Total Fat
Antoine's (Cont.)	∇ Fusilli Tricolore ∇ Gemelli ∇ Penne Rigote ∇ Radiatore Tricolore ∇ Radiatore ∇ Spicy Spirals		
BellaVie	Organic Pasta		
Betty Crocker	Hamburger Helper: ▲ Beef Noodle ▲ Beef Taco ▲ Cheesy Italian ▲ Chili Macaroni ▲ Homestyle Beef Stew ▲ Homestyle Italian Rigatoni ▲ Homestyle Salisbury ▲ Italian Rigatoni ▲ Lasagne ▲ Pizza Pasta ▲ Stroganoff ▲ Zesty Italian Suddenly Salad: Creamy Macaroni Tuna Helper: Tuna Salad	Hamburger Helper: ▲ Cheeseburger Macaroni ▲ Fettucini Alfredo Tuna Helper: ▲ Cheesy Noodles ▲ Creamy Broccoli ▲ Fettuccine Alfredo ▲ Garden Cheddar ▲ Tetrazzini	Dinner Sensations: ▲ Chicken Alfredo Hamburger Helper: ▲ Swedish Meatballs Tuna Helper: ▲ Creamy Noodles
Borden	Red Cross Pasta: ∇ All Varieties		
Casbah	Couscous Pilaf Mix		
Cortiella	Pasta: ∇ All Varieties		
Creamette	Pasta: ∇ All Varieties		

▲ High Sodium, 480 mg. or greater per serving.
∇ Low Sodium, 140 mg. or less per serving.

BRAND	BEST CHOICE	ACCEPTABLE CHOICE	OCCASIONAL CHOICE
	Fat Free or Low Fat AND Low Saturated Fat	Contains Greater Than 3 Grams But Less Than or Equal To 5 Grams Total Fat OR Contains Less Than or Equal to 5 Grams Total Fat and Greater Than 1 Gram Saturated Fat	Contains Greater Than 5 Grams Total Fat
DaVinci	Pasta: ▽ All Varieties	Tortellini: ▲ Multi-Color w/Parmesan Cheese Ravioletti ▲ Spinach ▲ w/Parmesan Cheese	
DeBole's	▽ Eggless Pasta Noodles Flavored Pasta: ▽ All Varieties ▽★ Whole Wheat Pasta		
DeCecco	Enriched Macaroni Products: ▽ All Shapes		
Dell' Alpe	Fine Italian Foods: ▽ All Flavors		
Delverde	Pasta: ▽ All Varieties		
Dino & David	Semolina Pasta: ▽ All Varieties		
Fantastic Foods	▽☆ Couscous Macaroni & Cheese: ▲★ Traditional Cheddar ▽★ Whole Wheat Couscous		
Ferrara	Pasta: ▽ All Shapes		
Golden Grain	Macaroni & Cheese: ▲ Cheddar		
Herb's	Pasta: ▽ All Varieties		
Hodgson Mill	▽ Veggie Bows		

▲ High Sodium, 480 mg. or greater per serving.
▽ Low Sodium, 140 mg. or less per serving.
☆ Good Source of Fiber, between 2.5 g. and 5 g. per serving.
★ High Fiber, 5 g. or greater per serving.

BRAND	BEST CHOICE	ACCEPTABLE CHOICE	OCCASIONAL CHOICE
	Fat Free or Low Fat AND Low Saturated Fat	Contains Greater Than 3 Grams But Less Than or Equal To 5 Grams Total Fat OR Contains Less Than or Equal to 5 Grams Total Fat and Greater Than 1 Gram Saturated Fat	Contains Greater Than 5 Grams Total Fat

Hodgson Mill (Cont.)	Whole Wheat:
	  ∇☆ Egg Noodles
	  ∇★ Fettuccine
	  ∇★ Lasagna
	  ∇★ Spaghetti
	  ∇★ Spinach Spaghetti
	  ∇★ Spirals		

Kaboodles	∇ Egg Noodles		

Kraft	Light Pasta Salad:
	  ▲ Italian
	Macaroni & Cheese:
	  ▲ Family Size
	  ▲ Mild White Cheddar
	  ▲ Original
	Macaroni & Cheese Dinner:
	  ▲ Premium Thick'n Creamy
	Spaghetti Dinner:
	  ▲ Tangy Italian
		Egg Noodle Dinner:
		  ▲ Cheddar Cheese
		  ▲ Chicken
		Macaroni & Cheese:
		  ▲ Dinosaurs
		  ▲ Spirals
		  ▲ Super Mario
		  ▲ The Flintstones
			Rotini & Cheese:
			  ▲ Broccoli
			Shells & Cheese:
			  ▲ Bacon
			Velveeta Rotini & Cheese:
			  ▲ Broccoli
			Velveeta Shells & Cheese:
			  ▲ Original
			  ▲ Salsa

La Rosa	Pasta: ∇ All Shapes		
Light n' Fluffy	Egg Noodles: ∇ Extra Wide		
Liguori	Macaroni Products: ∇ All Varieties		

Lipton	Golden Saute:
	  ▲ Penne Pasta Chicken Stir Fry
	Golden Saute Angel Hair Pasta:
	  ▲ Chicken/Broccoli
	Noodles and Sauce:
	  ▲☆ Chicken Broccoli
		Golden Saute Rotini Pasta:
		  ▲☆ Chicken Herb Parmesan
		Noodles and Sauce:
		  ▲☆ Beef Flavor
		  ▲ Chicken
		  ▲ Mild Cheddar Bacon
		  ▲ Stroganoff
		Pasta & Sauce:
		  ▲ 3 Cheese Rotini
		  ▲☆ Rotini Primavera
			Golden Saute Angel Hair Pasta:
			  ▲ Parmesan
			Noodles and Sauce:
			  ▲ Alfredo
			  ▲ Butter
			  ▲ Creamy Chicken
			  ▲ Parmesan
			  ▲ Romanoff
			  ▲ Sour Cream and Chives
			Pasta & Sauce:
			  ▲ Cheddar Broccoli

▲ High Sodium, 480 mg. or greater per serving.
∇ Low Sodium, 140 mg. or less per serving.
☆ Good Source of Fiber, between 2.5 g. and 5 g. per serving.
★ High Fiber, 5 g. or greater per serving.

BRAND	BEST CHOICE	ACCEPTABLE CHOICE	OCCASIONAL CHOICE
	Fat Free or Low Fat AND Low Saturated Fat	Contains Greater Than 3 Grams But Less Than or Equal To 5 Grams Total Fat OR Contains Less Than or Equal to 5 Grams Total Fat and Greater Than 1 Gram Saturated Fat	Contains Greater Than 5 Grams Total Fat
Maggi	Spaetzle		
Manischewitz	Passover Gold: ∇ Egg Noodles ∇ Yolk-Free Noodle-Style Pasta		
Mendocino Pasta Co.	Pasta: ∇★ All Flavors		
Mom's Choice	▲ Lasagna Dinner	▲ Cheeseburger Macaroni Dinner ▲ Stroganoff Dinner	
Mrs. Weiss	Kluski: ∇ Enriched Egg Noodles		
Mueller's	Yolk Free Noodles: ∇ All Varieties Egg Noodles: ∇ All Varieties Macaroni: ∇ All Varieties		
Near East	∇ Couscous Moroccan Pasta		
New Mill	Kluski		
No Yolks	∇☆ Cholesterol Free Egg Noodle Substitute		
Pasta DeFino	∇ No Boil Lasagna		
Pasta LaBella	Pasta: ∇ All Varieties		
Prince	Egg Noodles: ∇ All Varieties Macaroni Products: ∇ All Varieties		

▲ High Sodium, 480 mg. or greater per serving.
∇ Low Sodium, 140 mg. or less per serving.
☆ Good Source of Fiber, between 2.5 g. and 5 g. per serving.
★ High Fiber, 5 g. or greater per serving.

Pasta, Potatoes, Stuffings and Grains 159

BRAND	BEST CHOICE	ACCEPTABLE CHOICE	OCCASIONAL CHOICE
	Fat Free or Low Fat AND Low Saturated Fat	Contains Greater Than 3 Grams But Less Than or Equal To 5 Grams Total Fat OR Contains Less Than or Equal to 5 Grams Total Fat and Greater Than 1 Gram Saturated Fat	Contains Greater Than 5 Grams Total Fat
Pritikin	∇ Whole Wheat Spaghetti		
Racconto	Pasta: ∇ All Varieties		

Rice-A-Roni	Fast Cook:
	    ▲ Broccoli Cheese
	    ▲ Chicken
	    ▲ Oriental Style
	▲ Macaroni & Cheddar
	Pasta Roni:
	    ▲☆ Linguine Pasta w/
	        Chicken & Broccoli
		Pasta Roni:
		    ▲ Angel Hair Pasta w/
		        Parmesan Cheese
		    ▲ Corkscrew Pasta w/
		        Creamy Garlic Sauce
		    ▲ Corkscrew Pasta w/
		        Four Cheese Sauce
		    ▲ Fettuccine Pasta w/
		        Mild Cheddar
		    ▲☆ Linguine w/Creamy
		        Chicken Parmesan
		    ▲☆ Tender Thin Pasta w/
		        Broccoli & Mushroom
		    ▲ Tender Thin Pasta w/
		        Parmesano
			Pasta Roni:
			    ▲ Fettuccine Pasta w/
			        Alfredo
			    ▲ Fettuccine Pasta w/
			        Stroganoff Sauce
			    ▲ Pasta Shells w/White
			        Cheddar Sauce
			    ▲ Rigatoni Pasta w/White
			        Cheddar & Broccoli Sauce

Romance	Pasta:
	    ∇ Linguine
			Pasta:
			    ▲ Meat Ravioli

Ronzoni	Enriched Macaroni Products: ∇ All Varieties		
San Giorgio	Pasta: ∇ All Varieties		
Silver Award	Pasta: ∇ All Varieties		

Terrazza	Florentine Red Beans &
	    Fusilli
	∇ Napoli Mixed Beans &
	    Radiatore
	Tuscan White Beans & Gemilli
		∇☆ Sicilian Red Lentils &
		    Bow Ties	

▲ High Sodium, 480 mg. or greater per serving.
∇ Low Sodium, 140 mg. or less per serving.
☆ Good Source of Fiber, between 2.5 g. and 5 g. per serving.

160   **Pasta, Potatoes, Stuffings and Grains**

BRAND	BEST CHOICE	ACCEPTABLE CHOICE	OCCASIONAL CHOICE
	Fat Free or Low Fat AND Low Saturated Fat	Contains Greater Than 3 Grams But Less Than or Equal To 5 Grams Total Fat OR Contains Less Than or Equal to 5 Grams Total Fat and Greater Than 1 Gram Saturated Fat	Contains Greater Than 5 Grams Total Fat
Wacky Mac	▽ Wacky Mac		
Westbrae Natural	Pasta: ▽ All Shapes		
POTATO AND POTATO MIXES			

Betty Crocker	▲ Au Gratin Potatoes
	Cheddar Classics:
	  ▲ Cheddar & Bacon
	    Potatoes
	  ▲ Cheddar & Sour Cream
	  ▲ Three Cheese Potatoes
	  ▲ White Cheddar Potatoes
	Hamburger Helper:
	  ▲ Potato Stroganoff
	▽ Hash Brown Potatoes
	▲ Julienne Potatoes
	Potato Buds:
	  ▲ Cheddar Cheese
	  ▽ Real Mashed Potatoes
	Potato Shakers:
	  ▲ Original Seasoned
	  ▲ Parmesan & Herb
	  ▲ Zesty Cheddar
	Potatoes Express:
	  ▲ Broccoli Au Gratin
	▲ Scalloped Potatoes
	Skin-On Homestyle Potatoes:
	  ▲ American Cheese
	  ▲ Broccoli Au Gratin
	  Cheddar Cheese
	  ▲ Cheesy Scalloped
	▲ Smokey Cheddar Flavored
	    Potatoes
	▲ Sour Cream 'n Chive
	    Potatoes
	Twice Baked Potatoes:
	  ▲ Bacon and Cheddar
		Potato Buds:
		  Sour Cream 'N Chives	

Cavendish			Hash Brown Patties

▲ High Sodium, 480 mg. or greater per serving.
▽ Low Sodium, 140 mg. or less per serving.

BRAND	BEST CHOICE	ACCEPTABLE CHOICE	OCCASIONAL CHOICE
	Fat Free or Low Fat AND Low Saturated Fat	Contains Greater Than 3 Grams But Less Than or Equal To 5 Grams Total Fat OR Contains Less Than or Equal to 5 Grams Total Fat and Greater Than 1 Gram Saturated Fat	Contains Greater Than 5 Grams Total Fat
Hormel			Scalloped Potatoes: ▲★ Flavored w/Ham
Idaho	▽ Idaho Spuds Mashed Potatoes		
Idahoan	Complete Mashed Potatoes Real Mashed Potatoes ☆ Scalloped Potatoes ☆ Western Style Potatoes		
Martha White	Spud Flakes: ▽ Instant Mashed Potatoes		
Panni	Potato Dumpling Mix: Shredded		
Pillsbury	Hungry Jack: ▲ Au Gratin Potatoes ▲ Cheesy Scalloped Potatoes ▽ Mashed Potatoes ▽ Mashed Potatoes Cheese ▽ Mashed Potatoes Parsley Butter ▽ Mashed Potatoes Sour Cream 'n Chives Potato Pancake Mix ▽ Sour Cream & Chives Potatoes		
Read	German Potato Salad		
STUFFING MIXES AND CROUTONS			
Arnold	Bread Crumbs: Italian ▽ Plain ▽ Corn Stuffing Crispy Croutons: Italian	▲ Cornbread Stuffing	

▲ High Sodium, 480 mg. or greater per serving.
▽ Low Sodium, 140 mg. or less per serving.
☆ Good Source of Fiber, between 2.5 g. and 5 g. per serving.
★ High Fiber, 5 g. or greater per serving.

162   **Pasta, Potatoes, Stuffings and Grains**

BRAND	BEST CHOICE	ACCEPTABLE CHOICE	OCCASIONAL CHOICE
	Fat Free or Low Fat AND Low Saturated Fat	Contains Greater Than 3 Grams But Less Than or Equal To 5 Grams Total Fat OR Contains Less Than or Equal to 5 Grams Total Fat and Greater Than 1 Gram Saturated Fat	Contains Greater Than 5 Grams Total Fat

Arnold (Cont.)	Crispy Croutons:
	  ∇ Onion & Garlic
	  ∇ Ranch
	Croutons:
	  ∇ Cheese Garlic Crispy
	  ∇ Fine Herb Crispy
	Stuffing:
	  ▲☆ Herb		

Brownberry	Bread Cubes:
	  ▲☆ Unseasoned Toasted
	  ▲☆ Sage and Onion Stuffing
	Stuffing:
	  ▲☆ Traditional Herb
	      Season		

Chatham Village	Croutons:
	  ∇ Caesar
	  ∇ Garlic & Butter
	  ∇ Lightly Seasoned		

Kellogg's	Croutettes: Stuffing Mix		

Kitchen Cupboard	Croutons:
	  ∇ Seasoned
	Toasted Croutons:
	  ∇ Unseasoned		

Koepplinger's	Stuffing Mixes:
	  Herb
	  Sage & Onion
	  Seasoned Croutons		

Marie Callender's	Croutons: ∇ All Varieties		
Nature's Harvest	Stuffing Croutons: ∇ All Varieties		
Old London	Restaurant Style Croutons: ∇ Seasoned Sourdough		

▲ High Sodium, 480 mg. or greater per serving.
∇ Low Sodium, 140 mg. or less per serving.
☆ Good Source of Fiber, between 2.5 g. and 5 g. per serving.

BRAND	BEST CHOICE	ACCEPTABLE CHOICE	OCCASIONAL CHOICE
	Fat Free or Low Fat AND Low Saturated Fat	Contains Greater Than 3 Grams But Less Than or Equal To 5 Grams Total Fat OR Contains Less Than or Equal to 5 Grams Total Fat and Greater Than 1 Gram Saturated Fat	Contains Greater Than 5 Grams Total Fat

Oven Fresh	Bread Crumbs:
	  Plain
	  ▲ Seasoned		

Pepperidge Farm	Distinctive Stuffing:
	  Apple & Raisin
	Stuffing:
	  ▲ Corn Bread
	  Cubed Country Style
	  ▲ Cubed Herb Seasoned
	  ▲☆ Herb Seasoned
	Stuffing For Poultry:
	  ▲ Sage & Onion
		Distinctive Stuffing:
		  Country Garden Herb
		  Honey Pecan Corn Bread	

Progresso	Bread Crumbs:
	  Italian Style
	  Plain		

Quality Hearth	Corn Bread Crumb Style Stuffing Seasoned Cube Style Stuffing Traditional Cube Style Stuffing		

Reese	Croutons:
	  ▽ Caesar Salad
	  ▽ Seasoned		

Rothbury Farms	Croutons: ▽ Cheese & Garlic		

Special Edition	Salad Nuggets:
	  ▽ Garlic 'N Cheese
	  ▽ Regular		

Stove Top	Lower Sodium Stuffing Mix:
	  Chicken Flavor
	Microwave Stuffing Mix:
	  ▲ Homestyle Cornbread
	Stuffing Mix:
	  Chicken Flavor
	  ▲ Corn Bread
		Microwave Stuffing Mix:
		  Chicken Flavor	

▲ High Sodium, 480 mg. or greater per serving.
▽ Low Sodium, 140 mg. or less per serving.
☆ Good Source of Fiber, between 2.5 g. and 5 g. per serving.

BRAND	BEST CHOICE	ACCEPTABLE CHOICE	OCCASIONAL CHOICE
	Fat Free or Low Fat AND Low Saturated Fat	Contains Greater Than 3 Grams But Less Than or Equal To 5 Grams Total Fat OR Contains Less Than or Equal to 5 Grams Total Fat and Greater Than 1 Gram Saturated Fat	Contains Greater Than 5 Grams Total Fat
Stove Top (Cont.)	Stuffing Mix: ▲ for Beef ▲ for Pork ▲ for Turkey Homestyle Herb ▲ Long Grain and Wild Rice Mushroom & Onion Flavor ▲ San Francisco Style ▲ Savory Herbs Stuffing Mix, Flexible Serving: Chicken Flavor Stuffing Mix, Twin Pack: Chicken Flavor		
Wonder	Crouton & Stuffing Mix: Seasoned		
YOUR FAVORITE PRODUCTS NOT LISTED IN THE *GUIDE*			

▲ High Sodium, 480 mg. or greater per serving.

Pasta, Potatoes, Stuffings and Grains   165

VEGETABLES

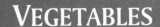

This food category contains a wide range of vegetable products that are either fresh, frozen, canned, or dried and have been subdivided into those classifications. Vegetables are major sources of vitamin C, vitamin E, beta-carotene, folate, other vitamins, minerals, and dietary fiber. They are cholesterol-free and are generally low in fat. A diet rich in fruits and vegetables is recommended by most health authorities because of its link to good health.

The *Food Guide Pyramid* suggests 3 to 5 servings of vegetables a day. One serving counts as 1 cup raw leafy vegetables, $1/2$ cup cooked, chopped, or raw vegetables, or $3/4$ cup vegetable juice. The FDA has established reference amounts or standardized serving sizes for use on the food label. The reference amounts for vegetables vary depending on type of processing. These reference amounts range from 85 grams (3 ounces) for fresh or frozen to 130 grams ($4^1/2$ ounces) for canned in liquid. Be sure to read the *Nutrition Facts* label for the serving size information of your vegetable choice. (See pages 51 and 52 for an explanation of reference amounts and the difference between serving sizes established by the FDA for food labeling and those recommended by the *Food Guide Pyramid*.)

At this time, nutrition information labeling is voluntary for fresh vegetables. As part of the FDA's voluntary point-of-purchase program, many supermarkets will display posters in the produce section detailing the nutrition content of the 20 most frequently eaten fresh vegetables. Free nutrition information pamphlets may also be available for the consumer.

This food category contains a variety of products ranging from those that have little or no fat or sodium to those prepared with buttery or creamy sauces or added salt. Criteria were therefore designed to distinguish those products lower in total fat, saturated fat, and sodium.

Criteria Key

▲ Best Choice: Fat Free or Low Fat, AND Low Saturated Fat, AND Less Than 480 mg Sodium

Products listed in this category meet the FDA definition for "Fat Free" (less than $1/2$ gram fat per serving), or "Low Fat" (3 grams or less fat per serving), and "Low Saturated Fat" (1 gram or less saturated fat per serving). These products contain less than 480 milligrams sodium per serving (less than 20% of the Daily Value).

▲ Acceptable Choice: Low Fat

Products listed in this category meet the FDA definition for "Low Fat."

▲ Occasional Choice: Contains Greater Than 3 Grams Total Fat

Vegetable products listed in this category **do not** meet the FDA's criteria for "Low Fat."

BRAND	BEST CHOICE	ACCEPTABLE CHOICE	OCCASIONAL CHOICE
	Fat Free or Low Fat AND Low Saturated Fat AND Less Than 480 mg. Sodium	Low Fat	Contains Greater Than 3 Grams Total Fat
	FRESH		

Dole	▽ Classic Salad
	Low Fat Complete Salads:
	  Herb Ranch
	  Raspberry Romaine
	  Tangy French
	Special Blend Salads:
	  ▽ California Blend
	  ▽ French Blend
	  ▽ Italian Blend
	  ▽ Romaine
			Complete Salads:
			  ▲ Caesar
			  Oriental
			  ▲☆ Spinach Bacon

Fresh	▽ Alfalfa Sprouts
	▽★ Artichoke
	▽ Asparagus
	▽ Bamboo Shoots
	▽ Bean Sprouts
	▽ Beets
	Bell Peppers:
	  ▽ All Varieties
	▽☆ Brocco-flower
	▽☆ Broccoli
	▽☆ Brussels Sprouts
	Cabbage:
	  ▽☆ All Varieties
	▽ Carrots
	▽ Cauliflower
	▽ Celery
	▽ Cherry Tomatoes
	▽ Collards
	Corn:
	  ▽☆ All Varieties
	▽ Cucumber
	▽ Eggplant
	▽ Endive
	▽ Fennel
	▽☆ Green Bean (snap)
	▽ Green Onion
	▽ Iceberg Lettuce
	▽ Jicama
	Kale:
	  ▽☆ All Varieties
	▽ Kohlrabi
	▽ Leaf Lettuce
	▽ Leeks		

▲ High Sodium, 480 mg. or greater per serving.
▽ Low Sodium, 140 mg. or less per serving.
☆ Good Source of Fiber, between 2.5 g. and 5 g. per serving.
★ High Fiber, 5 g. or greater per serving.

Vegetables 169

BRAND	BEST CHOICE Fat Free or Low Fat AND Low Saturated Fat AND Less Than 480 mg. Sodium	ACCEPTABLE CHOICE Low Fat	OCCASIONAL CHOICE Contains Greater Than 3 Grams Total Fat

Fresh (Cont.)	Mushrooms:
	  ∇ All Varieties
	∇ Mustard Greens
	Onion:
	  ∇☆ All Varieties
	Potato w/Skin:
	  ∇☆ All Varieties
	∇ Pumpkin
	∇ Radish
	∇ Rutabaga
	Squash:
	  ∇ All Varieties
	∇☆ Sweet Potato
	∇ Swiss Chard
	∇ Tomato
	∇ Turnip
	∇ Turnip Greens
	∇ Yam		

Mann's	∇☆ Broccoli Cole Slaw Sunny Shores: ∇☆ Vegetable Medley		
Pearson	∇ Cole Slaw Salad Mix		
Saco			Easy Ceasar Salad Kit Sassy Spinach
FROZEN			
Act II			∇★ Microwave French Fries
Basic Country Goodness	∇ Shredded Hashbrowns		

Birdseye	∇ Cut Green Beans
	Deluxe Vegetables:
	  ∇ "Sugar Snap" Peas
	  ∇★ Tender Tiny Peas
	Farm Fresh Mixtures:
	  ∇ Broccoli, Carrots and
	    Water Chestnuts
	  ∇☆ Broccoli, Cauliflower
	    and Carrots
	  ∇☆ Broccoli, Corn and
	    Red Peppers
		Broccoli w/Cheese Sauce
		International Recipe:
		  ▲ Stir-fry Chinese Style
			Easy Recipe:
			  ▲ Vegetable, Herb Sauce, &
			    Pasta for Chicken
			    Primavera
			  ▲☆ French Green Beans
			    w/Almonds
			International Recipe:
			  Bavarian Style Vegetables
			  ☆ New England Style
			    Vegetables
			  ▲ Rice & Broccoli Au Gratin

▲ High Sodium, 480 mg. or greater per serving.
∇ Low Sodium, 140 mg. or less per serving.
☆ Good Source of Fiber, between 2.5 g. and 5 g. per serving.
★ High Fiber, 5 g. or greater per serving.

BRAND	BEST CHOICE	ACCEPTABLE CHOICE	OCCASIONAL CHOICE
	Fat Free or Low Fat AND Low Saturated Fat AND Less Than 480 mg. Sodium	Low Fat	Contains Greater Than 3 Grams Total Fat
Birdseye (Cont.)	Farm Fresh Mixtures: ∇ Broccoli, Green Beans, Pearl Onions and Red Peppers ∇☆ Brussel Sprouts, Cauliflower & Carrots ∇ Cauliflower Nuggets, Carrots & Snow Peas ∇☆ Mixed Vegetables ★ Peas and Pearl Onions Peas and Potatoes w/Cream Sauce ∇ Sweet Corn		
Borden			∇ Cottage Fries

Freshlike	∇ Baby Vegetable Blend
	∇ Broccoli Cuts
	∇ Broccoli Stir Fry
	∇☆ Brussel Sprouts
	∇ California Blend
	∇ Classic Blend
	∇ Corn on the Cob
	∇ Cut Golden Corn
	∇ Cut Green Beans
	∇ Cut Leaf Spinach
	∇☆ Green Peas
	∇ Midwestern Blend
	∇ Mixed Vegetables
	∇ Oriental Blend
	∇ Pepper Stir Fry
	Select:
	  ∇ Cut Asparagus
	∇ Sliced Carrots
	∇ Sugar Snap Stir Fry
	∇ Summer Blend
	Sweet Corn:
	  ∇ Regular		

Green Giant	American Mixtures: ∇ California Style Broccoli Spears in Butter Sauce Cut Leaf Spinach in Butter Sauce ∇ Extra Sweet Niblets Corn	▲ Broccoli in Cheese Flavored Sauce ▲ Broccoli, Cauliflower and Carrots in Cheese Flavored Sauce ▲ Cauliflower in Cheese Flavored Sauce	

▲ High Sodium, 480 mg. or greater per serving.
∇ Low Sodium, 140 mg. or less per serving.
☆ Good Source of Fiber, between 2.5 g. and 5 g. per serving.
★ High Fiber, 5 g. or greater per serving.

Vegetables 171

BRAND	BEST CHOICE	ACCEPTABLE CHOICE	OCCASIONAL CHOICE
	Fat Free or Low Fat AND Low Saturated Fat AND Less Than 480 mg. Sodium	Low Fat	Contains Greater Than 3 Grams Total Fat
Green Giant (Cont.)	Family Size: 　▽ Niblets Corn Harvest Fresh: 　Cut Broccoli 　▽ Cut Green Beans 　▽☆ Niblets Corn Heartland Style: 　▽☆ Broccoli Cauliflower & Carrots Microwave: 　▽☆ Corn Niblets, No Sauce 　Cut Broccoli, No Sauce 　▽ Green Beans, No Sauce 　☆ Sweet Peas, No Sauce ▽☆ Mixed Vegetables Niblet Ears: 　▽☆ Corn on the Cob ▽ Niblets Corn One Serving: 　▽☆ Nibblers Corn on the Cob ▽ Select Broccoli Spears Sweet Peas: 　▽☆ Regular	Microwave: 　▲ Broccoli in Cheese Flavored Sauce 　▲ Cauliflower in Cheese Flavored Sauce 　☆ Niblets Corn in Butter Sauce One Serving: 　☆ Baby Peas in Butter ☆ Shoepeg White Corn in a Butter Sauce Valley Combination: 　Broccoli, Pasta	
Inland Valley	▽ Simply Shreds Potatoes		
J.R. Simplot	▽ Hashbrown Shreds		
McKenzie's	Garden Fresh Mixtures: 　▽ Broccoli, Cauliflower, Carrots		
Micro Magic			Microwave: 　▽ French Fries
Ore Ida	▽ Chopped Onions ▽ Dinner Fries Hash Browns: 　▽ Country Style 　▽ Regular 　▽ Southern Style Potatoes Mashed Potatoes: 　▽ Butter Flavor ▽ Potato Wedges w/Skins		Crispy Crunchies! Fast Fries: 　Original 　Ranch ▽ Golden Crinkles ▽ Golden Fries Golden Patties ▽☆ Golden Twirls Hot Tots

▲ High Sodium, 480 mg. or greater per serving.
▽ Low Sodium, 140 mg. or less per serving.
☆ Good Source of Fiber, between 2.5 g. and 5 g. per serving.

172   **Vegetables**

BRAND	BEST CHOICE	ACCEPTABLE CHOICE	OCCASIONAL CHOICE
	Fat Free or Low Fat AND Low Saturated Fat AND Less Than 480 mg. Sodium	Low Fat	Contains Greater Than 3 Grams Total Fat
Ore Ida (Cont.)	∇ Potatoes O'Brien w/Onions and Peppers		Microwave: ∇ Crinkle Cuts Hash Browns Tater Tots Onion Ringers Onion Rings ∇☆ Pixie Crinkles ∇ Shoestrings Tater Tots: ▲ Bacon Onion Texas Crispers! ▲ Toaster Hash Browns Topped Baked Potatoes: ☆ Broccoli & Cheese Twice Baked Potatoes: ☆ Butter Flavor ☆ Cheddar Cheese ☆ Ranch Flavor Sour Cream & Chives Zesties!
PictSweet	Chinese Stir-Fry ∇ Japanese Vegetables Oriental Stir-Fry ∇ Oriental Vegetables		
Stouffer's			★ Creamed Spinach
The Budget Gourmet			Side Dish: Cheddared Potatoes and Broccoli ▲ Spinach Au Gratin Spring Vegetables in Cheese Sauce ▲☆ Three-Cheese Potatoes
CANNED			
Aunt Nellie's	Harvard Beets: Sweet & Sour Pickled Beets: Sliced Whole Onions: Holland-Style	Red Cabbage: ▲ Sweet & Sour	

▲ High Sodium, 480 mg. or greater per serving.
∇ Low Sodium, 140 mg. or less per serving.
☆ Good Source of Fiber, between 2.5 g. and 5 g. per serving.
★ High Fiber, 5 g. or greater per serving.

BRAND	BEST CHOICE	ACCEPTABLE CHOICE	OCCASIONAL CHOICE
	Fat Free or Low Fat AND Low Saturated Fat AND Less Than 480 mg. Sodium	Low Fat	Contains Greater Than 3 Grams Total Fat
Brooks	Just For Chili Diced Tomatoes: Medium w/Onions Mild		
Bush's Best	Collard Greens: Chopped ☆ Cut Green & Shelly Beans Kale Greens: Chopped Mustard Greens: Chopped Turnip Greens: Chopped		
Contadina	Crushed Tomatoes in Puree		
Dei Fratelli	Crushed Tomatoes: ∇ Italian Style		
Del Monte	Asparagus Spears: All Varieties Beets: All Varieties Cream Style Corn Cut Green Beans Cut Wax Beans French Style Green Beans ☆ Italian Beans ☆ Lima Beans Mixed Vegetables: No Preservatives Original No Salt: ∇ Cut Green Beans ∇☆ Whole Kernel Corn Peas & Carrots ☆ Slice Carrots Spinach: Whole Leaf Stewed Tomatoes: Italian Recipe Original Recipe ☆ Summer Crisp Corn ☆ Summer Crisp Golden	▲ Chunky Tomatoes, Pasta Style Zucchini: ▲ With Italian-Style Tomato Sauce	

▲ High Sodium, 480 mg. or greater per serving.
∇ Low Sodium, 140 mg. or less per serving.
☆ Good Source of Fiber, between 2.5 g. and 5 g. per serving.

BRAND	BEST CHOICE	ACCEPTABLE CHOICE	OCCASIONAL CHOICE
	Fat Free or Low Fat AND Low Saturated Fat AND Less Than 480 mg. Sodium	Low Fat	Contains Greater Than 3 Grams Total Fat
Del Monte (Cont.)	Sweet Corn ☆ Sweet Peas ☆ Very Young Small Sweet Peas White Sweet Corn Whole Green Beans Whole Kernel Corn: ☆ Supersweet No Sugar Added Whole Leaf Spinach		
Dell' Alpe	Artichoke Hearts		
Flannagan's	Krrrrisp Kraut		
Frank's	Stewed Tomatoes		

Freshlike	☆ Baby Green Lima Beans
	Cut Green Beans:
	  ∇☆ No Salt Added
	  Regular
	☆ Cut Leaf Spinach
	Garden Peas:
	  ☆ Tender
	Green Beans:
	  ★ French Style
	  ∇★ French Style No Salt
	    Added
	Leaf Spinach:
	  ☆ Cut
	Mushrooms
	★ Petite Sweet Peas
	Sliced Carrots:
	  Crinkle
	Small Sliced Beets
	Sweet Corn:
	  Cream Style
	  Whole Kernel
	  with Peppers
	Sweet Corn, Whole Kernel:
	  ∇ No Salt or Sugar Added
	☆ Sweet Peas & Carrots
	☆ Sweet Peas & Tiny Onions
	Tender Garden Peas:
	  ∇☆ No Salt Added
	  ☆ Regular		

∇ Low Sodium, 140 mg. or less per serving.

☆ Good Source of Fiber, between 2.5 g. and 5 g. per serving.

★ High Fiber, 5 g. or greater per serving.

BRAND	BEST CHOICE	ACCEPTABLE CHOICE	OCCASIONAL CHOICE
	Fat Free or Low Fat AND Low Saturated Fat AND Less Than 480 mg. Sodium	Low Fat	Contains Greater Than 3 Grams Total Fat
Freshlike (Cont.)	Whole Beets: Small Whole Green Beans		

Green Giant	Asparagus Spears:
	  Extra Long Tender Green
	Cut Green Beans
	Mexicorn
	Niblets Golden Sweet Corn
	Sliced Mushrooms
	Sweet Corn:
	  Whole Kernel
	Sweet Peas:
	  ☆ Very Young Tender		

Hunt's	Choice Cut:
	  Diced Tomatoes
	Stewed Tomatoes:
	  ▽ No Salt Added
	  Regular
	Whole Tomatoes:
	  ▽ No Salt Added
	  Regular
		Choice Cut:
		  ▲ Diced Tomatoes in
		    Roasted Garlic
		  ▲ Diced Tomatoes w/
		    Italian Style Herbs	

International Bazaar		Hearts of Artichokes: ▲ All Varieties	

Kuner's	Chili Tomatoes
	Gold 'N White Corn:
	  ▽ Southwestern
	▽ Gold 'N White Extra Crispy
	  Two-Color Corn		

Le Sueur	☆ Small Young Peas		
Muir Glen	▽ Ground Peeled Tomatoes		

Pennsylvania Dutchman	Mushrooms:
	  All Varieties
	Mushrooms:
	  ▽ No Salt Added		

Pine Cone	Peeled Tomatoes Whole Peeled Tomatoes		

▲ High Sodium, 480 mg. or greater per serving.
▽ Low Sodium, 140 mg. or less per serving.
☆ Good Source of Fiber, between 2.5 g. and 5 g. per serving.

BRAND	BEST CHOICE	ACCEPTABLE CHOICE	OCCASIONAL CHOICE
	Fat Free or Low Fat AND Low Saturated Fat AND Less Than 480 mg. Sodium	Low Fat	Contains Greater Than 3 Grams Total Fat

Progresso	∇ Artichoke Hearts
	Crushed Tomatoes:
	  ∇ w/Added Puree
	∇ Eggplant Appetizer
	Peeled Tomatoes:
	  with Basil
	Recipe Ready:
	  ∇ Crushed Tomatoes		

Reese	Artichoke Bottoms
	Artichoke Hearts:
	  All Varieties
	Baby Carrots:
	  Extra Tiny Belgian
	Baby Corn on the Cob:
	  Whole Spears
	Hearts of Palm
			Artichoke Salad

Ro-tel	Diced Tomatoes w/Green Chiles ∇ Whole Tomatoes w/Green Chiles		

S & W	∇ Green and Wax Beans
	Julienne Beets:
	  Premium, French Style
	Julienne Carrots
	New Potatoes:
	  Premium Small Whole
	Sweet Peas
		▲☆ Peas w/Tiny Pearl Onions	

Sea Side	Mixed Vegetables: Original		
Silver Floss	Barrel Cured Sauerkraut	▲☆ Sauerkraut	
Star Cross	Stewed Tomatoes		
Stokely's	Stewed Tomatoes		
Thank You	Cut Asparagus		
The Allens	☆ Butterfield Sliced New Potatoes ☆ Cut Okra ∇☆ Popeye Low Salt Spinach		

▲ High Sodium, 480 mg. or greater per serving.
∇ Low Sodium, 140 mg. or less per serving.
☆ Good Source of Fiber, between 2.5 g. and 5 g. per serving.

BRAND	BEST CHOICE	ACCEPTABLE CHOICE	OCCASIONAL CHOICE
	Fat Free or Low Fat AND Low Saturated Fat AND Less Than 480 mg. Sodium	Low Fat	Contains Greater Than 3 Grams Total Fat
Veg All	Large Cut Vegetables: Homestyle Mixed Vegetables: ∇ No Salt Added Original		
DRIED			
Sonoma	∇ Marinated Dried Tomatoes		
YOUR FAVORITE VEGETABLES NOT LISTED IN THE GUIDE			

∇ Low Sodium, 140 mg. or less per serving.

FRUITS

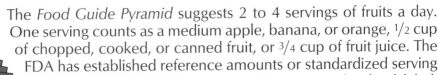

This food category contains a wide range of fruit products that are either fresh, frozen, canned, or dried and have been subdivided into those classifications. Fruits are major sources of vitamin C, beta-carotene, dietary fiber, potassium, and other minerals. They are naturally cholesterol-free and generally low in fat. A diet rich in fruits and vegetables is recommended by most health authorities because of its link to good health.

The *Food Guide Pyramid* suggests 2 to 4 servings of fruits a day. One serving counts as a medium apple, banana, or orange, 1/2 cup of chopped, cooked, or canned fruit, or 3/4 cup of fruit juice. The FDA has established reference amounts or standardized serving sizes for use on the food label. The reference amount for fruits varies, depending on type and use. The reference amount for most fruit (fresh, frozen, canned) is 140 grams (5 ounces). Be sure to read the *Nutrition Facts* label for the serving size information of your fruit choice. (See pages 51 and 52 for an explanation of reference amounts and the difference between serving sizes established by the FDA for food labeling and those recommended by the *Food Guide Pyramid*.)

At this time, nutrition information labeling is voluntary for fresh fruits. As part of the FDA's voluntary point-of-purchase program, many supermarkets will display posters in the produce section detailing the nutrition content of the 20 most frequently eaten fresh fruits. Nutrition information pamphlets may also be available for the consumer.

Most fruits are generally low in total fat and contain no saturated fat or cholesterol unless ingredients like coconut, coconut oil, or cream are added. Fruit contains natural sugars, but, in many cases, additional sugars or other sweeteners are added in processing. The criteria were therefore designed to distinguish those fruit products lower in fat and without added sugars.

Criteria Key

▲ **Best Choice:**   **Fat Free, AND No Added Sugars**

Products listed in this category meet the FDA's definition for "Fat Free" (less than $1/2$ gram fat per serving), and "No Added Sugars" (processing does not increase the sugar content above the amount naturally present in the fruit).

△ **Acceptable Choice:**   **Fat Free, AND With Added Sugars**

Fruits listed in this category meet the FDA's definition for "Fat Free" but have sugar added during processing. The *Dietary Guidelines for Americans*[11] recommend that foods high in sugar be consumed in moderation by most healthy people and sparingly by people who need to limit their calorie intake. (See pages 45-47 for discussion of this guideline.) Because of the wide variety of fruits available without additional sugars, we recommend that most fruits be consumed in their fresh state or processed without added sugars or fats.

▲ **Occasional Choice:**   **Total Fat Content Greater Than 1 Gram**

Fruits listed in this category do **not meet** the FDA's definition for "Fat Free." Some fruits (such as avocado, olives, and coconut) naturally contain fat. Other fruits may have certain fats (e.g., palm oil, coconut, cream, soybean oil) added during processing. While avocado and olives contain primarily monounsaturated fat, the fat in coconut is highly saturated, as are the fats typically added during processing. Because of the higher-fat nature of these fruits, they should only be consumed on occasion.

BRAND	BEST CHOICE	ACCEPTABLE CHOICE	OCCASIONAL CHOICE
	Fat Free AND No Added Sugars	Fat Free AND With Added Sugars	Total Fat Content Greater Than 1 Gram
FRESH			

Fresh	∇ Acerola
	∇☆ Apple
	∇☆ Apricots
	∇ Banana
	∇☆ Blackberries
	∇ Blueberries
	∇ Canteloupe
	∇ Carambola
	∇ Clementine
	∇☆ Cranberries
	Currants:
	   ∇☆ European Black
	∇★ Elderberries
	∇☆ Figs
	Grapefruit:
	   ∇★ Pink
	   ∇★ White
	Grapes:
	   ∇ American
	∇★ Guava
	∇ Honeydew
	∇☆ Kiwifruit
	∇ Kumquats
	∇ Lemon
	∇ Lime
	∇ Mango
	∇ Mineola
	∇☆ Nectarine
	∇☆ Orange
	∇☆ Papaya
	∇ Peach
	∇☆ Pear
	∇☆ Persimmon
	∇ Pineapple
	∇ Plum
	∇★ Pomegranate
	∇ Pricklypear
	∇ Quince
	∇★ Raspberries
	∇ Rhubarb
	∇☆ Strawberries
	∇☆ Sweet Cherries
	∇★ Tamarind
	∇ Tangerine
	∇ Uglifruit
	∇ Watermelon
			∇ Avocado
			∇ Coconut
			▲ Olives

∇ Low Sodium, 140 mg. or less per serving.
☆ Good Source of Fiber, between 2.5 g. and 5 g. per serving.
★ High Fiber, 5 g. or greater per serving.

BRAND	BEST CHOICE	ACCEPTABLE CHOICE	OCCASIONAL CHOICE
	Fat Free AND No Added Sugars	Fat Free AND With Added Sugars	Total Fat Content Greater Than 1 Gram
FROZEN			
Big Valley	∇ Blueberries ∇☆ Burst O'Berries ∇ California Fruit Collection ∇☆ Dark Sweet Cherries ∇ Strawberries		
Coloma	No Sugar Added Frozen Fruit: ∇ All Varieties		
Orville Kent		Chilled Selections: ∇ Fruit Salad	
Stillwell	Frozen Select Fruits: ∇ No Sugar Added All Varieties		
Stouffer's			∇ Escalloped Apples
CANNED			
3 Diamonds	Pineapple in Its Own Juice: ∇ All Varieties	Mandarin Orange Segments: ∇ in Light Syrup	
All Brands	Applesauce: ∇ Unsweetened ∇ Maraschino Cherries in Water ∇ Pineapple in its Own Juice	Applesauce: ∇ Sweetened ∇ Maraschino Cherries in Syrup ∇ Pineapple in Heavy Syrup	
Del Monte	Fruit Naturals: ∇ Chunky Mixed Fruit-No Sugar Added ∇ Fruit Cocktail in Fruit Juices ∇ Pear Halves in Pear Juice Fruit Naturals Cup: ∇ All Flavors Fruit Naturals Fruit Cocktail: ∇ in Fruit Juices Pineapple, Chunks: ∇ in Its Own Juice Pineapple, Crushed: ∇ in Its Own Juice Pineapple, Sliced: ∇ in Its Own Juice Pineapple, Spears: ∇ in Its Own Juice	Apricot Halves: ∇ in Heavy Syrup Cherries, Dark Pitted: ∇ in Heavy Syrup Cherries, Dark Whole Unpitted: ∇ in Heavy Syrup Chunky Mixed Fruits: ∇ in Heavy Syrup Fruit Cocktail: ∇ in Heavy Syrup Fruit Cup in Syrup: ∇ All Flavors Light Fruit Cup: ∇ All Flavors Lite Apricot Halves: ∇ in Extra Light Syrup Lite Chunky Mixed Fruits: ∇ in Extra Light Syrup	

∇ Low Sodium, 140 mg. or less per serving.
☆ Good Source of Fiber, between 2.5 g. and 5 g. per serving.

BRAND	BEST CHOICE	ACCEPTABLE CHOICE	OCCASIONAL CHOICE
	Fat Free AND No Added Sugars	Fat Free AND With Added Sugars	Total Fat Content Greater Than 1 Gram
Del Monte (Cont.)	Pineapple, Tidbits: ∇ in Its Own Juice Pineapple, Wedges: ∇ in Its Own Juice	Lite Fruit Cocktail: ∇ in Extra Light Syrup Lite Pear Halves: ∇ in Extra Light Syrup Lite Sliced Peaches: ∇ in Extra Light Syrup Mandarin Oranges: ∇ in Light Syrup Peaches, Halves: ∇ in Heavy Syrup Peaches, Lite Halves: ∇ in Extra Light Syrup Peaches, Lite Slices: ∇ in Extra Light Syrup Peaches, Melba Halves: ∇ in Heavy Syrup Peaches, Sliced: ∇ in Heavy Syrup Peaches, Spiced: ∇ in Heavy Syrup Pear, Halves: ∇ in Heavy Syrup Pears, Sliced: ∇ in Heavy Syrup Pineapple, Chunks: ∇ in Heavy Syrup Pineapple, Crushed: ∇ in Heavy Syrup Pineapple, Sliced: ∇ in Heavy Syrup	
Dole	Crushed Pineapple: ∇ in Unsweetened Juice Pineapple Chunks: ∇ in Unsweetened Juice Pineapple Slices: ∇ in Unsweetened Juice Pineapple Tidbits: ∇ in Unsweetened Juice	Mandarin Orange Segments: ∇ in Light Syrup Pineapple Chunks: ∇ in Heavy Syrup Pineapple Slices: ∇ in Heavy Syrup Tropical Fruit Salad: ∇ in Light Syrup	
Geisha	Pineapple: ∇ Sliced in Natural Juice Pineapple Chunk: ∇ in Its Own Juice		

∇ Low Sodium, 140 mg. or less per serving.

BRAND	BEST CHOICE	ACCEPTABLE CHOICE	OCCASIONAL CHOICE
	Fat Free AND No Added Sugars	Fat Free AND With Added Sugars	Total Fat Content Greater Than 1 Gram
Hunt's		∇ Peaches in Heavy Syrup	
International Bazaar		∇ Slice Kiwi in Syrup	
Libby's	Lite Chunky Mixed Fruit: ∇ No Sugar Added Lite Sliced Peaches: ∇ No Sugar Added		
Liberty Gold	Pineapple in Natural Juice: ∇ All Varieties		
Mott's	Applesauce: ∇ Natural	Applesauce: ∇ Cinnamon ∇ Original ∇ w/Mixed Fruit ∇ w/Strawberries Homestyle Chunky Applesauce: ☆ w/Brown Sugar & Cinnamon	
Musselman's	Applesauce: ∇ Natural ∇ Lite Applesauce	Applesauce: ∇ Cinnamon ∇ Regular	
Ocean Spray		Cran-Fruit for Chicken: ∇ Cranberry Orange Sauce ∇ Cranberry Raspberry ∇ Jellied Cranberry Sauce ∇ Whole Berry Cranberry Sauce	
Oregon		Blackberries: ∇★ in Heavy Syrup Blueberries: ∇ in Heavy Syrup Red Raspberries: ∇★ in Heavy Syrup Thompson Grapes: ∇ in Light Syrup	
Packers Pride	∇ Red Tart Pitted Cherries	Dark Sweet Pitted Cherries: ∇ in Heavy Syrup	

∇ Low Sodium, 140 mg. or less per serving.
☆ Good Source of Fiber, between 2.5 g. and 5 g. per serving.
★ High Fiber, 5 g. or greater per serving.

184 **Fruits**

BRAND	BEST CHOICE	ACCEPTABLE CHOICE	OCCASIONAL CHOICE
	Fat Free AND No Added Sugars	Fat Free AND With Added Sugars	Total Fat Content Greater Than 1 Gram
S & W	Grapefruit Sections: ∇ No Sugar Added	Bartlett Pears: ∇ in Heavy Syrup Freestone Peaches: ∇ in Heavy Syrup Old Fashioned Whole Yellow Cling Spice Peaches Yellow Cling Peach Halves: ∇ in Heavy Syrup	
Sunsweet		Prunes: ∇ Ready to Serve	
Thank You		Blackberries: ∇ in Heavy Syrup Dark Sweek Cherries: ∇ in Heavy Syrup Dessert Cherries: ∇ in Extra Heavy Syrup Figs: ∇ in Light Syrup Purple Plums: ∇ in Heavy Syrup Raspberries: ∇ in Heavy Syrup Royal Anne Cherries: ∇ in Heavy Syrup Seedless Grapes: ∇ in Heavy Syrup Strawberries: ∇ in Heavy Syrup	
White House		∇ Applesauce	
White Swan		∇ Maraschino Cherries in Corn Syrup	
Wilderness		Applesauce: ∇ Old Fashioned ∇ Peach ∇ Raspberry ∇ Strawberry	
DRIED			
All Brands	∇ Dates without Added Sugar ∇★ Prunes without Added Sugar ∇☆ Seedless Raisins without Added Sugar		

∇ Low Sodium, 140 mg. or less per serving.
☆ Good Source of Fiber, between 2.5 g. and 5 g. per serving.
★ High Fiber, 5 g. or greater per serving.

BRAND	BEST CHOICE	ACCEPTABLE CHOICE	OCCASIONAL CHOICE
	Fat Free AND No Added Sugars	Fat Free AND With Added Sugars	Total Fat Content Greater Than 1 Gram
Blue Ribbon	∇★ Calimyrna Figs ∇★ Misson Figlets ∇★ Misson Figs		
Champion	Raisins: ∇ No Sugar Added		
Dole	∇☆ Pitted Prunes ∇ Raisins	Dates: ∇☆ Chopped	
L'Esprit De Champagne		∇ Dried Cherries	
Nutra-Fig	∇☆ California Figs		
Pavitch	∇ Organically Grown Raisins		
Sun Maid	∇ Baking Raisins ∇ California Golden Raisins ∇ California Sun-Dried Raisins ∇★ Mission Figs ∇ Zanite Currants		
Sunsweet	∇☆ Breakfast Prunes International Style: ☆ Dried Apricots ∇☆ Dried Mixed Fruit ∇ Fruit Morsels ∇☆ Our Premium Prunes Pitted Prunes: ∇☆ Lemon Essence ∇☆ Orange Essence ∇☆ Regular		
YOUR FAVORITE FRUITS NOT LISTED IN THE *GUIDE*			

∇ Low Sodium, 140 mg. or less per serving.

☆ Good Source of Fiber, between 2.5 g. and 5 g. per serving.

★ High Fiber, 5 g. or greater per serving.

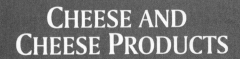

CHEESE AND CHEESE PRODUCTS

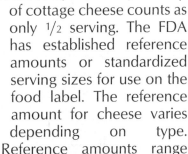

Historically, cheeses have had a reputation of being a major contributor of total fat and saturated fat to the American diet. However, due to consumer demands, food manufacturers have introduced many lower-fat versions of cheeses into the market. These lower-fat versions provide protein, calcium, vitamins, and minerals and can be included in the daily diet.

Cheeses are included in the "Milk, Yogurt, and Cheese Group" of the *Food Guide Pyramid*. Two to three servings from this group should be consumed each day to provide adequate calcium for adults as well as children and teenagers. One cup of milk or yogurt, 1¹/₂ ounces of natural cheese (e.g., Cheddar), or 2 ounces of processed cheese (e.g., American), make up one serving size. Cottage cheese is lower in calcium than most cheeses; therefore, one cup of cottage cheese counts as only ¹/₂ serving. The FDA has established reference amounts or standardized serving sizes for use on the food label. The reference amount for cheese varies depending on type. Reference amounts range from 5 grams (0.2 ounce) for grated hard cheeses such as Parmesan and Romano, to 30 grams (1 ounce) for most other cheeses (except cottage cheese, which is 110 grams, or 4 ounces). Be sure to read the *Nutrition Facts* label for the serving size information of your cheese choice. (See pages 51 and 52 for an explanation of reference amounts and the difference between serving sizes established by the FDA for food labeling and those recommended by the *Food Guide Pyramid*.)

Because regular cheese and cheese products can add a significant amount of saturated fat, which is the strongest contributor to increased blood cholesterol, the criteria were designed to distinguish those products that are lower in saturated fat content.

Criteria Key

▲ **Best Choice:**   **Low Saturated Fat**

Products listed in this category meet the FDA's definition for "Low Saturated Fat" (1 gram or less saturated fat per serving).

△ **Acceptable Choice:**   **Contains Greater Than 1 Gram, but
                             Less Than 4 Grams Saturated Fat**

Products listed in this category **do not** meet the FDA's definition for "Low Saturated Fat" but contain less than 4 grams saturated fat (less than 20% of the Daily Value). Although many of these products are reduced in fat, they can still contribute a substantial amount of saturated fat to the diet. Cheese from this category contains as much saturated fat as equal portions of meat.

▲ **Occasional Choice:**   **High Saturated Fat**

Products listed in this category are considered high in saturated fat because they contain 4 grams or more saturated fat per serving (20% or greater of the Daily Value). Foods in this category should be consumed only on occasion. If large amounts of food from this category were selected as part of a regular diet, it would be difficult to meet the *Dietary Guidelines for Americans*[11] for choosing a diet low in saturated fat.

BRAND	BEST CHOICE	ACCEPTABLE CHOICE	OCCASIONAL CHOICE
	Low Saturated Fat	Contains Greater Than 1 Gram but Less Than 4 Grams Saturated Fat	High Saturated Fat

All Brands	Cottage Cheese:
	  1% Low Fat
	  ∇ Dry Curd
	  ∇ Nonfat
	Ricotta:
	  ∇ Fat Free
		Cottage Cheese:
		  2% Low Fat
		  4% Fat Creamed
		∇ Jarlsberg Light
		Light Havarti
		Mozzarella:
		  Low Moisture, Part-Skim
		  ∇ Part-Skim
		  ∇ Regular
		Processed Cheese Spread:
		  American
		Ricotta:
		  ∇ Part Skim
			Blue
			Brick
			Brie
			Camembert
			Cheddar
			∇ Chevre Goat Cheese
			Colby
			∇ Cream Cheese
			Edam
			Farmer's Cheese
			Feta
			∇ Fontina
			Gjetost
			Gouda
			∇ Gruyere
			Havarti
			∇ Jalsberg
			Limburger
			Mozzarella:
			  ∇ Low Moisture
			Muenster
			∇ Neufchatel
			Parmesan
			Pinconning
			Port du Salut
			Provolone
			Ricotta:
			  ∇ Whole Milk
			Romano
			Roquefort:
			  ▲ Sheep's Milk
			Swiss:
			  ∇ Regular

Alouette		Light Soft Spreadable Cheese:
		  ∇ Herbs & Garlic
		  ∇ Spring Vegetables
			Soft Spreadable Cheese:
			  ∇ Garlic and Spices

Alpine Lace	Fat Free Cheese Spread:
	  All Flavors
	Fat Free Cream Cheese:
	  All Flavors
	Fat Free Shredded Cheese:
	  All Varieties
	Fat Free Sliced Cheese:
	  All Varieties
		Mozzarella Cheese:
		  ∇ Low Moisture Part-Skim
		∇ Reduced Fat Colby
		∇ Reduced Fat Smoked
		  Provolone
		∇ Reduced Sodium
		  Mozzarella
			∇ Reduced Sodium Muenster

Axelrod	Nonfat Cottage Cheese: Pineapple		

▲ High Sodium, 480 mg. or greater per serving.
∇ Low Sodium, 140 mg. or less per serving.

BRAND	BEST CHOICE	ACCEPTABLE CHOICE	OCCASIONAL CHOICE
	Low Saturated Fat	Contains Greater Than 1 Gram but Less Than 4 Grams Saturated Fat	High Saturated Fat
BelGioioso			∇ Mascarpone Sweet Cheese

Berne'A			∇ Amish Style Swiss Cheese
			Longhorn Colby Cheese:
			   ∇ No Salt Added
			   Regular

Black Diamond			Canadian Extra Old Cheddar

Borden	Fat Free Cheese Product:
	   Sharp
	   Swiss
	Low Fat American Cheese
	Low Fat Sharp Cheddar Cheese
	Low Fat Swiss Cheese
		American Singles
		Light American Cheese
		   Product
			American Cheese
			American Cheese Food
			American Cheese Spread
			American Sharp Cheese
			Cheddar Cheese Wheel
			Cold Pack Sharp Cheddar
			   Cheese Food
			Swiss Cheese
			Swiss Cheese Food

Breakstone's		Lowfat Cottage Cheese	∇ Temp-Tee Whipped Cream Cheese
Cheez Whiz		▲ Light Cheese Product	▲ Cheese Spread ▲ Hot Salsa Cheese Spread ▲ Mild Salsa Cheese Spread
Chi Chi's			Shredded Cheese: Mexican Blend

Country Fresh	Cottage Cheese:
	   1% Milkfat Lowfat
		Cottage Cheese:
		   4% Milkfat Large Curd	

County Line		100% Natural String Cheese:
		   Mozzarella Part-Skim
		Part-Skim Mozzarella:
		   (Regular)
		   (Shredded)
		Pasteurized Process Cheese
		Food:
		   American Single Slices
			Cheddar Cheese:
			   (Shredded)
			Colby Jack
			Cracker Backers:
			   Mild Cheddar
			Medium Sharp Cheddar
			Mild Colby Cheese:
			   (Block)
			Monterey Jack
			Sharp Cheddar:
			   (Shredded)
			Sharp Colby
			Shredded Taco Cheese

▲ High Sodium, 480 mg. or greater per serving.
∇ Low Sodium, 140 mg. or less per serving.

190 **Cheese and Cheese Products**

Brand	Best Choice	Acceptable Choice	Occasional Choice
	Low Saturated Fat	Contains Greater Than 1 Gram but Less Than 4 Grams Saturated Fat	High Saturated Fat
Cracker Barrel		Reduced Fat Sharp Cheddar	∇ Baby Swiss Cold Pack Cheese Food: Sharp Extra Sharp Cheddar Medium Cheddar ∇ New York Aged Cheddar Sharp Cheddar Vermont Sharp-White
Dairy Fresh	Fat Free Cream Cheese	Singles: American	Cream Cheese
Dean Foods	Cottage Cheese: ▲ Nonfat	Cottage Cheese: Small Curd	
Deli		Cheese Sauce: ▲ All Flavors Cheese Spread: All Flavors	
Di Giorno	All Varieties Parmesan Cheese: ∇ (2 teaspoon serving) All Varieties Romano Cheese: ∇ (2 teaspoon serving)		
Dorman's		Light Cheda-Jack	
Fleur-de-Lait		Light Cream Cheese: Garden Vegetable ∇ Garlic & Spices	
Formagg	∇ Mozzarella Cheese Alternative		
Friendship	Nonfat Cottage Cheese	Cottage Cheese: with Pineapple	
Frigo	Truly Lite: ∇ Fat Free Ricotta	Grated Parmesan: ∇ (1 tablespoon serving) Part-Skim Mozzarella Cheese Truly Lite: ∇ Ricotta	Crumbled Feta Cheese Part-Skim Ricotta
Healthy Choice	Fat Free: Pasteurized Process Cheese Product		

▲ High Sodium, 480 mg. or greater per serving.
∇ Low Sodium, 140 mg. or less per serving.

BRAND	BEST CHOICE	ACCEPTABLE CHOICE	OCCASIONAL CHOICE
	Low Saturated Fat	Contains Greater Than 1 Gram but Less Than 4 Grams Saturated Fat	High Saturated Fat

Healthy Choice (Cont.)	Fat Free Cream Cheese:
	    All Flavors
	Fat Free Shredded:
	    All Flavors
	Fat Free Singles:
	    All Flavors
	Fat Free String Cheese:
	    All Flavors		

Kaukauna		Lite 50: Port Wine Cheese	

Knudsen	Lowfat Cottage Cheese & Fruit:
	    Peach
	    Pineapple
	    Strawberry
	Nonfat Cottage Cheese
		Cottage Cheese
		Lowfat Cottage Cheese & Fruit:
		    Tropical Fruit	

Kraft	100% Grated Parmesan Cheese:
	    ∇ (1 tablespoon serving)
	Free:
	    ∇ Nonfat Grated Topping
	Free Singles:
	    All Flavors
	Healthy Favorites:
	    Fat Free, Shredded, Mild
	        Cheddar
	    Fat Free, Shredded,
	        Mozzarella
		⅓ Less Fat Naturals:
		    All Flavors
		⅓ Less Fat Singles:
		    American
		    Swiss
		Deluxe American Slices:
		    25% Less Fat
		Grated House Italian:
		    ∇ ⅓ Less Fat
		Pimento Single Slices
		Singles:
		    American
		    Swiss
		String Cheese:
		    Low Moisture Part Skim
		    Mozzarella w/Jalapeno
		        Peppers
		Velveeta Light:
		    (Brick)
		Velveeta Slices:
		    (Regular)
			Deli Thin:
			    Colby Slices
			    ∇ Swiss Slices
			Deluxe American Slices:
			    Regular
			Finely Shredded:
			    Mild Cheddar
			Handi Snacks:
			    Mozzarella String Cheese
			Mozzarella Cheese:
			    Part Skim
			Mozzarella Cheese Slices:
			    Low Moisture, Part Skim
			Natural:
			    Colby Cheese (Brick)
			    Colby/Monterey Jack
			        (Shredded)
			    Extra Sharp Cheddar Cheese
			    Longhorn Style Colby &
			        Monterey Jack Brick
			    Medium Cheddar Cheese
			    ∇ Mild Cheddar Brick
			    Mild Cheddar Reduced Fat
			        (Shredded)
			    Mild Cheddar (Shredded)
			    Monterey Jack (Brick)
			    New York Extra Sharp
			        Cheddar Cheese

∇ Low Sodium, 140 mg. or less per serving.

BRAND	BEST CHOICE	ACCEPTABLE CHOICE	OCCASIONAL CHOICE
	Low Saturated Fat	Contains Greater Than 1 Gram but Less Than 4 Grams Saturated Fat	High Saturated Fat
Kraft (Cont.)			Natural: Part-Skim Mozzarella Slices Sharp Cheddar Brick Shredded Sharp Cheddar ∇ Swiss Shredded ∇ Swiss Slices Pizza Cheese, Shredded: 4 Cheese Mozzarella and Cheddar Smoked Sharp Old English Slices Shredded Part-Skim: Mozzarella Shredded Taco Cheese Singles: Sharp Cheddar Spreadery Cheese Snack: Neufchatel Garden Vegetable Toppings, Finely Shredded: Sharp Cheddar Velveeta Processed Cheese Spread: ▲ Hot Mexican Mild Mexican Regular Velveeta Slices: ▲ Extra Thick
Land O Lakes		Low Moisture Part-Skim Mozzarella Cheese: (Shredded)	American Singles Chedarella Part-Skim Cheese: (Brick) (Shredded) Midget Longhorn Colby Cheese Mild Cheddar Cheese: (Shredded) Sharp Cheddar Cheese: (Brick)
Laughing Cow		Light Cheese Spread: Wedges	Baby Bel Bonbel Cheez Bits: Original Flavor Edam Gouda

▲ High Sodium, 480 mg. or greater per serving.
∇ Low Sodium, 140 mg. or less per serving.

BRAND	BEST CHOICE	ACCEPTABLE CHOICE	OCCASIONAL CHOICE
	Low Saturated Fat	Contains Greater Than 1 Gram but Less Than 4 Grams Saturated Fat	High Saturated Fat

Light N' Lively	Free Cottage Cheese
	Lowfat Cottage Cheese:
	  Peach & Pineapple
	  Regular		

London's	Cottage Cheese:
	  Lowfat
	  Nonfat
		Cottage Cheese:
		  Small Curd	

Melody Farms		Cottage Cheese:
		  4% Milkfat
		Low-Fat Cottage Cheese:
		  2% Milkfat	

Merkt's			Cheese Spread:
			  Almond Swiss Cheese
			  Port Wine
			  Sharp Cheddar

Miceli's		Lite Ricotta:
		  ∇ Low Fat
		∇ Part-Skim Ricotta
			Ricotta:
			  ∇ Traditional

Michigan	Lowfat Cottage Cheese:
	  1% Milkfat
	Nonfat Cottage Cheese
		Cottage Cheese:
		  Small and Large Curd 4%
		  Milkfat	

Milkhouse Cheese		American Singles	
Mohawk Valley			▲ Limburger Cheese
Nabisco			Easy Cheese: All Flavors
Norweigan		Jarlsberg: ∇ Lite Cheese	
Old European Style			∇ Farmers Cheese
Old Fashioned Foods			Old Fashioned Cheese: All Flavors
Organic Valley		Part-Skim Mozzarella	Colby Cheese ∇ Cream Cheese (Box) Mild Cheddar Muenster Cheese Provolone

▲ High Sodium, 480 mg. or greater per serving.
∇ Low Sodium, 140 mg. or less per serving.

BRAND	BEST CHOICE	ACCEPTABLE CHOICE	OCCASIONAL CHOICE
	Low Saturated Fat	Contains Greater Than 1 Gram but Less Than 4 Grams Saturated Fat	High Saturated Fat

Philadelphia	Cream Cheese:
	    Free (Tub & Boxed)
			Cream Cheese:
			    ∇ Chives and Onion
			    ∇ Original
			    ∇ Pineapple
			Light Cream Cheese
			∇ Neufchatel Cheese
			Soft Cream Cheese:
			    ∇ Chives and Onions
			    Herb & Garlic
			    Olive & Pimento
			    Smoked Salmon
			    ∇ Strawberry

Polly-O	∇ Nonfat Ricotta Cheese		
Quark	Spreadable Cheese: ∇ Nonfat		

Sargento	Shredded:
	    Part-Skim Mozzarella
	Shredded Imitation Cheddar
	Shredded Imitation Mozzarella
		∇ Light Ricotta
		MooTown Snackers:
		    Light Mozzarella String
		        Cheese
		    Mozzarella String Cheese
		Natural Part-Skim:
		    ∇ Ricotta Cheese
		Preferred Light:
		    Shredded Cheese for Tacos
		    Shredded Mild Cheddar
		    Shredded Part-Skim
		        Mozzarella
		    Sliced Mozzarella
		    ∇ Sliced Swiss Cheese
			Classic Supreme:
			    Montery Jack (Shredded)
			    Shredded Cheese for Tacos
			    Shredded Mild Cheddar
			    Shredded Part-Skim
			        Mozzarella
			Crumbled Blue Cheese
			Fancy Supreme:
			    Shredded Cheese for Nachos
			        and Tacos
			    Shredded Colby Jack Cheese
			    Shredded Mild Cheddar
			    Shredded Parmesan
			    Shredded Part-Skim
			        Mozzarella
			    Shredded Pizza Double
			        Cheese
			    Shredded Sharp Cheddar
			Italian, 6 Cheese:
			    Shredded Cheese
			Mexican (Shredded)
			MooTown Snackers:
			    Colby Jack Cheese
			    ∇ Mild Cheddar
			Natural Crumble:
			    Blue Cheese
			Natural Old Fashioned:
			    ∇ Ricotta Cheese
			Sliced Colby
			∇ Sliced Jarlsberg

∇ Low Sodium, 140 mg. or less per serving.

BRAND	BEST CHOICE	ACCEPTABLE CHOICE	OCCASIONAL CHOICE
	Low Saturated Fat	Contains Greater Than 1 Gram but Less Than 4 Grams Saturated Fat	High Saturated Fat
Sargento (Cont.)			Sliced Monterey Jack Sliced Mozzarella Sliced Muenster Sliced Provolone ∇ Sliced Swiss Swiss Cheese: ∇ Wafer Thin Style
Sealtest		Cottage Cheese Lowfat Cottage Cheese	
Smart Beat	Lactose Free: Non-Dairy Slices		

Sorrento	∇ Fat Free Ricotta Cheese		∇ Deli Style Part-Skim
			        Ricotta
			Pizza Cheese:
			    Mozzarella & Cheddar
			    Mozzarella, Romano &
			        Parmesan
			Whole Milk Mozzarella Cheese:
			    ∇ (Shredded)

Stella	∇ Fat Free Ricotta		

Weight Watchers	Fat Free:
	    Non Fat Slices
	    Swiss Slices
	Fat Free Grated Parmesan
	    Italian Topping:
	    ∇ (1 tablespoon serving)		

Win Schuler's		Bar-Scheeze:
		    Cheddar Cheese Spread
		Lite Bar-Scheeze:
		    All Flavors	

WisPride		Light: Port Wine Cheddar	
YOUR FAVORITE CHEESE AND CHEESE PRODUCTS NOT LISTED IN THE *GUIDE*			

∇ Low Sodium, 140 mg. or less per serving.

MILK AND MILK ALTERNATIVES

This food category contains a variety of dairy and non-dairy products. Dairy products such as milk are a significant source of the body's requirement for calcium, the mineral needed for the growth, maintenance, and repair of bones. Milk also provides protein, minerals, vitamin A, and vitamin D. Skim milk, 1/2% and 1% milk provide all of these nutrients with minimal amounts of fat.

Milk alternative-type products such as soy or rice beverages are also included in this category. Some of these products are fortified with calcium and may provide other nutritional benefits. These products are naturally low in saturated fat, are cholesterol-free, and may have other health benefits. However, because not all of these products are fortified with calcium, vitamin A and vitamin D, it is important for consumers to check the *Nutrition Facts* label, especially if the product is fed to children. These products (as well as skim milk) should **not** be used as a substitute for infant formulas or fed to children under two years of age.

Milk products are included as part of the "Milk, Yogurt, and Cheese Group" of the *Food Guide Pyramid*. In order to supply the body's daily requirements for the above nutrients, especially calcium, two to three servings of low-fat dairy products are recommended per day. Women who are pregnant or breast feeding, teenagers, and young adults to age 24 need three servings per day. One serving of milk is equal to 1 cup (8 ounces). The FDA has established reference amounts or standardized serving sizes for use on the food label. The reference amount for milk and milk-based drinks is 240 milliliters (8 ounces). Be sure to read the *Nutrition Facts* label for the serving size information of your milk choice. (See pages 51 and 52 for an explanation of reference amounts and the difference between serving sizes established by the FDA for food labeling and those recommended by the *Food Guide Pyramid*.)

The National Cholesterol Education Program Guidelines[35] recommend that Americans over the age of 2 reduce the amount of saturated fat in the diet to

less than 10% of total calories. Because whole milk, and whole-milk dairy products are significant contributors of saturated fat to the diet, the criteria for these categories were designed to distinguish those products that are lower in saturated fat from their higher saturated fat alternatives.

Criteria Key

▲ **Best Choice:**   **Low Saturated Fat**

Products listed in this category meet the FDA's definition for "Low Saturated Fat" (1 gram or less saturated fat per serving).

▲ **Acceptable Choice:**   **Contains Greater Than 1 Gram, but Less Than 4 Grams Saturated Fat**

Products listed in this category **do not** meet the FDA's definition for "Low Saturated Fat" but contain less than 4 grams saturated fat (less than 20% of the Daily Value).

▲ **Occasional Choice:**   **High Saturated Fat**

Products listed in this category are considered high in saturated fat because they contain 4 grams or more saturated fat per serving (20% or greater of the Daily Value). Foods in this category should be consumed only on occasion. If large amounts of food from this category were selected as part of a regular diet, it would be difficult to meet the *Dietary Guidelines for Americans*[11] for choosing a diet low in saturated fat.

BRAND	BEST CHOICE	ACCEPTABLE CHOICE	OCCASIONAL CHOICE
	Low Saturated Fat	Contains Greater Than 1 Gram but Less Than 4 Grams Saturated Fat	High Saturated Fat
All Brands	Buttermilk: ∇ Dry Lowfat: ∇ ½% Milk Nonfat Dry Milk ∇ Skim Milk ∇ Nonfat Chocolate Milk	∇ 2% Chocolate Milk ∇ 1% Chocolate Milk Buttermilk: Cultured ∇ Lowfat Egg Nog Lowfat: ∇ 1% Milk ∇ 2% Milk	∇ Chocolate Milk Egg Nog: ∇ Non Alcoholic ∇ Goat Milk ∇ Sheep Milk ∇ Whole Milk - 3.3%
Borden			∇ Egg Nog
C.F. Burger	∇ Fat Free Egg Nog Lactose Reduced: ∇ Nonfat	Lactose Reduced Creamery: ∇ 1% Milkfat	∇ Old Fashioned Egg Nog
Carnation	∇ Nonfat Dry Milk Powder		
Dairy Ease	Lactose Reduced: ∇ Nonfat Milk	Lactose Reduced: ∇ 1% Lowfat Milk	
Dean Foods	½% Cultured Buttermilk	Dairy Ease: ∇ Reduced Lactose Lowfat Milk	
Hershey		∇ Lowfat Milk in Drink Boxes	
Lactaid	Lactaid 100 Lactose Reduced: ∇ Nonfat Milk Lactose Reduced: ∇ Nonfat Milk ∇ Nonfat Milk, Calcium Fortified	Lactose Reduced: ∇ 1% Lowfat Milk	
Melody Farms		Cultured Lowfat Buttermilk	Vitamin D Chocolate Milk
Nestle		Quik Lowfat Milk: ∇ Banana	∇ Quik Chocolate Milk ∇ Quik Strawberry Milk
Parmalat	Long Life: ∇ Skim Milk	Long Life Lowfat Milk: ∇ 2% Shake A Shake Lowfat Milk: ∇ All Flavors	∇ Long Life Whole Chocolate Milk ∇ Long Life Whole Milk
Saco	Cultured Buttermilk Blend: Powdered		
Sanalac	∇ Nonfat Dry Milk		
Weight Watchers	∇ Nonfat Milk		

∇ Low Sodium, 140 mg. or less per serving.

BRAND	BEST CHOICE	ACCEPTABLE CHOICE	OCCASIONAL CHOICE
	Low Saturated Fat	Contains Greater Than 1 Gram but Less Than 4 Grams Saturated Fat	High Saturated Fat
EVAPORATED & CONDENSED MILK: 2 TABLESPOON SERVING			
All Brands	∇ Evaporated Skim Milk	∇ Evaporated Whole Milk	
Borden	Eagle Brand: ∇ Lowfat Sweetened Condensed Milk	Eagle Brand: ∇ Sweetened Condensed Milk	
Carnation	∇ Lite Evaporated Skimmed Milk	∇ Evaporated Milk ∇ Sweetened Condensed Milk	
Meadow Gold		∇ Sweetened Condensed Milk	
Meyenberg		∇ Evaporated Goat Milk	
Pet Inc.	∇ Evaporated Skimmed Milk	∇ Evaporated Milk	
MILK ALTERNATIVES			
All Brands	∇ Soy Milk		
Alta-Dena	Nonfat Liquid Yogurt Beverage: ∇ All Flavors		
Amazake	Light: ∇ Almond ∇ Original	∇ Almond Shake	
EdenBlend	Rice & Soy Beverage: ∇ Original		
EdenRice	Rice Beverage: ∇ Original		
EdenSoy	Dairy Free Soy Beverage Extra: ∇ Original ∇ Vanilla Organic Soy Beverage: ∇ Carob ∇ Original ∇ Vanilla		
Health Valley	∇ Fat Free Soy Moo		
Rice Dream	Enriched Non-Dairy Beverage: ∇ Chocolate ∇ Original		

∇ Low Sodium, 140 mg. or less per serving.

BRAND	BEST CHOICE	ACCEPTABLE CHOICE	OCCASIONAL CHOICE
	Low Saturated Fat	Contains Greater Than 1 Gram but Less Than 4 Grams Saturated Fat	High Saturated Fat
Rice Dream (Cont.)	Enriched Non-Dairy Beverage: ∇ Vanilla Lite Rice Beverage: ∇ All Flavors Rice Beverage: ∇ Original		
Westbrae Natural	Vitasoy Light Non-Dairy Beverage: ∇ All Flavors Vitasoy Natural Soy Drink: ∇ All Flavors ∇ Westsoy Lite Beverage Westsoy Low Fat Soy Beverage: ∇ All Flavors Westsoy Lunchbox Plus: ∇ Cocoa ∇ Plain ∇ Vanilla Westsoy Nonfat Soy Beverage: ∇ Plain ∇ Vanilla		
Wholesome and Hearty	Almond Mylk: All Flavors		
YOUR FAVORITE MILK AND MILK ALTERNATIVES NOT LISTED IN THE *GUIDE*			

∇ Low Sodium, 140 mg. or less per serving.

YOGURT AND NON-DAIRY ALTERNATIVES

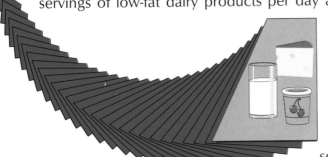

Foods in the yogurt category provide protein, calcium and other minerals, vitamin A, and vitamin D to the daily diet, as do other dairy products. Nonfat and low-fat yogurt provide as much of these nutrients as those made from whole milk, with minimal amounts of fat. Some yogurts are also high in sugar content. Those individuals monitoring their sugar or caloric intake may want to assess simple sugar as well as fat content of yogurt. Many low-calorie yogurts contain sugar substitutes such as NutraSweet®.

Yogurt products in this category are included as part of the "Milk, Yogurt, and Cheese Group" of the *Food Guide Pyramid*. In order to supply the body's daily requirements for the above nutrients, especially calcium, two to three servings of low-fat dairy products per day are recommended. Women who are pregnant or breast feeding, teenagers, and young adults to age 24 need three servings per day. One serving of yogurt is equal to 1 cup. The FDA has established reference amounts or standardized serving sizes for use on the food label. The reference amount for yogurt is 225 grams (8 ounces). Be sure to read the *Nutrition Facts* label for the serving size information of your yogurt choice. (See pages 51 and 52 for an explanation of reference amounts and the difference between serving sizes established by the FDA for food labeling and those recommended by the *Food Guide Pyramid*.)

Products in this category range from those that are made from skim milk and are fat-free, to those that are made from whole milk and provide a substantial amount of fat. The criteria were therefore designed to distinguish those products that are lowest in fat from their higher-fat alternatives.

Criteria Key

▲ **Best Choice:** **Fat Free**

Products listed in this category meet the FDA's definition for "Fat Free" (less than $1/2$ gram of fat per serving) and are the preferred choice.

△ **Acceptable Choice:** **Low Fat**

Products listed in this category meet the FDA's definition for "Low Fat" (3 grams or less fat per serving).

▲ **Occasional Choice:** **Contains Greater Than 3 grams Total Fat**

Products listed in this category **do not** meet the FDA's definition for "Low Fat." Because there are many other choices that will provide the same amount of nutrients with little or no saturated or total fat, the products listed in this category should be consumed only on occasion.

BRAND	BEST CHOICE	ACCEPTABLE CHOICE	OCCASIONAL CHOICE
	Fat Free	Low Fat	Contains Greater Than 3 Grams Total Fat

Alta-Dena	Nonfat Yogurt:
	  All Flavors
			Lowfat Yogurt:
			  All Flavors
			Maya Yogurt:
			  All Flavors

Axelrod	Nonfat Yogurt:
	  All Flavors
		Lowfat Yogurt:
		  All Flavors	

Breyers		Blended Lowfat Yogurt:
		  ∇ All Flavors
		Lowfat Yogurt:
		  ∇ All Flavors
		Mix 'N Crunch Yogurt:
		  Vanilla
			Mix 'N Crunch Yogurt:
			  ∇ Strawberry

Brown Cow Farm	Apricot Mango Nonfat Yogurt:
	  ∇ With Crunchy Granola
	Maple Walnut Nonfat Yogurt:
	  ∇ With Crunchy Granola
	Nonfat Yogurt:
	  ∇ Maple Walnut
	  ∇ Raspberry Popper
		Amaretto Nonfat Yogurt:
		  ∇ With Crunchy Granola
		Nonfat Yogurt:
		  ∇ Amaretto Topped w/
		    Crunchy Granola
			Whole Milk Yogurt:
			  ∇ Blueberry
			  ∇ Vanilla

Columbo	Fat Free Yogurt:
	  ∇ All Flavors
	Light 100:
	  ∇ All Flavors
			Regular Yogurt:
			  ∇ All Flavors

Cool Cups		Lowfat Yogurt: ∇ All Flavors	

Dannon	Blended Fat Free:
	  ∇ All Flavors
	Fat Free:
	  Plain
	Light:
	  All Flavors
		Danimals Lowfat Yogurt:
		  ∇ All Flavors
		Fruit on the Bottom:
		  ∇ All Flavors
		Premium Lowfat Yogurt:
		  Plain
		Sprinkl'ins:
		  ∇ All Flavors	

Gogurt		Gogurt: All Flavors	
Horizon	Nonfat Yogurt: ∇ All Flavors		

Knudsen	70 Calorie Nonfat Yogurt:
	  ∇ All Flavors
	Free Nonfat Yogurt:
	  ∇ All Flavors		

∇ Low Sodium, 140 mg. or less per serving.

BRAND	BEST CHOICE	ACCEPTABLE CHOICE	OCCASIONAL CHOICE
	Fat Free	Low Fat	Contains Greater Than 3 Grams Total Fat
La Yogurt	Light Yogurt: All Flavors	Sabor Latino Lowfat Yogurt: ∇ All Flavors	
Light N' Lively	Free: ∇ All Flavors	Kidpack Lowfat Yogurt: ∇ All Flavors Lowfat Yogurt: ∇ All Flavors	
Mountain High	Honey Light: ∇ All Flavors	Lowfat Yogurt: ∇ All Flavors	Whole Milk Yogurt: ∇ All Flavors
Stonyfield Farm	Nonfat Yogurt: ∇ All Flavors		Whole Milk Yogurt: ∇ All Flavors
TCBY	Nonfat Yogurt: All Flavors	Lowfat Yogurt: All Flavors	
Weight Watchers	Ultimate 90: ∇ All Flavors		
White Wave		Dairyless: ∇ Apricot-Mango ∇ Blueberry ∇ Lemon-Kiwi ∇ Peach ∇☆ Raspberry ∇☆ Strawberry ∇ Vanilla	Dairyless: ∇★ Plain
Yoplait	Crunch 'N Yogurt: Nonfat All Flavors Fat Free: Plain Extra Creamy Vanilla Extra Creamy Fat Free Fruit on the Bottom: ∇ All Flavors Fat Free Light Custard Style: ∇ All Flavors Fat Free Light Snack Pack: ∇ All Flavors Fat Free Light Yogurt: ∇ All Flavors	Breakfast Style Yogurt: ∇ All Flavors Crunch 'N Yogurt: ∇ Light All Flavors Vanilla w/Chocolate Crunchies Custard Style Yogurt: ∇ All Flavors Original Lowfat Yogurt: ∇ Fruit Flavors Trix Yogurt: ∇ All Flavors	
Yubi		Lowfat Yogurt: All Flavors	

∇ Low Sodium, 140 mg. or less per serving.
☆ Good Source of Fiber, between 2.5 g. and 5 g. per serving.
★ High Fiber, 5 g. or greater per serving.

BEEF, LAMB, PORK, AND VEAL

This category contains selections for standard cuts of fresh meats, including: beef, lamb, pork, and veal. Meats are especially good sources of high-quality proteins, highly-absorbable iron, zinc, vitamin B-12, niacin, potassium, phosphorous, and other minerals. However, some meats also provide significant amounts of fat, saturated fat, and cholesterol to the diet.

Meats are included as part of the "Meat, Poultry, Fish, Dry Beans, Eggs, and Nuts Group" of the *Food Guide Pyramid*. Since many foods from other food groups also contain protein, most Americans can obtain adequate protein by consuming 2 to 3 servings from this group per day. Two and one-half to three ounces of cooked lean meat, poultry, or fish, count as one serving from this food group. As a general rule, 3 ounces of cooked meat is approximately the size of a deck of cards or the size of the palm of a woman's hand. When preparing meats, it is recommended that you trim all visible fat and bake, broil, grill, or stir-fry using a small amount of monounsaturated oil (see Fats and Oils, pages 305-310).

For those who prefer to avoid or limit their intake of meat, equal amounts of protein can be obtained by substituting 1/2 cup of cooked beans, or 3 ounces of tofu, or 1 egg, or 2 tablespoons of nut butters for 1 ounce of meat (about 1/3 serving).

The criteria for the Beef, Lamb, Pork, and Veal product category are based on the Food Safety and Inspection Service (FSIS) of the U.S. Department of Agriculture's (USDA) nutrition labeling definitions for "Extra Lean" and "Lean." The criteria were therefore designed to distinguish those products lower in total fat, saturated fat, and cholesterol from their higher-fat and higher-cholesterol alternatives.

Criteria Key

▲ **Best Choice:** **Extra Lean**

Products listed in this category meet the USDA/FSIS definition for "Extra Lean" (less than 5 grams of fat, less than 2 grams of saturated fat, and less than 95 mg cholesterol per 100 grams or 3.5 ounces). Although lower in total fat and saturated fat than most other red meats, veal is higher in cholesterol, ranging from 103-158 milligrams per 100 grams or 3.5 ounces. Therefore, veal meets the "Extra Lean" definition for total fat and saturated fat but not for cholesterol. Veal cuts that contain 95 milligrams cholesterol or greater will be indicated by a ● symbol.

▲ **Acceptable Choice:** **Lean**

Products listed in this category meet the USDA/FSIS definition for "Lean" (less than 10 grams of fat, less than or equal to 4.5 grams of saturated fat, and less than 95 mg of cholesterol per 100 grams or 3.5 ounces). Although lower in total fat and saturated fat than most other red meats, veal is higher in cholesterol, ranging from 103-158 milligrams per 100 grams or 3.5 ounces. Therefore, veal meets the "Lean" definition for total fat and saturated fat but not for cholesterol. Veal cuts that contain 95 milligrams cholesterol or greater will be indicated by a ● symbol.

▲ **Occasional Choice:** **Contains Greater Than or Equal to 10 Grams Fat, or Greater Than 4.5 Grams Saturated Fat, or Greater Than or Equal to 95 mg Cholesterol per 100 Grams (3.5 ounces)**

Products listed in this category do not meet either definition for "Lean" or "Extra Lean." Choices from this category can add a significant amount of fat, saturated fat and cholesterol to the diet. For this reason, these meats should be consumed only on occasion.

Note
Nutrient data for the various cuts of meat were taken from "Nutri-Facts" and is based on USDA Handbook data for three-ounce cooked serving without added fat, salt, or sauces.[76]

BRAND	BEST CHOICE	ACCEPTABLE CHOICE	OCCASIONAL CHOICE
	Extra Lean	Lean	Contains Greater Than or Equal to 10 Grams Fat OR Greater Than 4.5 Grams Saturated Fat OR Greater Than or Equal to 95 mg. Cholesterol/100 g
BEEF			
Armour			▲ Homestyle Meatballs
Beef	▽ Eye of Round, Roast (trimmed of all visible fat) ▽ Top Round Steak (trimmed of all visible fat)	▽ Bottom Round Steak (trimmed of all visible fat) ▽ Chuck Arm Pot Roast (trimmed of all visible fat) ▽ Eye of Round, Roast (⅛" or more fat trim) ▽ Flank ▽ Ground Beef (91% Lean) ▽ Loin, Sirloin Steak (trimmed of all visible fat) ▽ Loin, Tenderloin Steak (trimmed of all visible fat) ▽ Round, Tip Roast (trimmed of all visible fat) ▽ Tip Round (trimmed of all visible fat) ▽ Top Loin, Steak (trimmed of all visible fat) ▽ Top Round, Steak (⅛" fat trim) ▽ Top Sirloin	▽ Bottom Round, Steak (⅛" or more fat trim) ▽ Chuck Blade Roast ▽ Ground Beef (10%-27% fat) ▽ Loin, Sirloin Steak (⅛" or more fat trim) ▽ Loin, Tenderloin Steak (⅛" or more fat trim) ▽ Rib Roast, Large-end ▽ Rib Roast, Small-end ▽ Round, Tip Roast (⅛" or more fat trim) ▽ Top Loin, Steak (⅛" or more fat trim) ▽ Whole Brisket
Beefalo		Beefalo: ▽ All Parts	
Coleman Natural Meats		▽ Bottom Round Roast ▽ Bottom Round Steak ▽ Eye of Round Steak ▽ Flank Steak ▽ Ground Beef (91% Lean) ▽ Kabobs ▽ London Broil ▽ New York Strip/Strip Loin ▽ Sirloin Tip Roast ▽ Tenderloin ▽ Top Round Steak ▽ Top Sirloin Steak	▽ Boneless Chuck Roast ▽ Brisket ▽ Ribeye Steak
Grobbel's	▲ Gourmet Corned Beef Brisket		

▲ High Sodium, 480 mg. or greater per serving.
▽ Low Sodium, 140 mg. or less per serving.

BRAND	BEST CHOICE	ACCEPTABLE CHOICE	OCCASIONAL CHOICE
	Extra Lean	Lean	Contains Greater Than or Equal to 10 Grams Fat OR Greater Than 4.5 Grams Saturated Fat OR Greater Than or Equal to 95 mg. Cholesterol/100 g
J.T.M.			▲ 8 ¼ Pound Beef Patties ▲ Hoagie Beef Patties
Laura's Lean Beef	∇ Eye of Round ∇ Ribeye Steak ∇ Sirloin Tip Round ∇ Sirloin Top Butt ∇ Strip Steak ∇ Top Round	∇ Flank Steak ∇ Ground Beef ∇ Ground Round ∇ Tenderloins	
Maverick Ranch	∇ Extra Lean Bottom Round Roast ∇ Extra Lean Chuck Arm Roast ∇ Extra Lean Cube Steak ∇ Extra Lean Eye of Round Roast ∇ Extra Lean Ground Round ∇ Extra Lean New York Strip ∇ Extra Lean Tenderloin Filet ∇ Extra Lean Top Round Steak or Roast ∇ Extra Lean Top Sirloin Steak	∇ Lean Flank Steak ∇ Lean Ground Chuck ∇ Lean Prime Rib or Rib Eye	
Plevalean		Burger Patty	
Thorn Apple Valley			▲ Corned Beef Brisket
L A M B			

Lamb		∇ Cubes For Stew
		∇ Loin Chop
		  (trimmed of all visible fat)
		∇ Shank
		  (trimmed of all visible fat)
		∇ Shoulder, Arm Chop
		  (trimmed of all visible fat)
		∇ Whole Leg
		  (trimmed of all visible fat)
			∇ Ground Lamb
			∇ Loin Chop
			  (⅛" or more fat trim)
			∇ Rib Roast
			∇ Shank
			  (⅛" or more fat trim)
			∇ Shoulder, Arm Chop
			  (⅛" or more fat trim)
			∇ Shoulder, Blade Chop
			∇ Whole Leg
			  (⅛" or more fat trim)

▲ High Sodium, 480 mg. or greater per serving.
∇ Low Sodium, 140 mg. or less per serving.

BRAND	BEST CHOICE	ACCEPTABLE CHOICE	OCCASIONAL CHOICE
	Extra Lean	Lean	Contains Greater Than or Equal to 10 Grams Fat OR Greater Than 4.5 Grams Saturated Fat OR Greater Than or Equal to 95 mg. Cholesterol/100 g
PORK			
Farmland		▲ Canned Ham	
Hormel	Light & Lean 97: ▲ Boneless Ham ▲ Smoked Pork Chops		
Patrick Cudahy	▲ Realean Ham		

Pork	▲ Boneless Smoked Ham
	  (95% Lean)
	∇ Loin, Tenderloin Roast
	  (trimmed of all visible fat)
		∇ Boneless Loin Chop
		  (trimmed of all visible fat)
		∇ Boneless Rib Roast
		  (trimmed of all visible fat)
		∇ Boneless Sirloin Chop
		  (trimmed of all visible fat)
		▲ Canadian Bacon
		∇ Center Chop Loin
		  (trimmed of all visible fat)
		∇ Loin, Rib Chop
		  (trimmed of all visible fat)
		∇ Loin, Sirloin Roast
		  (trimmed of all visible fat)
		∇ Loin, Tenderloin Roast
		  (⅛" fat trim)
		∇ Top Loin Chop
		  (trimmed of all visible fat)
		Top Loin Roast
		  (trimmed of all visible fat)
			∇ Center Chop, Loin
			  (⅛" or more fat trim)
			∇ Ground Pork
			∇ Loin, Country-Style Ribs
			∇ Loin, Rib Chop
			  (⅛" or more fat trim)
			∇ Loin, Sirloin Roast
			  (⅛" or more fat trim)
			∇ Shoulder, Blade Steak
			∇ Spareribs
			∇ Top Loin, Chop
			  (⅛" or more fat trim)
			∇ Top Loin, Roast
			  (⅛" or more fat trim)

Thorn Apple Valley	▲ Golden Classic Ham		
Tyson			▲ Ham Loaf
West Virginia Brand	▲ Old Fashioned Ham		
VEAL			

Veal	∇ Cutlets
	  (trimmed of all visible fat)
		∇ Cutlets
		  (⅛" fat trim)
		∇● Ground Veal
		∇ Loin Chop
		  (trimmed of all visible fat)
			∇ Loin Chop
			  (⅛" or more fat trim)
			∇● Rib Roast
			  (⅛" or more fat trim)

▲ High Sodium, 480 mg. or greater per serving.
∇ Low Sodium, 140 mg. or less per serving.
● Cholesterol, 95 mg. or greater per serving.

BRAND	BEST CHOICE	ACCEPTABLE CHOICE	OCCASIONAL CHOICE
	Extra Lean	Lean	Contains Greater Than or Equal to 10 Grams Fat OR Greater Than 4.5 Grams Saturated Fat OR Greater Than or Equal to 95 mg. Cholesterol/100 g
Veal (Cont.)		∇● Rib Roast (trimmed of all visible fat) ∇● Shoulder, Arm Steak ∇● Shoulder Blade Steak	
YOUR FAVORITE MEATS NOT LISTED IN THE *GUIDE*			

∇ Low Sodium, 140 mg. or less per serving.
● Cholesterol, 95 mg. or greater per serving.

POULTRY AND GAME

This category contains selections of fresh poultry and game, including: chicken, turkey, duck, goose, pheasant, quail, rabbit, venison, elk, and other game. Foods in this section are similar in nutrient composition to those in other meat categories. These foods are good sources of high-quality proteins, highly absorbable iron, zinc, vitamin B-12, niacin, potassium, phosphorous, and other minerals. However, unlike most red meats, many poultry and game products are lower in total fat and saturated fat.

Poultry and game products are included as part of the "Meat, Poultry, Fish, Dry Beans, Eggs, and Nuts Group" of the *Food Guide Pyramid*. Because many foods from other food groups also contain protein, most Americans can obtain adequate protein by consuming 2 to 3 servings from this group per day. Two and one half to three ounces of cooked lean meat, poultry, or fish count as one serving from this food group. Equal amounts of protein can be obtained by substituting $1/2$ cup of cooked beans, or 3 ounces of tofu, or 1 egg, or 2 tablespoons of nut butters for 1 ounce of meat (about $1/3$ serving). As a general rule, a three ounce serving of cooked poultry is equivalent to a half chicken breast or a thigh and leg. When preparing poultry or game products, it is recommended that you trim all visible fat, remove the skin, and bake, broil, grill or stir-fry using a small amount of monounsaturated oil (see Fats and Oils, pages 305-310).

The criteria for the Poultry and Game product category are based on the Food Safety and Inspection Service (FSIS) of the U.S. Department of Agriculture's (USDA) nutrition labeling definitions for "Extra Lean" and "Lean." The criteria were therefore designed to distinguish those products lower in total fat, saturated fat, and cholesterol from their higher-fat and higher-cholesterol alternatives.

Criteria Key

▲ **Best Choice:**   **Extra Lean**

Products listed in this category meet the USDA/FSIS definition for "Extra Lean" (less than 5 grams of fat, less than 2 grams of saturated fat, and less than 95 mg cholesterol per 100 grams or 3.5 ounces).

▲ **Acceptable Choice:**   **Lean**

Products listed in this category meet the USDA/FSIS definition for "Lean" (less than 10 grams of fat, less than or equal to 4.5 grams of saturated fat, and less than 95 mg of cholesterol per 100 grams or 3.5 ounces).

▲ **Occasional Choice:**   **Contains Greater Than or Equal to 10 Grams Fat, or Greater Than 4.5 Grams Saturated Fat, or Greater Than or Equal to 95 mg Cholesterol per 100 Grams (3.5 ounces)**

Products listed in this category do not meet either definition for "Lean" or "Extra Lean." Choices from this category can add a significant amount of fat, saturated fat, and cholesterol to the diet. For this reason, these meats should be consumed only on occasion.

Note
Nutrient data for the various cuts of meat were taken from "Nutri-Facts" and is based on USDA Handbook data for three-ounce cooked serving without added fat, salt, or sauces.[76]

---

214   Poultry and Game

Brand	Best Choice	Acceptable Choice	Occasional Choice
	Extra Lean	Lean	Contains Greater Than or Equal to 10 Grams Fat OR Greater Than 4.5 Grams Saturated Fat OR Greater Than or Equal To 95 mg. Cholesterol/100 g
Buffalo	▽ Buffalo Meat		
Butter Moist		Turkey Roast: ▲ Boneless White	Turkey Roast: ▲ Boneless White & Dark
Butterball	▲ Hickory Smoked Skinless Breast of Turkey Portion ▲ Oven Roasted Skinless Breast of Turkey Portion		▽ Whole Turkey
Chicken	▽ Skinless Breast ▽ Skinless Drumstick ▽ Skinless Whole Chicken (without neck or giblets)	▽ Breast w/Skin ▽ Drumsticks w/Skin ▽ Skinless Thigh ▽ Skinless Wings	▽ Thigh w/Skin ▽ Whole Chicken w/Skin (without neck or giblets) ▽ Wings w/Skin
Duck	Wild Duck without Skin: ▽ Breast	▽ Domesticated Duck without Skin	▽ Duck w/Skin
Elk	Elk: ▽ All Parts		
Empire		Chicken Patty Nuggets	Fried Chicken Drumsticks & Thighs Turkey Patties
Frankenmuth Poultry Company	Frankenmuth Chicken: ▽ Whole Chicken		
Goose		▽ Domesticated Goose without Skin	
Guinea	Guinea without Skin		
Hormel	Light & Lean 97: ▲ Boneless Turkey		
Lloyds	Chicken Fillet: ▲ With Barbeque Sauce		
Louis Rich		▲ Original Turkey Sausage	▽ Pure Ground Turkey ▲ Turkey Nuggets ▲ Turkey Sticks
Mr. Turkey			▽ Frozen Ground Turkey Turkey Breakfast Sausage

▲ High Sodium, 480 mg. or greater per serving.
▽ Low Sodium, 140 mg. or less per serving.

BRAND	BEST CHOICE	ACCEPTABLE CHOICE	OCCASIONAL CHOICE
	Extra Lean	Lean	Contains Greater Than or Equal to 10 Grams Fat OR Greater Than 4.5 Grams Saturated Fat OR Greater Than or Equal To 95 mg. Cholesterol/100 g
Ostrich	▲ Gourmet Ham ∇ Ostrich Steak Smoked, Peppered Ostrich	∇ Fillet Mignon	

Pheasant	Pheasant without Skin:
	   ∇ Breast
	   ∇ Leg		

Quail	Quail without Skin:
	   ∇ Breast
			Quail Flesh and Skin:
			   ∇ All Other Parts

Rabbit	Wild Rabbit:
	   All Parts
		Domesticated Rabbit:
		   All Parts	

Squab (Pigeon)			Squab Flesh and Skin: All Parts
Swift Premium			Turkey Roast: ▲ White & Dark

The Turkey Store	∇ Boneless Breast Tenderloins
	∇ Breast Slices
	▲ Hickory Seasoned Turkey
	   Breast Steaks
	▲ Italian Seasoned Turkey
	   Breast Filets
	Premium Fresh Turkey:
	   ∇ Extra Lean Ground Breast
		∇ Lean Burger Patties
		Premium Fresh Cooked Turkey:
		   ∇ Lean Ground	

Turkey	∇ Ground Turkey Breast
	   (all meat, no skin)
	∇ Skinless Breast
	∇ Skinless Drumstick
	∇ Skinless Whole Turkey
	   (without neck or giblets)
	∇ Skinless Wings
		∇ Breast w/Skin
		∇ Drumstick w/Skin
		∇ Ground Turkey
		∇ Skinless Turkey Thigh
		∇ Thigh w/Skin
		∇ Whole Turkey w/Skin
		   (without neck or giblets)
			∇ Wings w/Skin

Tyson	∇ Boneless Skinless Chicken
	   Breast Portions
	Roasted Chicken:
	   ▲ Ready to Eat
		Breast Fillets
		Drums:
		   Hot Barbecue Style Chicken
		   Drumsticks
			Boneless Chicken Breast
			Breast Patties:
			   Regular
			   Southern Fried
			Breast Tenders
			Chicken Half Breasts
			Chicken Patties

▲ High Sodium, 480 mg. or greater per serving.
∇ Low Sodium, 140 mg. or less per serving.

BRAND	BEST CHOICE	ACCEPTABLE CHOICE	OCCASIONAL CHOICE
	Extra Lean	Lean	**Contains Greater Than or Equal to 10 Grams Fat OR Greater Than 4.5 Grams Saturated Fat OR Greater Than or Equal To 95 mg. Cholesterol/100 g**
Tyson (Cont.)			Wings: ▽ Barbecue Style Chicken Wings ▲ Hot 'n Spicy Chicken Wings Roasted Chicken Wings ▲ Wings of Fire
Venison	Venison: ▽ All Parts		
YOUR FAVORITE POULTRY AND GAME NOT LISTED IN THE *GUIDE*			

▲ High Sodium, 480 mg. or greater per serving.
▽ Low Sodium, 140 mg. or less per serving.

FISH

This category contains selections of fresh fish and shellfish. Similar to meat, fish and shellfish are good sources of high-quality protein, vitamins, and minerals; but **unlike** meat, most are usually low in fat and particularly low in saturated fat. More importantly, some fish are high in a type of polyunsaturated fat called omega-3 fatty acids.

Omega-3 fatty acids are thought to protect against heart disease in three ways: (1) thinning the blood, making platelets less sticky and, therefore, less likely to cause a blood clot; (2) by lowering blood triglycerides; and (3) by decreasing the tendency of **certain** blood cells to stick to the linings of arteries, therefore inhibiting the incorporation of fat into the walls of the arteries.

At this time, it is not known how much Omega-3 fatty acids are needed in order to have a beneficial effect. However, research has shown that men who eat as little as 8 ounces of fish per week are half as likely to die from heart disease as those who do not eat fish.[76] Many health authorities recommend regular consumption of fish.

On the other hand, fish oil capsules taken as supplements to lower cholesterol are generally not recommended without medical monitoring. Health risks of using fish oil supplements may include:

◆ Undesirable effects on blood clotting

◆ Possible toxic amounts of vitamin A and vitamin D

◆ Possible presence of environmental contaminants such as lead or mercury.

Newer, more sophisticated analytical methods for measuring the cholesterol content of shellfish have revealed that shellfish are lower in cholesterol than previously thought. Most shellfish (e.g., lobster, clams, oysters, scallops, crab), on average, contain lower amounts of cholesterol than equal portions of lean red

meat or poultry. Although shrimp contains twice the amount of cholesterol as equal portions of lean meats, it is 91% lower in saturated fat. As discussed on page 37, saturated fat is more likely to elevate blood cholesterol than is dietary cholesterol. Therefore, shrimp can be judiciously included as part of a low-cholesterol, low-saturated fat diet. Cholesterol is not used to evaluate fish and shellfish in this section, but those products with 95 mg or more of cholesterol per 3^1/$_2$ ounce serving will be indicated by a ● symbol.

Fish and shellfish products are included as part of the "Meat, Poultry, Fish, Dry Beans, Eggs, and Nuts Group" of the *Food Guide Pyramid*. Because many foods from other food groups also contain protein, most Americans can obtain adequate protein by consuming 2 to 3 servings from this group per day. Two and one-half to three ounces of cooked lean meat, poultry, or fish count as one serving from this food group. As a general rule, a three-ounce serving of cooked fish is equivalent to the size of a deck of cards or the size of the palm of a woman's hand. When preparing fish or shellfish products, it is recommended that you remove the fatty skin and boil, steam, poach, bake, broil, grill or stir-fry using a small amount of monounsaturated oil (see Fats and Oils, pages 305-310).

The criteria for the Fish product category are based on the Food Safety and Inspection Service (FSIS) of the U.S. Department of Agriculture's (USDA) nutrition labeling definitions for "Extra Lean" and "Lean," **with one exception**: Because fish and shellfish are low in saturated fat, which is known to have a greater effect on blood cholesterol levels than is cholesterol itself, the cholesterol descriptor of these definitions was removed. However, those fish that contain greater than 95 mg of cholesterol per 3.5 ounce serving will be indicated by a ● symbol.

Criteria Key

▲ **Best Choice:** **Contains Less Than 5 Grams Total Fat AND Less Than 2 Grams Saturated Fat per 100 Grams (3.5 oz)**

Fish products listed in this category meet the USDA/FSIS "Extra Lean" definition for total fat and saturated fat but may not for cholesterol. Those fish that contain 95 milligrams of cholesterol or greater per 3.5 ounce serving will be indicated by a ● symbol.

▲ **Acceptable Choice:** **Contains Greater Than or Equal to 5 Grams, but Less Than 10 grams of Total Fat, AND Greater Than or Equal to 2 Grams, but Less Than or Equal to 4.5 Grams Saturated Fat per 100 Grams (3.5 oz)**

Fish products listed in this category meet the USDA/FSIS "Lean" definition for total fat and saturated fat but may not for cholesterol. Those fish that contain 95 milligrams of cholesterol or greater per 3.5 ounce serving will be indicated by a ● symbol.

▲ **Occasional Choice:** **Contains Greater Than or Equal to 10 Grams Total Fat or Greater Than 4.5 Grams Saturated Fat per 100 Grams (3.5 oz)**

Fish products listed in this category **do not** meet either the "Lean" or "Extra Lean" definition for total fat and saturated fat. Choices from this category can add a significant amount of total fat and saturated fat to the diet. For this reason, only occasional consumption is recommended. Those fish selections that contain 95 milligrams of cholesterol or greater per 3.5 ounce serving will be indicated by a ● symbol.

BRAND	BEST CHOICE	ACCEPTABLE CHOICE	OCCASIONAL CHOICE
	Contains Less Than 5 Grams Total Fat AND Less Than 2 Grams Saturated Fat per 100 grams (3.5 oz)	Contains Greater Than or Equal to 5 Grams but Less Than 10 Grams Total Fat AND Greater Than or Equal to 2 Grams but Less Than or Equal to 4.5 Grams Saturated Fat per 100 grams (3.5 oz.)	Contains Greater Than or Equal to 10 Grams Total Fat OR Greater Than 4.5 Grams Saturated Fat per 100 grams (3.5 oz)
Crustaceans	▲ Crab, Alaska King Crab, Blue Crab, Dungeness ▲ Crab, Queen ∇● Crayfish, Unspecified Lobster, Northern ● Shrimp, Boiled Spiny Lobster Mixed Species		
Finfish	∇ Anchovy, European ∇ Bass, Freshwater ∇ Bass, Striped ∇ Bluefish ∇ Burbot ∇ Catfish, Channel ∇ Cisco ∇ Cod, Atlantic ∇ Cod, Pacific ∇ Croaker, Atlantic ∇ Dolphinfish ∇ Flounder ∇ Grouper, Mixed Species ∇ Haddock ∇ Halibut, Atlantic & Pacific ∇ Mackerel, King ∇ Mullet, Striped ∇ Ocean Perch, Atlantic ∇ Pike, Northern ∇ Pike, Walleye ∇ Pollock, Atlantic ∇ Pollock, Walleye ∇ Rockfish, Pacific, Mixed Species ∇ Roughy, Orange ∇ Salmon, Chum ∇ Salmon, Pink ∇ Sea Bass, Mixed Species ∇ Seatrout, Mixed Species ∇ Shark ∇ Sheepshead ∇ Smelt, Rainbow	∇ Carp ∇ Drum, Freshwater ∇ Herring, Atlantic ∇ Mackerel, Spanish ∇ Pompano, Florida ● Roe, Mixed Species ∇ Salmon, Atlantic ∇ Salmon, Coho ∇ Salmon, Sockeye ∇ Whitefish, Mixed Species ∇ Yellowtail	Sardine, Atlantic: ▲● Packed in Oil and Drained

▲ High Sodium, 480 mg. or greater per serving.
∇ Low Sodium, 140 mg. or less per serving.
● Cholesterol, 95 mg. or greater per serving.

BRAND	BEST CHOICE	ACCEPTABLE CHOICE	OCCASIONAL CHOICE
	Contains Less Than 5 Grams Total Fat AND Less Than 2 Grams Saturated Fat per 100 grams (3.5 oz)	Contains Greater Than or Equal to 5 Grams but Less Than 10 Grams Total Fat AND Greater Than or Equal to 2 Grams but Less Than or Equal to 4.5 Grams Saturated Fat per 190 grams (3.5 oz.)	Contains Greater Than or Equal to 10 Grams Total Fat OR Greater Than 4.5 Grams Saturated Fat per 100 grams (3.5 oz)
Finfish (Cont.)	∇ Snapper, Mixed Species ∇ Spot ∇ Sturgeon, Mixed Species ∇ Sunfish, Pumpkinseed Surimi ∇ Swordfish ∇ Trout, Rainbow ∇ Tuna, Bluefin ∇ Tuna, Skipjack ∇ Tuna, Yellowfin Turbot, European ∇ Whiting, Mixed Species ∇ Wolffish, Atlantic		
Mollusks	Abalone, Mixed Species ● Cuttlefish Mussel, Blue ∇ Octopus, Common ∇ Oyster, Eastern ∇ Oyster, Pacific Scallop, Mixed Species ∇● Squid, Mixed Species Whelk, Mixed Species		
FROZEN			
Aqua Star	∇ Cod Fillets		
Contessa	● Cooked Shrimp Scallops		
Delta-Pride		Catfish: ▲ Breaded Fillet Strips ∇ Catfish Nuggets	
Fisher Boy		Crispy Batter Dip Fish Portions	▲ Crunchy Fish Sticks
Gorton's		Grilled Fillets: Italian Herb Lemon Pepper	Batter Dipped Fish Portions ▲ Crispy Fish Fillets in Batter

▲ High Sodium, 480 mg. or greater per serving.
∇ Low Sodium, 140 mg. or less per serving.
● Cholesterol, 95 mg. or greater per serving.

224 **Fish**

BRAND	BEST CHOICE	ACCEPTABLE CHOICE	OCCASIONAL CHOICE
	Contains Less Than 5 Grams Total Fat AND Less Than 2 Grams Saturated Fat per 100 grams (3.5 oz)	Contains Greater Than or Equal to 5 Grams but Less Than 10 Grams Total Fat AND Greater Than or Equal to 2 Grams but Less Than or Equal to 4.5 Grams Saturated Fat per 100 grams (3.5 oz.)	Contains Greater Than or Equal to 10 Grams Total Fat OR Greater Than 4.5 Grams Saturated Fat per 100 grams (3.5 oz)
Gorton's (Cont.)			Crunchy Breaded Fish Fillets: ▲ Garlic and Herb ▲ Hot & Spicy ▲ Regular Crunchy Breaded Fish Sticks Potato Breaded Fish Fillets Potato Breaded Fish Sticks
Mrs. Paul's	Healthy Treasures: Breaded Fish Fillets Breaded Fish Sticks	▲ Crispy Crunchy Breaded Fish Sticks	Batter Dipped Fish Fillets ▲ Crispy Crunchy Breaded Fish Fillets Premium Fillets: ▲ Cod ▲ Flounder
Northern King	▲● Cooked Shrimp		
Schooner	∇ Cod Fillets	∇ Alaska Pollock Fillets ∇ Ocean Pearch Fillets Shrimp Crunchies	
Sea Harvest	Cape Capensis Loins		
SeaPak	∇ Ocean Perch Fillets		▲ Popcorn Shrimp ▲ Shrimp Poppers
Taste O'Sea	∇ Cod Fillets		
Van de Kamp's	Crisp & Healthy: Baked, Breaded Fish Fillets Baked, Breaded Fish Sticks		Breaded Fish Fillets Breaded Fish Sticks ▲ Breaded Whole Popcorn Shrimp ▲ Breaded Whole Shrimp
YOUR FAVORITE FISH NOT LISTED IN THE *GUIDE*			

▲ High Sodium, 480 mg. or greater per serving.
∇ Low Sodium, 140 mg. or less per serving.
● Cholesterol, 95 mg. or greater per serving.

LUNCHMEATS, CURED MEATS, AND CANNED MEATS, FISH, POULTRY

This food category contains a variety of processed lunchmeats such as bologna, salami, sausage, and frankfurters, along with other canned and cured meats, fish and poultry. Processed meats can contain large quantities of "hidden fat," saturated fat, and sodium. There are many new processed lunchmeat-type products on the market that are lower in saturated fat, total fat, and cholesterol. It is important for consumers to check the nutrition label to see how much total fat, saturated fat, cholesterol, and sodium each product provides per serving.

These processed meat products are included as part of the "Meat, Poultry, Fish, Dry Beans, Eggs, and Nuts Group" of the *Food Guide Pyramid*. Because many foods from other food groups also contain protein, most Americans can obtain adequate protein by consuming 2 to 3 servings from this group per day. Two and one-half to three ounces of cooked lean meat, poultry, or fish count as one serving from this food group. As a general rule, three ounces of canned meat is equivalent to 3/4 cup. Serving size for processed lunchmeats varies according to the thickness of the slice. Consumers are encouraged to read product labels to determine the appropriate serving size. (See pages 51 and 52 for an explanation of reference amounts and the difference between serving sizes established by the FDA for food labeling and those recommended by the *Food Guide Pyramid*.)

Meat products fall under the food labeling jurisdiction of the Food Safety and Inspection Service (FSIS) of the U.S. Department of Agriculture (USDA). USDA/FSIS has formally adopted the FDA's definitions for "Low Fat" and "Low Saturated Fat." The criteria were, therefore, designed to distinguish those products lower in total fat and saturated fat from their higher-fat alternatives.

Criteria Key

▲ **Best Choice:** **Low Fat AND Low Saturated Fat**

Products listed in this category meet the FDA's definition for "Low Fat" (3 grams or less fat per serving) and "Low Saturated Fat" (1 gram or less per serving).

▲ **Acceptable Choice:** **Contains Greater Than 3 Grams but Less Than or Equal to 5 Grams Total Fat AND Low Saturated Fat**

Products listed in this category **do not** meet the FDA's definition for "Low Fat," but **do** meet the definition for "Low Saturated Fat." The 5 grams of total fat cut-off was used in order to be consistent with the amount of fat equal to one diabetes diet fat exchange and is also equivalent to 1 teaspoon of added fat.[75] These products are therefore higher in total fat than those listed in the "Best Choice" category but are equally as low in saturated fat.

▲ **Occasional Choice:** **Contains Greater Than 5 Grams Total Fat, or Greater Than 1 Gram Saturated Fat**

Products listed in this category **do not** meet the FDA's definition for either "Low Fat," or "Low Saturated Fat." Those products that contain greater than 5 grams of total fat per serving are also listed in this category. These products can contribute a significant amount of fat to the overall daily diet and should be consumed only on occasion.

BRAND	BEST CHOICE	ACCEPTABLE CHOICE	OCCASIONAL CHOICE
	Low Fat AND Low Saturated Fat	Contains Greater Than 3 Grams but Less Than or Equal to 5 Grams Total Fat AND Low Saturated Fat	Contains Greater Than 5 Grams Total Fat OR Greater Than 1 Gram Saturated Fat
All Brands (per 55 grams)			▲ Bacon ▲ Beer Salami ▲ Bologna ▲ Bratwurst ▲ Braunschweiger ▲ Breakfast Strips ▲ Corned Beef Brisket ▲ Frankfurter/Hot Dog ▲ Pastrami ▲ Pepperoni ▲ Salami ▲ Sausage
Armour	Canadian Style Bacon: ▲ 95% Fat Free ▲ Sliced Dried Beef		Premium Pepperoni: ▲ Italian Style ▲ Treet Luncheon Loaf Vienna Sausage
Best's Kosher			▲ Bagel Dog Beef Frankfurters: ▲ Jumbo Size Lower Fat Lower Sodium ▲ More Beef Than Bun Regular Beef Knackwurst: ▲ Lower Fat ▲ Regular ▲ Beef Polish Sausage ▲ Cooked Corned Beef ▲ Mini Bagel Dogs
Bob Evans			Brown & Serve Country Lite Sausage Links Grillin' Sausage: ▲ Italian ▲ Homestyle Sausage Gravy & Biscuits ▲ Italian Sausage Pork Sausage: ▲ All Flavors Small Casing Links Patties ▲ Sausage & Biscuits
Butterball	Chicken Breast-Smoked		▲ Bun Size Turkey Franks

▲ High Sodium, 480 mg. or greater per serving.

Lunchmeats, Cured Meats, and Canned Meat, Fish, Poultry 229

BRAND	BEST CHOICE	ACCEPTABLE CHOICE	OCCASIONAL CHOICE
	Low Fat AND Low Saturated Fat	Contains Greater Than 3 Grams but Less Than or Equal to 5 Grams Total Fat AND Low Saturated Fat	Contains Greater Than 5 Grams Total Fat OR Greater Than 1 Gram Saturated Fat

Butterball (Cont.)	Cooked Turkey Salami
	Deli Thin Sliced:
	  Honey Roasted & Smoked Turkey
	  ▲ Oven Roasted Turkey Breast
	  Smoked Chicken Breast
	  Smoked Turkey Breast
	▲ Fat Free Franks
	Fat Free Oven Roasted Chicken Breast
	Fat Free Turkey Breast:
	  Honey Roasted & Smoked
	  Oven Roasted
	▲ Smoked White Turkey
	Turkey Breast:
	  Honey Roasted
	  Oven Roasted
	  Smoked
	Turkey Ham:
	  Honey Cured
	  ▲ Regular
			Lean Fresh Turkey:
			  ▲ Bratwurst
			  ▲ Polish Sausage
			Turkey Bacon
			▲ Turkey Bologna
			▲ Turkey Salami
			▲ Turkey Smoked Sausage

Carl Buddig			▲ Chicken ▲ Corned Beef ▲ Ham ▲ Honey Ham ▲ Honey Roasted Turkey ▲ Pastrami ▲ Smoked Beef
Country Club Brand			▲ Sliced Corned Beef ▲ Sliced Smoked Beef ▲ Sliced Smoked Chicken ▲ Sliced Smoked Ham ▲ Sliced Smoked Turkey

Eckrich	▲ Cooked Ham
	Ham and Cheese Loaf
	Honey Style Loaf
	▲ Lower Sodium Cooked Ham
		Lean Slender Sliced:
		  ▲ Smoked Chicken
			Beef Bologna
			Beef Franks
			▲ Beef Lebanon Bologna
			Beef Smoky Links
			Bologna
			Bun Size Franks:
			  ▲ Reduced Fat
			  ▲ Beef Franks
			▲ Cotto Beef Salami

▲ High Sodium, 480 mg. or greater per serving.

230 **Lunchmeats, Cured Meats, and Canned Meat, Fish, Poultry**

BRAND	BEST CHOICE	ACCEPTABLE CHOICE	OCCASIONAL CHOICE
	Low Fat AND Low Saturated Fat	Contains Greater Than 3 Grams but Less Than or Equal to 5 Grams Total Fat AND Low Saturated Fat	Contains Greater Than 5 Grams Total Fat OR Greater Than 1 Gram Saturated Fat

Eckrich (Cont.)			Country Sausage
			Franks
			Garlic Bologna
			German Brand Bologna
			▲ Hard Salami
			Jumbo Polska Kielbasa
			Lean Slender Sliced:
			  ▲ Beef
			  ▲ Corned Beef
			  ▲ Smoked Ham
			  ▲ Smoked Turkey
			Macaroni & Cheese Loaf
			Old Fashioned Loaf
			Olive Loaf
			Reduced Fat:
			  ▲ Polska Kielbasa
			  ▲ Smoked Sausage
			Sandwich Bologna
			Smok-Y-Links Sausage:
			  Beef
			  Cheese
			  ▲ Ham
			  ▲ Maple
			  Original
			  ▲ Reduced Fat
			Smoked Sausage:
			  ▲ Reduced Fat
			  Regular
			▲ Thin Sliced Bologna

Empire	Smoked Turkey Breast Turkey Breast	Turkey Salami	Chicken Bologna
Farmer Peet's	▲ Ham Steak		
Farmland			▲ Salt Pork Belly

Healthy Choice	▲ Baked Cooked Ham
	Beef Bologna
	Bologna
	▲ Cooked Ham
	▲ Lowfat Beef Franks
	Deli Thin Sliced:
	  ▲ Baked Cooked Ham
	  ▲ Cooked Ham
	  ▲ Honey Ham		

▲ High Sodium, 480 mg. or greater per serving.

BRAND	BEST CHOICE	ACCEPTABLE CHOICE	OCCASIONAL CHOICE
	Low Fat AND Low Saturated Fat	Contains Greater Than 3 Grams but Less Than or Equal to 5 Grams Total Fat AND Low Saturated Fat	Contains Greater Than 5 Grams Total Fat OR Greater Than 1 Gram Saturated Fat

Healthy Choice (Cont.)	Deli Thin Sliced:
	   Oven Roasted Chicken Breast
	   ▲ Oven Roasted Turkey Breast
	   ▲ Roast Beef
	Franks:
	   Lowfat
	Honey Roasted & Smoked
	   Turkey Breast
	▲ Low Fat Polska Kielbasa
	▲ Low Fat Smoked Sausage
	Oven Roasted Chicken Breast
	Oven Roasted Turkey Breast
	▲ Polska Kielbasa
	Smoked Chicken Breast
	▲ Smoked Ham
	▲ Smoked Sausage
	Smoked Turkey Breast		

Hebrew National			Lean Beef Bologna Reduced Fat Beef Franks
Hereford			Corned Beef

Hillshire Farm	▲ Brown Sugar Baked Ham
	Deli Select:
	   ▲ Corned Beef
	   ▲ Cured Beef
	   ▲ Honey Ham
	   ▲ Honey Roasted Turkey
	      Breast
	   ▲ Oven Roasted Chicken
	      Breast
	   ▲ Oven Roasted Turkey Breast
	   ▲ Pastrami
	   ▲ Smoked Beef
	   ▲ Smoked Chicken Breast
	   ▲ Smoked Ham
	   ▲ Smoked Turkey Breast
	▲ Honey Ham
	▲ Oven Roasted Turkey Breast
	▲ Smoked Chicken Breast
			▲ Lit'l Smokies
			▲ Lit'l Wieners
			▲ Lite Polska Kielbasa
			▲ Lite Smoked Sausage
			Polska Kielbasa
			Smoked Sausage

Hormel	Light & Lean 97:
	   ▲ Deli Bologna
	   ▲ Deli Corned Beef
	   ▲ Deli Cotto Loaf
	   ▲ Deli Ham
			Pepperoni Slices
			SPAM:
			   ▲ Lite
			   ▲ Regular
			   ▲ Smoke Flavored

▲ High Sodium, 480 mg. or greater per serving.

Brand	Best Choice	Acceptable Choice	Occasional Choice
	Low Fat AND Low Saturated Fat	Contains Greater Than 3 Grams but Less Than or Equal to 5 Grams Total Fat AND Low Saturated Fat	Contains Greater Than 5 Grams Total Fat OR Greater Than 1 Gram Saturated Fat
Hormel (Cont.)	Light & Lean 97: ▲ Deli Pastrami ▲ Dinner Link ▲ Honey Turkey Breast ▲ Meat Franks ▲ Sliced Ham ▲ Sliced Turkey Smoked Ham Cuts Smoked Turkey Cuts Turkey Cuts		Vienna Sausage
HyGrade's	Ball Park: ▲ Fat Free Classic Frank		Ball Park: Bologna ▲ Bun Size Beef Franks ▲ Bun Size Franks ▲ Corn Dogs ▲ Franks ▲ Lite Franks ▲ Beef Franks Black Label Bacon: Original Bologna: Beef Garlic Regular Grill Master: Chicken Bologna Grill Master: ▲ Chicken Cheese Franks ▲ Chicken Franks ▲ Turkey Franks ▲ Hot Dogs Salami
Jefferson	▲ Jellied Pot Roast Beef Loaf		
Jennie O		▲ Turkey Ham	
Jimmy Dean			▲ Hot Pork Sausage Regular Light: ▲ Turkey and Pork Sausage ▲ Regular Pork Sausage
Johnsonville			▲ Beddar w/Cheddar ▲ Beef Bratwurst ▲ Cheesy Beer & Bratwurst

▲ High Sodium, 480 mg. or greater per serving.

Lunchmeats, Cured Meats, and Canned Meat, Fish, Poultry 233

BRAND	BEST CHOICE	ACCEPTABLE CHOICE	OCCASIONAL CHOICE
	Low Fat AND Low Saturated Fat	Contains Greater Than 3 Grams but Less Than or Equal to 5 Grams Total Fat AND Low Saturated Fat	Contains Greater Than 5 Grams Total Fat OR Greater Than 1 Gram Saturated Fat
Johnsonville (Cont.)			▲ Cooked Bratwurst ▲ Hot Italian Sausage ▲ Original Bratwurst ▲ Polish Sausage ▲ Smoked Bratwurst ▲ Smoked Sausage ▲ Texas Brand Hot Links
Jones Dairy Farm	Canadian Style Bacon		
Koegel			Bologna ▲ Braunschweiger Pickled Bologna ▲ Ring Bologna Skinless Frankfurters Viennas Natural Casing
Kowalski	Baked Krakowska		Bologna Fresh Liver Sausage Garlic Bologna Garlic Ring Bologna Keilbasa Loaf Natural Casing Franks ▲ Natural Casing Stadium Keilbasa Polish Keilbasa Ring Bologna Skinless Franks ▲ Skinless Stadium Kielbasa Smoked Liver Sausage Smoked Sausage
Land O Frost			▲ Thin Sliced Beef ▲ Thin Sliced Chicken ▲ Thin Sliced Ham ▲ Thin Sliced Honey Turkey ▲ Thin Sliced Turkey
Louis Rich	Carving Board Meats: ▲ Honey Glazed Ham ▲ Oven Roasted Turkey Breast ▲ Smoked Ham Cooked Turkey Salami: 50% Less Fat	Turkey Bologna: 50% Less Fat	Bun Length Franks: ▲ 50% Less Fat Franks: ▲ 50% Less Fat

▲ High Sodium, 480 mg. or greater per serving.

BRAND	BEST CHOICE	ACCEPTABLE CHOICE	OCCASIONAL CHOICE
	Low Fat AND Low Saturated Fat	Contains Greater Than 3 Grams but Less Than or Equal to 5 Grams Total Fat AND Low Saturated Fat	Contains Greater Than 5 Grams Total Fat OR Greater Than 1 Gram Saturated Fat
Louis Rich (Cont.)	Deli-Thin: ▲ Hickory Smoked Turkey Breast ▲ Oven Roasted Chicken Breast ▲ Oven Roasted Turkey Breast Hickory Smoked Turkey: Fat Free Oven Roasted Turkey Breast: 98% Fat Free Fat Free Turkey Bacon Turkey Cotto Salami Turkey Ham		
Mr. Turkey	Deli Cuts: ▲ Hardwood Smoked Turkey Breast ▲ Hardwood Smoked Turkey Ham ▲ Hardwood Smoked Turkey Pastrami ▲ Roast Turkey Breast ▲ Smoked Chicken Breast ▲ Hardwood Smoked Turkey Ham Oven Roasted Turkey Breast Turkey Bacon Turkey Cotto Salami ▲ Turkey Ham		▲ Cheese Franks Hearty Blend: ▲ Polish Kielbasa Hearty Blend Smoked Sausage: ▲ Lean Turkey: ▲ Bun Size Franks Turkey Bologna ▲ Turkey Franks ▲ Turkey Italian Style Smoked Sausage ▲ Turkey Polish Kielbasa ▲ Turkey Smoked Sausage
Oscar Mayer	▲ Baked Cooked Ham ▲ Boiled Ham Deli Thin: ▲ Boiled Ham ▲ Honey Glazed Chicken Breast ▲ Honey Ham ▲ Roast Turkey Breast Free: ▲ Bologna ▲ Chicken Hot Dogs ▲ Smoked Turkey ▲ Turkey		Bacon: America's Favorite Center Cut Thick Cut Beef Bologna: Light Regular Beef Franks: ▲ Bun Length Regular Big & Juicy Hot Dogs: ▲ Deli Style Beef ▲ Original

▲ High Sodium, 480 mg. or greater per serving.

Lunchmeats, Cured Meats, and Canned Meat, Fish, Poultry 235

BRAND	BEST CHOICE	ACCEPTABLE CHOICE	OCCASIONAL CHOICE
	Low Fat AND Low Saturated Fat	Contains Greater Than 3 Grams but Less Than or Equal to 5 Grams Total Fat AND Low Saturated Fat	Contains Greater Than 5 Grams Total Fat OR Greater Than 1 Gram Saturated Fat
Oscar Mayer (Cont.)	Healthy Favorites: ▲ Bologna ▲ Hot Dogs ▲ Smoked Cooked Ham ▲ Honey Ham ▲ Smoked Cooked Ham		Bologna: Light Regular ▲ Braunschweiger ▲ Cotto Salami ▲ Hard Salami Liver Cheese Wieners: ▲ Bun Length Regular
Ostrich	Salami ▲ Summer Sausage		
Pavone			▲ Pepperoni
Plum Rose			Premium Bacon
Rath Black Hawk			Breakfast Beef Hickory Smoked Bacon Hot Dogs: ▲ Bigger Than The Bun Polska Kielbasa: ▲ Skinless Smoked Sausage: ▲ Skinless
Swift Premium	▲ Dried Beef		Brown 'N Serve Sausage: Original Microwave ▲ Pizza Size 'Peperoni'
The Turkey Store	Gobble Stix: All Flavors		Breakfast Sausage Links Italian Sausage: ▲ Sweet Lean Lean Italian Sausage: ▲ Hot Turkey Italian Sausage: ▲ Mild
Thorn Apple Valley	▲ Boneless Ham Premium Sliced Turkey Breast Turkey Ham		Beef Bologna ▲ Braunschweiger Cooked Salami Hickory Smoked Bacon ▲ Liverwurst Pickle Loaf ▲ Red Hots

▲ High Sodium, 480 mg. or greater per serving.

236 **Lunchmeats, Cured Meats, and Canned Meat, Fish, Poultry**

BRAND	BEST CHOICE	ACCEPTABLE CHOICE	OCCASIONAL CHOICE
	Low Fat AND Low Saturated Fat	Contains Greater Than 3 Grams but Less Than or Equal to 5 Grams Total Fat AND Low Saturated Fat	Contains Greater Than 5 Grams Total Fat OR Greater Than 1 Gram Saturated Fat

Thorn Apple Valley (Cont.)			▲ Skinless Polish Sausage
			Skinless Smoked Sausage:
			    ▲ Regular
			    ▲ Spicy
			    ▲ w/Italian Seasonings
			Smoky Links Sausage:
			    Regular
			∇ Spiral Sliced Ham

Tyson			Chicken Bologna ▲ Chicken Franks

West Virginia Brand	Cooked Ham		Bacon:
			    Real Smoked Flavor
			    ▲ Thick Sliced
			▲ Boneless Golden Ham

CANNED			
Beach Cliff			Kippered Snacks
Breast O' Chicken	Chunk Light Tuna: in Water		
Brunswick			Kippered Snacks
Bulldog			▲ Maine Sardines in Soybean Oil

Bumble Bee	Chunk Light Tuna:
	    in Water
	Chunk Pink Salmon:
	    in Water
	Chunk White Tuna:
	    in Water
	Solid White Tuna:
	    in Water
		Alaska Pink Salmon
		Skinless Boneless Pink Salmon:
		    in Water
			Chunk Light Tuna:
			    in Vegetable Oil
			▲ Red Salmon

Chicken of the Sea	Chunk Light Tuna in Spring Water Chunk White Tuna in Spring Water: ∇ Very Low Sodium	Pink Salmon	Chunk Light Tuna in Canola Oil
Deming's		Alaska Pink Salmon	Alaska Red Sockeye Salmon

▲ High Sodium, 480 mg. or greater per serving.
∇ Low Sodium, 140 mg. or less per serving.

Lunchmeats, Cured Meats, and Canned Meat, Fish, Poultry   237

BRAND	BEST CHOICE	ACCEPTABLE CHOICE	OCCASIONAL CHOICE
	Low Fat AND Low Saturated Fat	Contains Greater Than 3 Grams but Less Than or Equal to 5 Grams Total Fat AND Low Saturated Fat	Contains Greater Than 5 Grams Total Fat OR Greater Than 1 Gram Saturated Fat
Doxsee	Chopped Clams		
Empress			▲ Jack Mackerel
Featherweight	Chunk Light Tuna: ▽ in Water	Tuna Combo Kit	
Harris	Fancy Lump Crab Meat Fancy White Crab Meat		

Hyde Park	Chunk Light Tuna:
	  in Water
			Chunk Light Tuna:
			  in Oil

Iceland Waters			Kippered Herring
International Bazaar	Claw Crab Meat ▲ Fancy White Crab Meat		Kipper Snacks
MW Polar	Broken Shrimp Crab Meat Fancy Whole Baby Clams ▽ Fancy Whole Smoked Oysters Minced Clams Tiny Whole Shrimp		Fancy Whole Oysters Smoked Clams
Orleans	▲ Deveined Medium Shrimp Fancy Whole Baby Clams ▽ Fancy Whole Oysters		Fancy Smoked Baby Clams Fancy Smoked Oysters Kipper Snacks
Pillar Rock			Red Salmon
Reese	▲ Anchovies Deep Sea Clams Precooked French Helix Snails		▽ Skinless & Boneless Sardines in Water

Roland			Sardines:
			  Lightly Smoked in Soybean
			    Oil

Seasons	▲ Flat Fillets of Anchovies		Skinless Boneless Sardines
Singleton	▽ Peeled & Deveined Shrimp		
Spirit of Norway			King Oscar Sardines in Mustard Sauce

▲ High Sodium, 480 mg. or greater per serving.
▽ Low Sodium, 140 mg. or less per serving.

238   **Lunchmeats, Cured Meats, and Canned Meat, Fish, Poultry**

BRAND	BEST CHOICE	ACCEPTABLE CHOICE	OCCASIONAL CHOICE
	Low Fat AND Low Saturated Fat	Contains Greater Than 3 Grams but Less Than or Equal to 5 Grams Total Fat AND Low Saturated Fat	Contains Greater Than 5 Grams Total Fat OR Greater Than 1 Gram Saturated Fat
Spirit of Norway (Cont.)			Kipper Snacks Sardines by King Oscar: in Soybean Oil
StarKist	Chunk Light Tuna in Spring Water ∇ Chunk White Tuna in Pure Distilled Water Solid White Tuna in Spring Water		Chunk Light Tuna in Vegetable Oil
Swanson	White Chicken in Water		Mixin' Chicken in Broth
Underwood			Chicken Spread Deviled Ham Spread
Valley Fresh	Premium Chunk: ∇ White Chicken in Water		
YOUR FAVORITE MEAT PRODUCTS NOT LISTED IN THE *GUIDE*			

∇ Low Sodium, 140 mg. or less per serving.

Lunchmeats, Cured Meats, and Canned Meat, Fish, Poultry 239

EGG SUBSTITUTES AND EGG PRODUCTS

This category contains a variety of egg substitutes and other egg products. Most egg substitutes are made from egg whites with added flavorings, colorings, preservatives, and salt. Some egg products may or may not have added fat, cheese, egg yolks, or other ingredients. Egg whites are an excellent source of protein and contain no cholesterol. The yolk is particularly rich in phosphorous, sulfur, iron and vitamin A, but unfortunately, provides the single most concentrated source of cholesterol (213 mg per yolk) in the American diet. The American Heart Association recommends that healthy Americans consume no more than four egg yolks per week, including those used in cooking. It is, therefore, not necessary to consume these egg substitute products in order to maintain a healthful diet; however, many people prefer to do so.

Products in this food category can be included as part of the "Meat, Poultry, Fish, Dry Beans, Eggs, and Nuts Group" of the *Food Guide Pyramid*. Two to three servings from this group are recommended per day. Two and one-half to three ounces of cooked lean meat, poultry, or fish, count as one serving from this food group. One egg, which is often equivalent to 1/4 cup of an egg substitute product, can substitute for one ounce of lean meat (about 1/3 serving). The FDA has established reference amounts or standardized serving sizes for use on the food label. The reference amount for an egg or egg substitute is 50 grams (amount to equal one large egg). Be sure to read the *Nutrition Facts* label for the serving size information of your egg product choice. (See pages 51 and 52 for an explanation of reference amounts and the difference between serving sizes established by the FDA for food labeling and those recommended by the *Food Guide Pyramid*.)

Criteria for these products are designed to distinguish those products lower in total fat, saturated fat, and cholesterol from their higher-fat and higher- cholesterol alternatives.

Criteria Key

▲ **Best Choice:**   **Fat Free or Low Fat, AND Cholesterol Free, AND Low Saturated Fat**

Products listed in this category meet the FDA's definitions for "Fat Free" (less than ½ gram fat per serving) or "Low Fat" (3 grams or less fat per serving), and are "Cholesterol free" (less than 5 mg of cholesterol), and "Low Saturated Fat" (1 gram or less saturated fat).

▲ **Acceptable Choice:**   **Low Fat, AND Low Cholesterol, or Greater Than 1 Gram Saturated Fat**

Products listed in this category meet the FDA's definitions for "Low Fat" (3 grams or less total fat) and "Low Cholesterol" (20 mg or less cholesterol). They **do not**, however, meet the definition for "Low Saturated Fat."

▲ **Occasional Choice:**   **Contains Greater Than 3 Grams Total Fat**

Products listed in this category **do not** meet the FDA's definition for "Low Fat."

BRAND	BEST CHOICE	ACCEPTABLE CHOICE	OCCASIONAL CHOICE
	Fat Free or Low Fat AND Cholesterol Free AND Low Saturated Fat	Low Fat AND Low Cholesterol OR Greater Than 1 Gram Saturated Fat	Contains Greater Than 3 Grams Total Fat
Fleischmann's	∇ Frozen Egg Beaters ∇ Refrigerated Egg Beaters		
Healthy Choice	∇ Cholesterol Free Egg Product		
Morningstar Farms	∇ Better 'n Eggs ∇ Scramblers		

Papetti's	100% Fat Free:
	  ∇ Liquid Egg Product
	  ∇ Liquid Egg Product w/ Skim Milk
	Healthy Morn:
	  ∇ Frozen Egg Substitute		

Quick Eggs	∇ Quick Eggs		
Second Nature	∇ No Cholesterol Real Egg Product		
YOUR FAVORITE EGG SUBSTITUTES AND PRODUCTS NOT LISTED IN THE GUIDE			

∇ Low Sodium, 140 mg. or less per serving.

LEGUMES AND MEAT ALTERNATIVES

This category contains a wide variety of legumes (dry beans and peas) that are processed either dry, frozen, or canned. Legumes are excellent sources of complex carbohydrate (starch), fiber, protein, potassium, phosphorous, and iron. Like all plant-based foods, legumes contain no cholesterol and only minimal amounts of saturated fat. They are also high in water-soluble fiber, which has been shown to help lower cholesterol levels and to stabilize blood sugar.[50-53]

Products in the Legumes and Meat Alternatives category are included as part of the "Meat, Poultry, Fish, Dry Beans, Eggs, and Nuts Group" of the *Food Guide Pyramid*. Because many foods from other food groups also contain protein, most Americans can obtain adequate protein by consuming 2 to 3 servings from this group per day. Two and one-half to three ounces of cooked lean meat, poultry, or fish count as one serving from this food group. For those who prefer to avoid or limit their intake of meat, equal amounts of protein can be obtained by substituting 1/2 cup of cooked beans, or 1 egg, or 2 tablespoons of nut butter for 1 ounce of lean meat (about 1/3 serving).

Legumes are protein-rich and are a low-fat, cholesterol-free alternative to meat. Because of their excellent nutritional quality and health benefits, regular consumption of legumes is recommended. Legumes can be substituted for, or combined with, smaller amounts of lean meat, fish, or poultry for a tasty main dish that can provide less fat and calories.

The Legumes and Meat Alternatives category contains a wide range of products, ranging from those that have little or no fat or sodium, to those processed with substantial amounts of fat and salt. The criteria were, therefore, designed to distinguish those products lower in total fat, saturated fat, and sodium from their higher-fat and higher-sodium alternatives.

Criteria Key

▲ **Best Choice:**   **Fat Free or Low Fat, AND Low Saturated Fat, AND Less Than 480 mg Sodium**

Products listed in this category meet the FDA definition for "Fat Free" (less than $1/2$ gram fat per serving) or "Low Fat" (3 grams or less fat per serving), and "Low Saturated Fat" (1 gram or less saturated fat per serving). These products contain less than 480 milligrams sodium per serving (less than 20% of the Daily Value).

△ **Acceptable Choice:**   **Contains Greater Than 3 Grams, but Less Than or Equal to 5 Grams Total Fat, OR Greater Than 1 Gram Saturated Fat, OR Greater than 480 mg Sodium**

Products listed in this category either **do not** meet the FDA's definition for "Low Fat," or for "Low Saturated Fat," or may contain greater than 20% (480 milligrams) of the Daily Value for sodium. The 5 grams of total fat cut-off was used in order to be consistent with the amount of fat equal to one diabetes diet fat exchange and is also equivalent to 1 teaspoon of added fat.[75]

▲ **Occasional Choice:**   **Contains Greater Than 5 Grams Total Fat**

Those products that contain greater than 5 grams of total fat per serving are listed in this category. These products can contribute a significant amount of fat to the overall daily diet and should be consumed only on occasion.

BRAND	BEST CHOICE	ACCEPTABLE CHOICE	OCCASIONAL CHOICE
	Fat Free or Low Fat AND Low Saturated Fat AND Less Than 480 mg. Sodium	Contains Greater Than 3 Grams but Less Than or Equal to 5 Grams Total Fat OR Low Fat and Greater Than 1 Gram Saturated Fat OR Greater Than 480 mg. Sodium	Contains Greater Than 5 Grams Total Fat
CANNED			
American Prairie	Beans: ∇☆ Black Beans ∇☆ Garbanzo Beans ∇☆ Kidney Beans		
Aunt Nellie's		▲★ Reber Butter Beans	
B & M	★ Brick Oven Baked Beans KC Masterpiece: ★ Barbeque Baked Beans		
Bearitos		Fat Free Refried Black Beans: ▲☆ Traditional ▲☆ Vegetarian	
Brooks		▲★ Chili Hot Beans in Chili Sauce ▲★ Chili Mix ▲★ Dark Red Kidney Beans ▲★ Mild Chili Beans	
Bush's Best	★ Dark Red Kidney Beans	Baked Beans: ▲★ Bacon ▲★ Onions ▲★ Original ▲★ Vegetarian ▲★ Baked Beans in Homestyle Sauce ▲★ Blackeye Peas ▲★ Chili Hot Beans	
Campbell's	Baked Beans: ☆ Barbecue ★ New England Style ★ Pork and Beans Vegetarian Beans: ★ in Tomato Sauce	Baked Beans: ▲★ Brown Sugar & Bacon ▲★ Chili Beans	

▲ High Sodium, 480 mg. or greater per serving.
∇ Low Sodium, 140 mg. or less per serving.
☆ Good Source of Fiber, between 2.5 g. and 5 g. per serving.
★ High Fiber, 5 g. or greater per serving.

BRAND	BEST CHOICE	ACCEPTABLE CHOICE	OCCASIONAL CHOICE
	Fat Free or Low Fat AND Low Saturated Fat AND Less Than 480 mg. Sodium	Contains Greater Than 3 Grams but Less Than or Equal to 5 Grams Total Fat OR Low Fat and Greater Than 1 Gram Saturated Fat OR Greater Than 480 mg. Sodium	Contains Greater Than 5 Grams Total Fat
Chi Chi's		Restaurant Refried Beans: ▲☆ Fat Free	▲☆ Refried Beans Restaurant Refried Beans: ▲☆ Vegetarian
DaVinci	∇☆ Chick Peas		
Eden	∇★ Organic Adzuki Beans ∇★ Organic Black Beans ∇★ Organic Garbanzo Beans ∇★ Organic Kidney Beans ∇★ Organic Navy Beans ∇★ Organic Pinto Beans		
Green Giant		▲★ Baked Beans	
Hain	★ Black Turtle Beans ★ Chick Peas		
Hanover	★ Chick Peas ★ Dark Red Kidney Beans ★ Redskin Kidney Beans	▲★ Brown Sugar and Bacon Baked Beans	
Health Valley	∇★ Fat Free Honey Baked Beans Vegetarian Cuisine: ★ Amaranth & Vegetables ★ Lentil Garden Vegetable ★ Tofu Baked Beans ★ Tofu Black Beans ★ Tofu Lentil ★ Western Black Bean & Veggies		
Heartland		▲★ Iron Kettle Baked Beans	
Heinz		▲★ Vegetarian Beans in Tomato Sauce	
Hunt's		▲★ Big John's Beans 'n Fixins Homestyle: ▲★ Chili Fixin's	

▲ High Sodium, 480 mg. or greater per serving.
∇ Low Sodium, 140 mg. or less per serving.
☆ Good Source of Fiber, between 2.5 g. and 5 g. per serving.
★ High Fiber, 5 g. or greater per serving.

Brand	Best Choice	Acceptable Choice	Occasional Choice
	Fat Free or Low Fat AND Low Saturated Fat AND Less Than 480 mg. Sodium	Contains Greater Than 3 Grams but Less Than or Equal to 5 Grams Total Fat OR Low Fat and Greater Than 1 Gram Saturated Fat OR Greater Than 480 mg. Sodium	Contains Greater Than 5 Grams Total Fat
Jack Rabbit	∇★ Black Turtle Beans ∇★ Red Kidney Beans		
Joan of Arc	★ Dark Red Kidney Beans	▲★ Spicy Chili Beans	
Kuner's	Black Beans: ★ Regular ∇★ Southwestern		
La Preferida	∇★ Black Beans ★ Garbanzos/Chick Peas ★ Pinto Beans Refried Beans: ☆ Vegetarian	Refried Beans: ☆ Authentic	Refried Beans: ▲★ Spicy Ranchero
Margaret Holmes	★ Black Eyed Peas ★ Great Northern Beans ★ Pinto Beans		
Old El Paso		▲★ Fat Free Refried Beans Refried Beans: ▲★ Original ▲★ With Green Chilies ▲★ Vegetarian Refried Beans	Refried Beans: ★ w/Sausage
Ortega		▲★ Refried Beans	
Progresso	★ Black Beans ★ Cannellini ★ Chick Peas ★ Fava Beans ★ Pinto Beans ★ Red Kidney Beans		
Randall	★ Deluxe Pinto Beans ★ Great Northern Beans ★ Mixed Beans		
Read	☆ Three Bean Salad		
Reber		▲★ Butter Beans California Butter Beans: ▲★ Seasoned w/Molasses	

▲ High Sodium, 480 mg. or greater per serving.
∇ Low Sodium, 140 mg. or less per serving.
☆ Good Source of Fiber, between 2.5 g. and 5 g. per serving.
★ High Fiber, 5 g. or greater per serving.

Legumes and Meat Alternatives 249

BRAND	BEST CHOICE	ACCEPTABLE CHOICE	OCCASIONAL CHOICE
	Fat Free or Low Fat AND Low Saturated Fat AND Less Than 480 mg. Sodium	Contains Greater Than 3 Grams but Less Than or Equal to 5 Grams Total Fat OR Low Fat and Greater Than 1 Gram Saturated Fat OR Greater Than 480 mg. Sodium	Contains Greater Than 5 Grams Total Fat
S & W		Brick Oven: ▲★ All Natural Baked Beans ▲ Chili Beans in a Zesty Sauce Chili Makin's: ▲★ Black Bean ▲★ Homestyle ▲★ Original ▲★ Santa Fe ▲★ Maple Sugar Baked Beans	
Sea Side	☆ Butter Beans ★ Dark Red Kidney Beans	▲☆ Garbanzo Beans	
Taco Bell	★ Refried Beans		
The Allens	★ Blackeye Peas w/Bacon ★ Green and White Lima Beans ★ Purple Hull Peas ★ Tiny Tender Field Peas w/ Snaps		
Trappey's	★ Jalapeno Navy Beans ★ Navy Beans ★ Pinto Beans	▲★ Jalapeno Pinto Beans ▲★ Jalapeno Pork & Beans	
Van Camp's	★ New Orleans Style Red Kidney Beans	▲★ Pork and Beans	
Vigo		▲★ Black Beans & Rice ▲☆ Red Beans & Rice	
Westbrae Natural	Canned Beans: ▽★ All Varieties		
Wiley's	★ Precious Purple Hull Peas		
DRIED			
All Brands	▽☆ Anasazi Beans ▽★ Black Beans ▽☆ Black Eyed Peas		

▲ High Sodium, 480 mg. or greater per serving.
▽ Low Sodium, 140 mg. or less per serving.
☆ Good Source of Fiber, between 2.5 g. and 5 g. per serving.
★ High Fiber, 5 g. or greater per serving.

BRAND	BEST CHOICE	ACCEPTABLE CHOICE	OCCASIONAL CHOICE
	Fat Free or Low Fat AND Low Saturated Fat AND Less Than 480 mg. Sodium	Contains Greater Than 3 Grams but Less Than or Equal to 5 Grams Total Fat OR Low Fat and Greater Than 1 Gram Saturated Fat OR Greater Than 480 mg. Sodium	Contains Greater Than 5 Grams Total Fat
All Brands (Cont.)	∇☆ Black Turtle Beans ∇★ Cranberry Beans ∇☆ Garbanzo Beans ∇★ Great Northern Beans ∇☆ Green Split Peas ∇★ Lentils ∇☆ Lima Beans ∇★ Navy Beans ∇★ Pinto Beans ∇★ Red Kidney Beans ∇★ Soybeans ∇☆ Whole Green Peas ∇☆ Yellow Split Peas		

Arrowhead Mills	Dried Legumes:
	  ∇☆ Anasazi Beans
	  ∇☆ Black Turtle Beans
	  ∇☆ Chickpeas
	  ∇★ Kidney Beans
	  ∇★ Pinto Beans
	  ∇★ Soybeans
	  ∇☆ Split Peas-Green		

Bascam's	∇☆ Dried Black Beans ∇☆ Dried Lentils		
Bean Cuisine	∇☆ Anasazi Beans ∇☆ Black Turtle Beans ∇☆ Cranberry Beans ∇☆ Garbanzo Beans ∇☆ Great Northern Beans ∇☆ Pinto Beans ∇☆ Small Red Beans ∇☆ Soldier Beans ∇☆ Steuben Yellow Eye Beans		

Carlson-Arbogast Farm	Bean Appetit:
	  ∇★ Black Turtle Beans
	  ∇★ Cranberry Beans
	  ∇★ Dark Red Kidney Beans
	  ∇★ Yellow Eye Beans		

∇ Low Sodium, 140 mg. or less per serving.
☆ Good Source of Fiber, between 2.5 g. and 5 g. per serving.
★ High Fiber, 5 g. or greater per serving.

BRAND	BEST CHOICE	ACCEPTABLE CHOICE	OCCASIONAL CHOICE
	Fat Free or Low Fat AND Low Saturated Fat AND Less Than 480 mg. Sodium	Contains Greater Than 3 Grams but Less Than or Equal to 5 Grams Total Fat OR Low Fat and Greater Than 1 Gram Saturated Fat OR Greater Than 480 mg. Sodium	Contains Greater Than 5 Grams Total Fat
Fantastic Foods	★ Instant Black Beans ★ Instant Refried Beans		
Martha White	▽☆ Black Eyed Peas ▽☆ Dry Baby Lima Beans ▽☆ Garbanzo Beans ▽★ Lentils ▽★ Red Kidney Beans		
MEAT ALTERNATIVES			
Amy's	☆ California Veggie Burger		
Azumaya	▽ Regular Firm Tofu	▽ Extra Firm Tofu ▽ Soft Tofu	

Boca Burger	98% Fat Free Boca Burger:
	  ☆ Chef Max's Favorite
	Meatless Boca Burger:
	  ★ Original		

Casbah		▲ Falafel Mix	
Chiecko	▽ Tofu		
Fantastic Foods	★ Nature's Burger Tofu Burger	▲★ Falafel Tofu Classics: ▲☆ Mandarian Chow Mein	
Frieda's	Tofu: ▽ Firm or Soft		
Green Giant		Harvest Burgers: ★ Original	
Ken & Robert's	Veggie Burger		
Lightlife	Fat Free Meatless Smart Dogs ▽ Meatless Lean Links Meatless Light Burgers Meatless Smart Deli Slices: All Varieties		

▲ High Sodium, 480 mg. or greater per serving.
▽ Low Sodium, 140 mg. or less per serving.
☆ Good Source of Fiber, between 2.5 g. and 5 g. per serving.
★ High Fiber, 5 g. or greater per serving.

BRAND	BEST CHOICE	ACCEPTABLE CHOICE	OCCASIONAL CHOICE
	Fat Free or Low Fat AND Low Saturated Fat AND Less Than 480 mg. Sodium	Contains Greater Than 3 Grams but Less Than or Equal to 5 Grams Total Fat OR Low Fat and Greater Than 1 Gram Saturated Fat OR Greater Than 480 mg. Sodium	Contains Greater Than 5 Grams Total Fat
Lightlife (Cont.)	Meatless Smart Dog to Go! Savory Seitan: All Varieties ∇ Tofu Pups Wonderdogs		
Mori-Nu	∇ Lite Silken Tofu ∇ Silken Tofu		
Morningstar Farms		Meatless Breakfast Links Meatless Breakfast Patties ☆ Meatless Garden Vege Patties ☆ Meatless Prime Patties	▲ Meatless Chick Patties ▲ Meatless Deli Franks ☆ Meatless Grillers
Mudpie		★ Veggie Burger	
Near East		Falafel Mix: ▲★ Vegetable Burger Mix	
Soy Boy	Meatless Leaner Wieners Veggie Sizzler	Not Dogs	
Today's Menu		Veggie Pattie: ☆ Original ☆ Zesty Italian	
White Wave	Meatless Healthy Franks Meatless Sandwich Slices: Beef-Style Chicken-Style Pastrami-Style Turkey-Style Tempeh: ∇★ Sea Veggie Veggie Burger: ★ Tempeh ★ Teriyaki Tempeh Veggie Life	▲ Meatless Jumbo Franks ∇ Reduced Fat Tofu Tempeh: ∇☆ 5-Grain ∇★ Soy Rice ∇★ Wild Rice	Baked Tofu: Italian Garlic Herb Mexican Jalapeno Oriental Teriyaki Thai Sesame Peanut ★ Meatless Healthy Links Meatless Sandwich Slices: ★ Bologna-Style Tempeh: ∇★ Original Soy Veggie Burger: ☆ Lemon Broil
Wholesome and Hearty	★ Garden Burger Garden Dogs	★ Garden Mexi Burger	

▲ High Sodium, 480 mg. or greater per serving.
∇ Low Sodium, 140 mg. or less per serving.
☆ Good Source of Fiber, between 2.5 g. and 5 g. per serving.
★ High Fiber, 5 g. or greater per serving.

BRAND	BEST CHOICE	ACCEPTABLE CHOICE	OCCASIONAL CHOICE
	Fat Free or Low Fat AND Low Saturated Fat AND Less Than 480 mg. Sodium	Contains Greater Than 3 Grams but Less Than or Equal to 5 Grams Total Fat OR Low Fat and Greater Than 1 Gram Saturated Fat OR Greater Than 480 mg. Sodium	Contains Greater Than 5 Grams Total Fat
Wholesome and Hearty (Cont.)	▽☆ Garden Sausage ★ Garden Veggie Burger		

Worthington	Natural Touch:
	   ☆ Fat Free Vegan Burger
	Vegetarian Burger
	Veja-Links
		Natural Touch:
		   ☆ Garden Vege Pattie
		Wham:
		   Vegetable Protein Roll
			▲ Meatless Salami
			Natural Touch:
			   Garden Grain Pattie
			   ☆ Lentil Rice Loaf
			   ★ Nine Bean Loaf
			   ☆ Okara Patty
			   ☆ Vege Burger
			   Vege-Frank
			Prosage Links
			Prosage Patties
			Sliced Chik
			▲☆ Smoked Beef Slices
			▲ Smoked Turkey Slices

Yves Veggie Cuisine	☆ Burger Burgers Chili Dogs Deli Slices ★ Garden Vegetable Patties ☆ Tofu Weiners Veggie Pepperoni Veggie Weiners	▲ Canadian Veggie Bacon	
YOUR FAVORITE PRODUCTS NOT LISTED IN THE *GUIDE*			

▲ High Sodium, 480 mg. or greater per serving.
▽ Low Sodium, 140 mg. or less per serving.
☆ Good Source of Fiber, between 2.5 g. and 5 g. per serving.
★ High Fiber, 5 g. or greater per serving.

254 **Legumes and Meat Alternatives**

MEALS AND MAIN DISHES

This category contains meal-type products such as frozen and canned entrées and dinners. Under FDA rules, a **Main Dish** must weigh at least 6 ounces and contain at least two different foods from at least two specified food groups. A **Meal** must weigh at least 10 ounces and have at least three different foods from at least two specified food groups. The specific food groups that the FDA has identified are: Bread, Cereal, Rice, and Pasta Group; Fruit and Vegetable Group; Milk, Yogurt, and Cheese Group; and Meat, Poultry, Fish, Dry Beans, Eggs, and Nuts Group. This grouping is similar to that of the *Food Guide Pyramid* (see Authors' Note below). Meals and Main Dishes, therefore, offer variety to the diet by providing servings from two or more food groups. Some processed meal-type products, however, have the potential of contributing excessive amounts of fat and sodium to the diet.

Claims that a meal or main dish is "Low Fat" can be made if the product contains no more than 3 grams of fat per 3.5 ounces (100 grams) of product and less than 30% of calories from fat. Similarly, a low-saturated-fat claim can be made if the meal or main dish contains no more than 1 gram of saturated fat per 3.5 ounces (100 grams) of product and no more than 10% of calories from fat. Additionally, in order to meet the FDA's/USDA's definition for "Healthy" these products must also contain no more than 90 mg of cholesterol and no more than 600 mg of sodium per labeled serving size and contain at least 10% of the Daily Value of two or more of the following nutrients: vitamin A, vitamin C, iron, calcium, protein, and fiber.

The Dietary Guidelines for Americans[11] recommend that most people choose a diet lower in fat, saturated fat, and cholesterol in order to maintain a healthy weight and to reduce the risk of cardiovascular disease and certain types of cancer. Criteria were, therefore, designed to reflect these current health recommendations by distinguishing those products that are lower in total fat, saturated fat, sodium, and cholesterol from their higher-fat, higher-cholesterol, higher-sodium alternatives. Additionally, those products that are high in sodium (greater than 600 mg per serving) are marked with a ▲ symbol.

Authors' Note

*While the FDA endorses the **five** food groups recommended in current Food Guide Pyramid (namely, Bread, Cereal, Rice and Pasta group, Fruit group, Vegetable group, Milk, Yogurt, and Cheese group, Meat, Poultry, Fish, Dry Beans, Eggs, and Nuts group, Fats, Oils, and Sweets group), the agency believes treating fruits and vegetables as separate groups in this situation would allow the inappropriate classification of a fruit and a vegetable product to be labeled as a Main Dish.*

Criteria Key

▲ **Best Choice:**
**30% or Less Calories from Total Fat, AND
10% or Less Calories from Saturated Fat, AND
No More Than 90 mg Cholesterol, AND
No More Than 600 mg Sodium**

Products listed in this category meet the "Healthy" definition of the FDA/USDA for total fat, saturated fat, cholesterol, and sodium content as described above. These products were not evaluated based on their vitamin, mineral, or fiber content.

△ **Acceptable Choice:**
**30% or Less Calories from Total Fat, AND
10% or Less Calories from Saturated Fat**

Products listed in this category meet the "Healthy" definition of the FDA/USDA for total fat and saturated fat but not for sodium or cholesterol. These products were not evaluated based on their vitamin, mineral, or fiber content.

▲ **Occasional Choice:**
**Contains Greater Than 30% Calories from
Total Fat OR Greater Than 10% Calories from
Saturated Fat**

Products listed in this category do not meet the FDA's/USDA's definition for "Healthy." These products are higher in total fat or saturated fat and should only be consumed on occasion.

BRAND	BEST CHOICE	ACCEPTABLE CHOICE	OCCASIONAL CHOICE
	30% or Less Calories From Fat AND 10% or Less Calories From Saturated Fat AND No More Than 90 mg. Cholesterol AND No More Than 600 mg. Sodium	30% or Less Calories From Fat AND 10% or Less Calories From Saturated Fat	Contains Greater Than 30% Calories From Fat OR Greater Than 10% Calories From Saturated Fat
Armour			▲★ Chili ▲ Chili No Beans ▲★ Chili w/Beans
Bean Cuisine	▽☆ Barcelona Red Beans w/ Radiatore ▽☆ Country French Beans w/ Gemelli ▽☆ Florentine Beans w/ Bowties ▽☆ Mediterranean Black Beans w/Fusilli		
Broccoli Time	☆ Stir Fry Broccoli w/ Noodles	▲ Fettucini Alfredo w/ Broccoli	☆ Broccoli Pasta Salad
Castleberry's			▲☆ Premium Beef Stew
Chef Boyardee	Sesame Street: 　☆ Pasta Shapes in Tomato and Meat Sauce 　☆ Pasta Shapes in Tomato Sauce 　☆ Pasta Shapes w/Mini Meatballs in Tomato Sauce 　Pasta Shapes w/Vegetables and Chicken	▲☆ ABC's & 123's ▲☆ Beef Ravioli Cheese Ravioli: 　▲☆ in Tomato Sauce w/ Beef ▲★ Cheese Tortellini Chomps-a-Lot: 　▲☆ Bite Size Beef Ravioli in Tomato and Meat Sauce 　▲ Bite Size Cheese Ravioli ▲☆ Complete Lasagna Dinner Dinosaurs: 　▲☆ Cheese ▲☆ Fettuccine in Hearty Meat Sauce ▲ Macaroni and Cheese Main Meals: 　▲★ Beef Ravioli Suprema 　▲★ Cheese Ravioli Suprema 　▲ Classic Noodles & Chicken w/Vegetables	▲☆ Beefaroni Dinosaurs: 　▲☆ w/Meatballs ▲★ Lasagna Pasta and Beef in Sauce Main Meals: 　▲★ Fettuccine in Meat Sauce 　▲ Hearty Lasagna 　▲★ Spaghetti Suprema Microwave Meals: 　▲ Beef Stew 　▲☆ Lasagna 　▲ Macaroni & Cheese 　▲☆ Spaghetti & Meatballs in Tomato Sauce Roller Coasters: 　▲☆ w/Mini Meatballs in Tomato Sauce Sharks: 　▲ w/Meatballs 　▲☆ Spaghetti and Meatballs

▲ High Sodium, 600 mg. or greater per serving.
▽ Low Sodium, 140 mg. or less per serving.
☆ Good Source of Fiber, between 2.5 g. and 5 g. per serving.
★ High Fiber, 5 g. or greater per serving.

Meals and Main Dishes 257

BRAND	BEST CHOICE	ACCEPTABLE CHOICE	OCCASIONAL CHOICE
	30% or Less Calories From Fat AND 10% or Less Calories From Saturated Fat AND No More Than 90 mg. Cholesterol AND No More Than 600 mg. Sodium	30% or Less Calories From Fat AND 10% or Less Calories From Saturated Fat	Contains Greater Than 30% Calories From Fat OR Greater Than 10% Calories From Saturated Fat
Chef Boyardee (Cont.)		Main Meals: ▲★ Hearty Beans and Pasta ▲★ Meat Tortellini ▲★ Pasta and Peas ▲★ Ziti in Tomato Sauce ▲★ Meat Tortellini Microwave Meals: ▲☆ Beef Ravioli in Tomato and Meat Sauce ▲☆ Beefaroni ▲☆ Cheese Ravioli in Tomato and Meat Sauce Mini Ravioli: ▲☆ Beef in Tomato and Meat Sauce Pizza Mix: ▲ Cheese ▲ Pepperoni Sharks: ▲☆ Cheese Flavor ▲ Spaghetti Dinner ▲☆ Tic Tac Toe in Spaghetti Sauce w/Cheese Flavor Turtles: ▲☆ Pasta Shapes in Tomato and Cheese Sauce	
Chilli Man			2-Time World Champion: ▲★ Chili w/Beans ▲★ Chili w/Beans - Hot ▲★ Vegetarian Chili w/ Beans
Derby			▲ Beef Tamales w/Sauce
Dinty Moore		American Classics: ▲ Chicken Breast & Gravy ▲☆ Lasagna Noodles w/ Meat and Sauce ▲ Chicken & Dumplings	American Classics: ▲☆ Beef Stew ▲ Chicken & Noodles ▲☆ Salisbury Steak ▲☆ Chicken Stew ▲ Corned Beef Hash ▲☆ Hearty Burger Stew

▲ High Sodium, 600 mg. or greater per serving.
☆ Good Source of Fiber, between 2.5 g. and 5 g. per serving.
★ High Fiber, 5 g. or greater per serving.

BRAND	BEST CHOICE	ACCEPTABLE CHOICE	OCCASIONAL CHOICE
	30% or Less Calories From Fat AND 10% or Less Calories From Saturated Fat AND No More Than 90 mg. Cholesterol AND No More Than 600 mg. Sodium	30% or Less Calories From Fat AND 10% or Less Calories From Saturated Fat	Contains Greater Than 30% Calories From Fat OR Greater Than 10% Calories From Saturated Fat
Dinty Moore (Cont.)			▲ Beef Stew
Franco American		Garfield Pizza O's: 　▲ Pasta in Pizza Sauce Gargoyles: 　▲ w/Tomato & Cheese Sauce Shnookums & Meat: 　▲ w/Tomato & Cheese Sauce ▲☆ Spaghetti in Tomato Sauce w/Cheese Spaghetti O's in Tomato & Cheese Sauce: 　▲ Adventure #1-Deep Sea 　▲ Adventure #2-Meanie Genie ▲ Spaghetti O's in Tomato and Cheese Sauce Where's Waldo?: 　▲ Pasta in Tomato & Cheese Sauce	▲☆ Beef Ravioli O's in Meat Sauce Garfield Ravioli: 　▲☆ in Meat Sauce ▲☆ Macaroni and Cheese Shnookums & Meat: 　▲★ w/Meatballs in Tomato Sauce ▲★ Spaghetti O's w/Meatballs in Tomato Sauce ▲☆ Spaghetti O's w/Sliced Franks in Tomato Sauce ▲☆ Spaghetti w/Meatballs in Tomato Sauce Where's Waldo?: 　▲★ Pasta w/Meatballs in Tomato Sauce
Health Valley	Fast Menu: 　★ Vegetarian Cuisine All Varieties		
Hormel		Kid's Kitchen: 　▲ Noodle Rings & Chicken ▲☆ Turkey Chili No Beans ▲★ Turkey Chili w/Beans	Chili: 　▲☆ No Beans ▲ Chili Mac ▲★ Chili w/Beans ▲★ Chunky Chili w/Beans Hot Chili: 　▲☆ No Beans Kid's Kitchen: 　▲★ Beans & Wieners ▲ Beefy Mac ▲ Cheesy Mac'N Cheese ▲☆ Mini Beef Ravioli ▲ Spaghetti and Mini Meatballs

▲ High Sodium, 600 mg. or greater per serving.
☆ Good Source of Fiber, between 2.5 g. and 5 g. per serving.
★ High Fiber, 5 g. or greater per serving.

Meals and Main Dishes　259

BRAND	BEST CHOICE	ACCEPTABLE CHOICE	OCCASIONAL CHOICE
	30% or Less Calories From Fat AND 10% or Less Calories From Saturated Fat AND No More Than 90 mg. Cholesterol AND No More Than 600 mg. Sodium	30% or Less Calories From Fat AND 10% or Less Calories From Saturated Fat	Contains Greater Than 30% Calories From Fat OR Greater Than 10% Calories From Saturated Fat
Hormel (Cont.)			Kid's Kitchen: ▲☆ Spaghetti Rings & Franks in Tomato Sauce ▲ Lasagna & Beef ▲★ Microwave Chili w/Beans ▲ Noodles & Chicken ▲ Scalloped Potatoes-Ham ▲ Spaghetti and Meatballs
Johnsonville	Table for Two: Chicken Coronado w/Rice Oriental Beef w/Vegetables & Rice ☆ Santa Fe Style Chicken w/Rice	Table for Two: ▲ Beef Francais w/Linguine ▲ Ham, Shrimp & Sausage Jambalaya Kit	Table for Two: ☆ Chicken Italiano w/ Vegetables & Linguine ▲☆ Italian Sausage & Sauce w/Linguine
Mary Kitchen			▲ Corned Beef Hash ▲ Roast Beef Hash
Nautilus		Lite 'n Luscious Lunch: ▲☆ Tuna Salad w/Garden Vegetables	
Starkist			Charlie's Lunch Kit: ▲ Chunk Light Tuna ▲ Chunk White Tuna
Swanson			Chicken Salad Lunch Kit
Win Schuler's			Mild Chili Sauce: ▲ w/Smoked Sausages ▲ Original Barbecue Sauce w/Meatballs
Worthington			Natural Touch: ▲ Vegetarian Chili

▲ High Sodium, 600 mg. or greater per serving.
☆ Good Source of Fiber, between 2.5 g. and 5 g. per serving.
★ High Fiber, 5 g. or greater per serving.

BRAND	BEST CHOICE	ACCEPTABLE CHOICE	OCCASIONAL CHOICE
	30% or Less Calories From Fat AND 10% or Less Calories From Saturated Fat AND No More Than 90 mg. Cholesterol AND No More Than 600 mg. Sodium	30% or Less Calories From Fat AND 10% or Less Calories From Saturated Fat	Contains Greater Than 30% Calories From Fat OR Greater Than 10% Calories From Saturated Fat
BREAKFAST			
Bob Evans			▲☆ Ham Burritos ▲☆ Sausage Burritos
Libby's			Morning Classics: ▲ All Flavors

Swanson			Breakfast Blasts:
			  5 Waffle Sticks w/Syrup
			  Mini French Toast Sticks
			    w/Syrup
			Great Starts:
			  Breakfast Burrito Bacon
			  Breakfast Burrito Sausage
			  Cinnamon Swirl French
			    Toast w/Sausage
			  ▲ Egg, Canadian Style Bacon
			    and Cheese on a
			    Muffin
			  ☆ French Toast w/Sausages
			  ▲ Pancakes w/Bacon
			  ▲☆ Pancakes w/Sausages
			  ▲☆ Sausage, Egg, and
			    Cheese on a Biscuit
			  ▲☆ Scrambled Eggs and
			    Sausage w/Hashed
			    Brown Potatoes
			  ▲ Scrambled Eggs, & Bacon
			    w/Home Fried
			    Potatoes
			Great Starts-Budget:
			  ▲ 6 Silver Dollar Pancakes
			    w/Sausage
			  Scrambled Eggs and Home
			    Fried Potatoes

Weight Watchers	Breakfast On-The-Go!:
	  Ham & Cheese Bagel
			Breakfast On-The-Go!:
			  ☆ Handy Ham & Cheese
			    Omelet
			  ☆ Sausage Biscuit

▲ High Sodium, 600 mg. or greater per serving.
☆ Good Source of Fiber, between 2.5 g. and 5 g. per serving.

BRAND	BEST CHOICE	ACCEPTABLE CHOICE	OCCASIONAL CHOICE
	30% or Less Calories From Fat AND 10% or Less Calories From Saturated Fat AND No More Than 90 mg. Cholesterol AND No More Than 600 mg. Sodium	30% or Less Calories From Fat AND 10% or Less Calories From Saturated Fat	Contains Greater Than 30% Calories From Fat OR Greater Than 10% Calories From Saturated Fat
FROZEN			
Amy's	Burrito: ★ Bean & Rice ★ Bean Rice & Cheese ★ Black Bean Ranchero Enchilada: Black Bean Vegetable ★ Mexican Tamale Pie ★ Shepherd's Pie	▲★ Tofu Vegetable Lasagna	▲☆ Broccoli Cheese Pot Pie ★ Cheese Ravioli Cheese Enchilada Macaroni & Cheese ☆ Macaroni & Soy Cheeze ☆ Pizza Pocket ▲★ Vegetable Lasagna ☆ Vegetable Pot Pie
Bagel Bites			Bagel Bites: ▲☆ Cheese and Pepperoni ★ Cheese, Sausage, & Pepperoni ▲ Queso Grande
Banquet			▲☆ Barbecue Style Chicken Meal ▲★ Beef Enchilada Meal ▲☆ Chicken Fried Beef Steak Meal ▲☆ Chicken Nugget Meal ▲☆ Chicken Parmesan Meal Chicken Parmigiana: ▲ Italian-Style Extra Helping: ▲★ Chicken Fried Beef Steak Dinner ▲★ Meat Loaf Dinner ▲★ Southern Fried Chicken ▲★ Turkey & Gravy w/ Dressing Dinner ▲☆ Oriental Syle Chicken Meal ▲★ Salisbury Steak Meal ▲☆ Sliced Beef Meal ▲☆ Turkey & Gravy w/Dressing Meal ▲★ Veal Parmigiana Meal ▲★ White Meat Fried Chicken Meal

▲ High Sodium, 600 mg. or greater per serving.
☆ Good Source of Fiber, between 2.5 g. and 5 g. per serving.
★ High Fiber, 5 g. or greater per serving.

BRAND	BEST CHOICE	ACCEPTABLE CHOICE	OCCASIONAL CHOICE
	30% or Less Calories From Fat AND 10% or Less Calories From Saturated Fat AND No More Than 90 mg. Cholesterol AND No More Than 600 mg. Sodium	30% or Less Calories From Fat AND 10% or Less Calories From Saturated Fat	Contains Greater Than 30% Calories From Fat OR Greater Than 10% Calories From Saturated Fat
Barber Foods			▲ Chicken Breasts Cordon Bleu ▲ Chicken Breasts w/Broccoli & Cheese Stuffing Chicken Kiev
Cedar Lane	∇☆ Low Fat Hearty Vegetable Stew		
Chung's		▲ Beef & Broccoli ▲★ Chicken Fried Rice	
El Monterey			Burritos: ☆ Bean & Cheese ☆ Beef & Bean ☆ Beef & Bean, Mild Red Chili
Empire Kosher	Classic: Beef Broccoli Beijing Potato Onion Pierogies		▲ Chicken Pie
Freezer Queen	Chicken Noodle Meal w/Gravy Gravy & Sliced Beef: Cook-in-Pouch	Deluxe Family Entree: ▲★ Lasagna in Meat Sauce ▲ Gravy & Sliced Turkey ▲ Macaroni & Cheese ▲ Veal Parmigiana	Deluxe Family Entree: ▲ Gravy & Sliced Beef ▲ Gravy & 6 Salisbury Steaks Gravy & Salisbury Steak: ▲ Cook-in-Pouch ▲★ Salisbury Steak Meal
Grecian Delight			Beef Gyros ▲ Gyros
Green Giant	Create A Meal: ★ Sweet & Sour Stir Fry	Create A Meal: ▲★ Lo Mein Stir Fry ▲★ Szechuan Style ▲☆ Teriyaki Stir Fry	Pasta Accents: ☆ Alfredo ▲★ Creamy Cheddar ▲★ Garden Herb Seasoning ▲★ Garlic Seasoning ★ Primavera
Healthy Choice	★ Beef & Peppers Cantonese ★ Beef Broccoli Bejing		★ Manicotti w/3 Cheeses

▲ High Sodium, 600 mg. or greater per serving.
∇ Low Sodium, 140 mg. or less per serving.
☆ Good Source of Fiber, between 2.5 g. and 5 g. per serving.
★ High Fiber, 5 g. or greater per serving.

Meals and Main Dishes 263

BRAND	BEST CHOICE	ACCEPTABLE CHOICE	OCCASIONAL CHOICE
	30% or Less Calories From Fat AND 10% or Less Calories From Saturated Fat AND No More Than 90 mg. Cholesterol AND No More Than 600 mg. Sodium	30% or Less Calories From Fat AND 10% or Less Calories From Saturated Fat	Contains Greater Than 30% Calories From Fat OR Greater Than 10% Calories From Saturated Fat

Healthy Choice (Cont.)	Beef Burrito Ranchero:
	  ★ Medium
	  ★ Mild
	Beef Enchiladas Rio Grande
	☆ Beef Pepper Steak Oriental
	★ Beef Tips w/BBQ Sauce
	★ Cacciatore Chicken
	☆ Chicken and Vegetable
	    Marsala
	★ Chicken Broccoli Alfredo
	★ Chicken Cantonese
	▲★ Chicken Con Queso
	    Burritos
	★ Chicken Dijon
	★ Chicken Enchilada Suiza
	★ Chicken Enchilada Suprema
	☆ Chicken Fettucini Alfredo
	★ Chicken Francesca
	★ Chicken Parmigiana
	★ Chicken Picante
	★ Chicken Teriyaki
	☆ Country Glazed Chicken
	★ Country Herb Chicken
	★ Country Inn Roast Turkey
	☆ Country Roast Turkey
	    w/Mushrooms
	★ Country Turkey and Pasta
	★ Fiesta Chicken Fajitas
	★ Garden Potato Casserole
	★ Ginger Chicken Hunan
	☆ Honey Mustard Chicken
	★ Lasagna Roma
	★ Lemon Pepper Fish Dinner
	★ Mesquite Beef w/Barbecue
	    Sauce
	★ Mesquite Chicken Barbeque
	★ Pasta Shells Marinara
	★ Salisbury Steak w/Mushroom
	    Gravy
	★ Sesame Chicken Shanghai
	★ Shrimp & Vegetables Maria		

▲ High Sodium, 600 mg. or greater per serving.
☆ Good Source of Fiber, between 2.5 g. and 5 g. per serving.
★ High Fiber, 5 g. or greater per serving.

264   **Meals and Main Dishes**

BRAND	BEST CHOICE	ACCEPTABLE CHOICE	OCCASIONAL CHOICE
	30% or Less Calories From Fat AND 10% or Less Calories From Saturated Fat AND No More Than 90 mg. Cholesterol AND No More Than 600 mg. Sodium	30% or Less Calories From Fat AND 10% or Less Calories From Saturated Fat	Contains Greater Than 30% Calories From Fat OR Greater Than 10% Calories From Saturated Fat
Healthy Choice (Cont.)	Shrimp Marinara ★ Smokey Chicken Barbeque ★ Southwestern Glazed Chicken ★ Supreme French Bread Pizza ★ Sweet & Sour Chicken ★ Traditional Beef Tips ★ Traditional Breast of Turkey ★ Traditional Salisbury Steak Dinner ★ Turkey Fettuccine Alla Crema Yankee Pot Roast		
Hormel			Cheeseburger Chicken Sandwich ▲ Chili Dog Mini Corn Dogs Premium Corn Dogs
Hot Pockets			▲ Beef & Cheddar ▲★ Beef Fajita ▲☆ Ham & Cheese ▲ Pepperoni & Sausage Combo Pizza ▲ Pepperoni Pizza ▲ Sausage Pizza ▲ Turkey & Ham w/Cheese
Jenos			Crisp'n Tasty Pizza: ▲ Canadian Style Bacon ▲☆ Combination ▲ Pepperoni ▲☆ Sausage
Ken & Robert's	Veggie Pockets: ★ Bar B Que Style ☆ Broccoli & Cheddar Style ☆ Greek Style ★ Indian Style ★ Oriental Style		

▲ High Sodium, 600 mg. or greater per serving.
☆ Good Source of Fiber, between 2.5 g. and 5 g. per serving.
★ High Fiber, 5 g. or greater per serving.

Meals and Main Dishes 265

BRAND	BEST CHOICE	ACCEPTABLE CHOICE	OCCASIONAL CHOICE
	30% or Less Calories From Fat AND 10% or Less Calories From Saturated Fat AND No More Than 90 mg. Cholesterol AND No More Than 600 mg. Sodium	30% or Less Calories From Fat AND 10% or Less Calories From Saturated Fat	Contains Greater Than 30% Calories From Fat OR Greater Than 10% Calories From Saturated Fat
Ken & Robert's (Cont.)	Veggie Pockets: ☆ Pizza Style ★ Tex-Mex Style		
Kid Cuisine	★ Pirate Pizza w/Cheese	▲☆ Magical Macaroni & Cheese	★ Beef Patty Sandwich w/Cheese ★ Cosmic Chicken Nuggets ▲★ High Flying Fried Chicken
La Choy	Restaurant Style Egg Rolls: ☆ Shrimp Sweet & Sour Chicken	Mini Egg Rolls: ▲★ Chicken ▲★ Pork & Shrimp ▲★ Shrimp	
Lean Pockets	▲ Glazed Chicken Supreme	▲☆ Chicken Fajita ▲ Chicken Parmesan Sausage & Pepperoni: ▲ Pizza Deluxe ▲☆ Turkey, Broccoli & Cheese	
Linda McCartney's		▲★ Bavarian Goulash ▲★ Pasta Provencale	▲★ Fettuccine Alfredo ▲☆ Pasta Primavera ▲★ Rigatoni Marinara ★ Spaghetti Milano
Marie Callender's			▲☆ Beef Stroganoff and Noodles ▲★ Breaded Chicken Parmigiana Dinner ☆ Cheese Raivoli in Marinara Sauce ▲ Chicken & Broccoli Pot Pie ▲ Chicken Pot Pie ▲★ Country Fried Chicken and Gravy Fettucini Alfredo Fettucini Primavera w/Tortellini ☆ Fettucini w/Broccoli & Chicken ▲☆ Lasagna w/Meat Sauce ▲★ Meatloaf & Gravy w/Mashed Potatoes

▲ High Sodium, 600 mg. or greater per serving.
☆ Good Source of Fiber, between 2.5 g. and 5 g. per serving.
★ High Fiber, 5 g. or greater per serving.

BRAND	BEST CHOICE	ACCEPTABLE CHOICE	OCCASIONAL CHOICE
	30% or Less Calories From Fat AND 10% or Less Calories From Saturated Fat AND No More Than 90 mg. Cholesterol AND No More Than 600 mg. Sodium	30% or Less Calories From Fat AND 10% or Less Calories From Saturated Fat	Contains Greater Than 30% Calories From Fat OR Greater Than 10% Calories From Saturated Fat
Marie Callender's (Cont.)			☆ Spaghetti and Meat Sauce w/Garlic Bread ▲ Turkey Pot Pie ▲ Turkey w/Gravy & Dressing
Michelina's	☆ Penne Primavera	International Recipes: ▲ Chicken a la King w/ Noodles ▲ Minestrone w/Penne Pasta ▲ Linguini w/Clams & Sauce ▲☆ Spaghetti Bolognese ▲☆ Spaghetti Marinara	▲☆ Chili-Mac ☆ Fettucine Alfredo w/ Broccoli ▲☆ Fettucini Alfredo International Recipes: ▲☆ Creamed Sauce-Beef w/Croutons ▲☆ Egg Noodles w/Rich Gravy and Swedish Meatballs ▲ Marinara Sauce w/Penne Pasta, Italian Sausage & Peppers ▲ Noodles Romanoff ▲ Noodles Stroganoff ▲ Noodles w/Chicken, Peas, & Carrots ▲ Risotto Parmesano ▲ Tuna Noodle Casserole ▲ Lasagna Alfredo ▲ Lasagna w/Meat Sauce ▲ Lasagna w/Vegetables ▲☆ Macaroni & Cheese ☆ Penne Pollo ▲ Shells & Cheese w/Jalapeno Peppers ▲ Spaghetti w/Three Meatballs & Pomodoro Sauce
Mrs. T's	Pierogies: Potato and Cheddar Potato and Onion		
Nancy's			French Baked Quiche: ▲ Broccoli Cheddar ▲ Classic French Florentine

▲ High Sodium, 600 mg. or greater per serving.
☆ Good Source of Fiber, between 2.5 g. and 5 g. per serving.

Meals and Main Dishes 267

BRAND	BEST CHOICE	ACCEPTABLE CHOICE	OCCASIONAL CHOICE
	30% or Less Calories From Fat AND 10% or Less Calories From Saturated Fat AND No More Than 90 mg. Cholesterol AND No More Than 600 mg. Sodium	30% or Less Calories From Fat AND 10% or Less Calories From Saturated Fat	Contains Greater Than 30% Calories From Fat OR Greater Than 10% Calories From Saturated Fat
Pappalo's			Deep Dish Pizza: ▲ Pepperoni ▲ Sausage and Pepperoni ▲ Supreme Pizza For One: ▲☆ Deep Dish Pepperoni ▲☆ Deep Dish Supreme ▲☆ Pepperoni ▲☆ Supreme Pizzeria Style Crust: ▲ Pepperoni ▲ Sausage and Pepperoni ▲ Supreme
Patio		Burrito: ▲★ Beef & Bean, Green Chili Mild ▲★ Beef & Bean, Hot Red Chili ▲★ Beef & Bean, Medium ▲★ Beef & Bean, Red Hot	
Pepperidge Farm			Croissant Crust Pizza: ▲ Pepperoni
Red Baron			Deep Dish Singles: ▲ All Varieties Oven Stuffs: Turkey Swiss ▲ Turkey, Cheddar & Bacon
Rosetto	Ravioli: w/Beef Filling w/Chicken Filling Salad & Soup Tortellini		Ravioli: w/Ricotta Cheese Filling
Rotanelli's	∇ Cannelloni w/Meat		Manicotti
SeaPak		Shrimp Sensations: ▲☆ Oriental Stir Fry ▲☆ Shrimp Fajita ▲☆ Shrimp Primavera	

▲ High Sodium, 600 mg. or greater per serving.
∇ Low Sodium, 140 mg. or less per serving.
☆ Good Source of Fiber, between 2.5 g. and 5 g. per serving.
★ High Fiber, 5 g. or greater per serving.

BRAND	BEST CHOICE	ACCEPTABLE CHOICE	OCCASIONAL CHOICE
	30% or Less Calories From Fat AND 10% or Less Calories From Saturated Fat AND No More Than 90 mg. Cholesterol AND No More Than 600 mg. Sodium	30% or Less Calories From Fat AND 10% or Less Calories From Saturated Fat	Contains Greater Than 30% Calories From Fat OR Greater Than 10% Calories From Saturated Fat
Stouffer's	Lean Cuisine: ☆ Angel Hair Pasta ☆ Baked Chicken ☆ Beef Pot Roast w/ Whipped Potatoes ☆ Cheddar Bake w/Pasta and Vegetables Chicken a L'Orange ★ Chicken and Vegetables w/Vermicelli Chicken Chow Mein ★ Chicken Enchiladas Suiza Chicken Fettucini Chicken in Honey Barbecue Sauce Chicken Italiano w/Fettucini and Vegetables ☆ Chicken Mediterranean ☆ Chicken Oriental ★ Chicken Parmesan ☆ Chicken Pie ★ Classic Cheese Lasagne Fettucini Alfredo ☆ Fettucini Primavera Fiesta Chicken Glazed Chicken ☆ Grilled Chicken Salsa ☆ Homestyle Turkey ☆ Honey Mustard Chicken Breast ★ Lasagna w/Meat Sauce ☆ Macaroni & Beef Marinara Twist ★ Meatloaf w/Gravy and Whipped Potatoes Rigatoni ☆ Sirloin Beef Peppercorn ☆ Spaghetti w/Meat Sauce ★ Stuffed Cabbage ☆ Swedish Meatballs	▲☆ Chicken a la King w/Rice ▲☆ Green Pepper Steak Homestyle: ▲☆ Chicken Breast Parmigiana Lean Cuisine Lunch Express: ▲ Oriental Beef w/ Vegetables and Pasta	▲ Beef Pie ▲ Beef Stroganoff w/Parsley Noodles ▲★ Cheese Manicotti w/Tomato Sauce ▲★ Cheese Shells w/Tomato Sauce ▲☆ Chicken Enchilada and Mexican-Style Rice ▲☆ Chicken Pie Corn Souffle ▲ Creamed Chipped Beef ▲ Creamy Chicken & Broccoli ▲ Escalloped Chicken & Noodles ▲☆ Fettucini Alfredo ▲☆ Four Cheese Lasagna French Bread Pizza: ▲☆ All Varieties Green Bean Mushroom Casserole ▲ Ham & Asparagus Bake Homestyle: ▲ Baked Chicken Breast in Gravy w/Whipped Potatoes ▲☆ Beef Pot Roast ▲☆ Breaded Chicken Fillets ▲ Chicken & Noodles ▲ Chicken Fettucini ▲☆ Chicken Monterey w/Mexican-Style Rice ▲ Fish Filet w/Macaroni & Cheese ▲☆ Fried Chicken Breast ▲☆ Meatloaf in Gravy & Whipped Potatoes Roast Turkey Breast ▲ Salisbury Steak in Gravy & Macaroni and Cheese ▲★ Veal Parmigiana

▲ High Sodium, 600 mg. or greater per serving.
☆ Good Source of Fiber, between 2.5 g. and 5 g. per serving.
★ High Fiber, 5 g. or greater per serving.

BRAND	BEST CHOICE	ACCEPTABLE CHOICE	OCCASIONAL CHOICE
	30% or Less Calories From Fat AND 10% or Less Calories From Saturated Fat AND No More Than 90 mg. Cholesterol AND No More Than 600 mg. Sodium	30% or Less Calories From Fat AND 10% or Less Calories From Saturated Fat	Contains Greater Than 30% Calories From Fat OR Greater Than 10% Calories From Saturated Fat

Stouffer's (Cont.)	Lean Cuisine French Bread Pizza:
	    Cheese
	    ★ Deluxe
	    ☆ Pepperoni
	Lean Cuisine Lunch Express:
	    ★ Cheese Lasagne Casserole
	Chicken Oriental w/
	    Vegetables and Rice
	Mandarin Chicken
	☆ Mexican Style Rice w/
	    Chicken
	☆ Pasta and Chicken
	    Marinara
	☆ Pasta and Tuna Casserole
	Pasta w/Turkey in a
	    Dijon Sauce
	Spaghetti w/Meat Sauce
	☆ Teriyaki Stir Fry
	Spaghetti w/Meat Sauce
			★ Lasagne w/Meat & Sauce
			Lean Cuisine:
			    ☆ Cheese Cannelloni
			    ☆ Deluxe Cheddar Potato
			    Macaroni & Cheese
			    ☆ Oriental Beef
			Salisbury Steak w/
			    Macaroni & Cheese
			Lean Cuisine Lunch Express:
			    ★ Broccoli & Cheddar Cheese
			    Baked Potato
			    ▲ Cheese Ravioli w/
			    Tomato Sauce
			    ▲ Chicken Alfredo
			    ☆ Chicken Fettucini w/
			    Broccoli
			    ★ Macaroni & Cheese
			    ▲☆ Macaroni & Beef w/
			    Tomatoes
			    ▲ Macaroni & Cheese
			    ▲ Noodles Romanoff
			Potatoes Au Gratin
			Scalloped Potatoes
			    ▲★ Spaghetti w/Meatballs in
			    Sauce
			Spinach Souffle
			    ▲ Stuffed Peppers
			    ▲☆ Stuffed Peppers w/Beef in
			    Tomato Sauce
			    ▲☆ Swedish Meatballs in
			    Gravy w/Parsley Noodles
			    ▲☆ Tuna Noodle Casserole
			    ▲☆ Turkey Pie
			    ▲ Turkey Tetrazzini
			    ▲☆ Vegetable Lasagne

Swanson	Fun Feast:
	    ★ Chilin' Cheese Pizza
		Grilled Chicken:
		    ▲★ White Meat
		▲★ Grilled Chicken in Garlic
		    Sauce w/Almonds
		    Dinner
			Beef and Broccoli in Sauce:
			    ▲☆ w/Brownie
			▲☆ Beef Pot Pie
			▲☆ Chicken Nuggets

▲ High Sodium, 600 mg. or greater per serving.
☆ Good Source of Fiber, between 2.5 g. and 5 g. per serving.
★ High Fiber, 5 g. or greater per serving.

BRAND	BEST CHOICE	ACCEPTABLE CHOICE	OCCASIONAL CHOICE
	30% or Less Calories From Fat AND 10% or Less Calories From Saturated Fat AND No More Than 90 mg. Cholesterol AND No More Than 600 mg. Sodium	30% or Less Calories From Fat AND 10% or Less Calories From Saturated Fat	Contains Greater Than 30% Calories From Fat OR Greater Than 10% Calories From Saturated Fat

Swanson (Cont.)		▲☆ Turkey Dinner (mostly white meat)	▲ Chicken Parmigiana Dinner
			▲☆ Chicken Pot Pie
			▲☆ Chopped Sirloin Beef Dinner
			▲★ Deluxe Chicken Pie
			▲★ Fish 'n Chips Dinner
			Fried Chicken Dinner:
			  ▲☆ Dark Portions
			  ▲★ White Portions
			Fun Feast:
			  ▲☆ Chompin' Chicken Drumlets
			  ▲☆ Frenzied Fish Sticks
			  ▲★ Growlin' Grilled Cheese
			  ★ Roarin' Ravioli
			  ★ Wobblin' Wheels and Cheese
			Hungry-Man:
			  ▲☆ Chicken Pot Pie
			  ▲★ Fried Chicken (mostly white meat)
			  ▲★ Salisbury Steak
			  ▲★ Turkey (mostly white meat)
			▲★ Meat Loaf Dinner
			▲★ Mexican Style Combination Dinner
			▲★ Salisbury Steak Dinner
			▲☆ Scalloped Potatoes w/Ham
			★ Sirloin Beef Tips
			▲ Turkey Pot Pie
			▲★ Veal Parmigiana Dinner

Taj Cuisine of India	★ Channa Masala Chicken Curry w/Brown Rice ★ Raj Mah	▲★ Chicken Masala w/Brown Rice ▲ Mushrooms and Green Peas Curry	Asparagus and Baby Carrots Curry ▲★ Palak Paneer ▲★ Shahi Paneer ▲★ Vegetable Korma

▲ High Sodium, 600 mg. or greater per serving.
☆ Good Source of Fiber, between 2.5 g. and 5 g. per serving.
★ High Fiber, 5 g. or greater per serving.

BRAND	BEST CHOICE	ACCEPTABLE CHOICE	OCCASIONAL CHOICE
	30% or Less Calories From Fat AND 10% or Less Calories From Saturated Fat AND No More Than 90 mg. Cholesterol AND No More Than 600 mg. Sodium	30% or Less Calories From Fat AND 10% or Less Calories From Saturated Fat	Contains Greater Than 30% Calories From Fat OR Greater Than 10% Calories From Saturated Fat
The Budget Gourmet	Light and Healthy: ★ Penne Pasta w/Chunky Tomato Sauce & Italian Sausage Special Recipe Sirloin of Beef Teriyaki Beef Light and Healthy Dinner: Beef Sirloin Meatballs and Gravy ★ Beef Sirloin Salisbury Steak w/Red Skinned Potatoes ★ Chicken in Mesquite Barbecue Sauce ★ Chicken Parmigiana ★ Honey Mustard Chicken Breast ★ Yankee Pot Roast	Light and Healthy: ▲ Chicken Oriental w/ Vegetables ▲☆ Chinese Style Vegetables & Chicken ▲ Glazed Turkey ▲☆ Italian Style Vegetables & Chicken ▲☆ Mandarin Chicken ▲ Orange Glazed Chicken Breast ▲★ Rigatoni in Cream Sauce w/Broccoli & Chicken Light and Healthy Dinner: ▲☆ Roast Chicken Breast and Herb Gravy ▲★ Stuffed Turkey Breast ▲☆ Teriyaki Chicken Breast w/Oriental Style Vegetables ▲☆ Pepper Steak w/Rice Special Selections: ▲★ Spicy Szechwan Style Vegetables w/Chicken	▲☆ Chicken and Egg Noodles ▲ Chicken Marsala ▲☆ Chicken w/Fettucini ▲ Italian Sausage Lasagna Light and Healthy: ▲☆ Beef Sirloin Salisbury Steak ☆ Beef Stroganoff ▲☆ French Recipe Chicken ▲☆ Lasagna w/Meat Sauce ▲☆ Macaroni & Cheese ▲☆ Oriental Beef ▲☆ Sirloin of Beef in Herb Sauce ▲☆ Linguini w/Bay Shrimp & Clams Marinara ▲ Linguini w/Tomato Sauce & Italian Sausage ▲ Macaroni and Cheese w/ Aged Sharp Cheddar ▲ Manicotti w/Meat Sauce ▲☆ Roast Sirloin Supreme Side Dish: New England Recipe Vegetables Oriental Rice w/Vegetables Rice Pilaf w/Green Beans Spring Vegetables in Cheese Sauce ▲☆ Sirloin Cheddar Melt ▲☆ Sirloin Tips w/Country Style Vegetables Special Selections: ▲ Escalloped Noodles and Turkey ▲☆ Fettucini Alfredo w/ 4 Cheese ▲☆ Homestyle Macaroni and Cheese ▲ Wide Ribbons Pasta w/Ricotta and Chunky Tomato Sauce

▲ High Sodium, 600 mg. or greater per serving.
☆ Good Source of Fiber, between 2.5 g. and 5 g. per serving.
★ High Fiber, 5 g. or greater per serving.

BRAND	BEST CHOICE	ACCEPTABLE CHOICE	OCCASIONAL CHOICE
	30% or Less Calories From Fat AND 10% or Less Calories From Saturated Fat AND No More Than 90 mg. Cholesterol AND No More Than 600 mg. Sodium	**30% or Less Calories From Fat AND 10% or Less Calories From Saturated Fat**	**Contains Greater Than 30% Calories From Fat OR Greater Than 10% Calories From Saturated Fat**
The Budget Gourmet (Cont.)			▲☆ Swedish Meatballs ★ Three Cheese Lasagna
Tina's	▲★ Bean & Cheese Burrito Chicken Burrito		
Tombstone	☆ Light Vegetable Pizza	For One - ½ Less Fat: ▲★ Vegetable Pizza	Double Top Pizza: ▲ Pepperoni w/Double Cheese ▲ Sausage & Pepperoni w/Double Cheese For One - ½ Less Fat: ▲☆ Pepperoni Pizza ▲☆ Light Supreme Pizza Original Pizza: ▲ Deluxe ▲ Extra Cheese ▲ Pepperoni & Sausage ▲ Pepperoni ▲ Supreme Special Order Pizza: ▲☆ Four Meat ▲ Pepperoni ▲ Super Supreme Pizza Thin Crust: ▲ Four Meat Combo Pizza ▲ Supreme Pizza ▲ Supreme Taco Pizza
Tony's			Pizza: ▲ Pepperoni ▲ Taco Style Pizza D'Primo: ▲ Meat Trio ▲ Sausage & Pepperoni ▲ Super Pepperoni ▲ Supreme
Totino's			Party Pizza: ▲ All Varieties

▲ High Sodium, 600 mg. or greater per serving.
☆ Good Source of Fiber, between 2.5 g. and 5 g. per serving.
★ High Fiber, 5 g. or greater per serving.

BRAND	BEST CHOICE	ACCEPTABLE CHOICE	OCCASIONAL CHOICE
	30% or Less Calories From Fat AND 10% or Less Calories From Saturated Fat AND No More Than 90 mg. Cholesterol AND No More Than 600 mg. Sodium	30% or Less Calories From Fat AND 10% or Less Calories From Saturated Fat	Contains Greater Than 30% Calories From Fat OR Greater Than 10% Calories From Saturated Fat

Totino's (Cont.)			Pizza Rolls:
			    Combination
			    Pepperoni & Cheese

Tyson	Beef Fajita Kit
	★ Chicken Marsala
	★ Chicken Mesquite
	Chicken Picante
	Chicken Picatta
	Chicken Stir Fry Kit
	Chicken w/Broccoli & Cheese
	Healthy Portion:
	    Chicken Marinara Meal
	    ★ Herb Chicken Meal
	    ★ Honey Mustard Chicken Meal
	Honey Roasted Chicken
	Sweet & Sour Chicken Kit
		▲ Blackened Chicken Dinner
		▲★ Glazed Chicken w/Sauce
		Healthy Portion:
		    ▲★ BBQ Chicken Meal
		    ▲★ Italian Style Chicken Meal
		    ▲★ Mesquite Chicken Meal
			Chicken Fajita Kit
			▲★ Chicken Pie
			☆ Chicken Supreme
			▲★ Turkey Pie

Van de Kamp's			Fish 'N Fries
Vigo			Spinach Pasta Tortellini w/Cheese

Weight Watchers	Baked Potato:
	    ★ Broccoli and Cheese
	Barbecue Glazed Chicken
	☆ Chicken Cordon Bleu
	Chicken Fettuccini
	★ Fettuccini Alfredo
	★ Garden Lasagna
	★ Macaroni & Cheese
	Smart Ones:
	    ☆ Chicken Chow Mein
	    ☆ Chicken Francais
	    ★ Fiesta Chicken
	    ★ Honey Mustard Chicken
	    ★ Lasagna Florentine
	    ☆ Lemon Herb Chicken Piccata
	    ★ Ravioli Florentine
	    ☆ Roast Turkey Medallions
		▲☆ Pepperoni Pizza	☆ Chicken Enchiladas Suiza
			Chicken Parmigiana
			☆ Roast Glazed Chicken
			Stuffed Turkey Breast

▲ High Sodium, 600 mg. or greater per serving.
☆ Good Source of Fiber, between 2.5 g. and 5 g. per serving.
★ High Fiber, 5 g. or greater per serving.

Brand	Best Choice	Acceptable Choice	Occasional Choice
	30% or Less Calories From Fat AND 10% or Less Calories From Saturated Fat AND No More Than 90 mg. Cholesterol AND No More Than 600 mg. Sodium	30% or Less Calories From Fat AND 10% or Less Calories From Saturated Fat	Contains Greater Than 30% Calories From Fat OR Greater Than 10% Calories From Saturated Fat
Weight Watchers (Cont.)	☆ Swedish Meatballs ★ Tuna Noodle Casserole		
White Castle			★ Microwaveable Cheeseburgers ★ Microwaveable Hamburgers
Wolfgang Puck's	★ 3 Mushrooms & Spinach Pizza ★ Vegetarian Pizza		☆ Artichoke Hearts Pizza ★ Spicy Chicken Pizza

World Cafe	Egg Rolls:
	   Chicken
	   Pork & Shrimp
	   Vegetable
			▲☆ Beef & Bean Sanchos
			▲☆ Beef & Bean Supreme Sanchos
			Egg Rolls:
			   ☆ Pork & Vegetables
			   Spicy Hunan Style
			▲ Red Hot Chili Beef Sanchos

Yu Sing	Egg Roll Snacks:
	   ☆ Sweet & Sour Chicken
	Sweet & Sour Chicken w/ Rice
		▲☆ Chicken & Almonds
		▲☆ Chicken & Almonds w/Rice
		▲ Chicken Fried Rice
		Egg Roll Snacks:
		   ▲☆ Pork & Shrimp
		▲ Oriental Beef & Peppers
		▲ Pork & Shrimp Fried Rice
		▲ Pork Chop Suey
			Egg Roll Snacks:
			   Chicken

YOUR FAVORITE MEALS AND MAIN DISHES NOT LISTED IN THE *GUIDE*			

▲ High Sodium, 600 mg. or greater per serving.
☆ Good Source of Fiber, between 2.5 g. and 5 g. per serving.
★ High Fiber, 5 g. or greater per serving.

BRAND	BEST CHOICE	ACCEPTABLE CHOICE	OCCASIONAL CHOICE
	30% or Less Calories From Fat AND 10% or Less Calories From Saturated Fat AND No More Than 90 mg. Cholesterol AND No More Than 600 mg. Sodium	30% or Less Calories From Fat AND 10% or Less Calories From Saturated Fat	Contains Greater Than 30% Calories From Fat OR Greater Than 10% Calories From Saturated Fat

SOUPS

The Soup category presents a wide variety of choices that are dry, canned ready-to-serve, or canned condensed. Soups provide an excellent means to incorporate wholesome vegetables, grains, and legumes into the diet. Although nutritious, commercially-prepared soups can also provide substantial amounts of sodium.

Depending on the primary ingredient or ingredients, soups can be considered as part of several food groups in the *Food Guide Pyramid* such as: "Meat, Poultry, Fish, Dry Beans, Eggs, and Nut Group," "Milk, Yogurt, and Cheese Group," "Vegetable Group," and "Bread, Cereal, Rice, and Pasta Group." The FDA has established reference amounts or standardized serving sizes for use on the food label. The reference amount for soups is 245 grams (8.5 ounces). Be sure to read the *Nutrition Facts* label for the serving size information of your soup choice. (See pages 51 and 52 for an explanation of reference amounts and the difference between serving sizes established by the FDA for food labeling and those recommended by the *Food Guide Pyramid*.)

Typically, broth-based soups contain a small amount of fat, whereas cream-based soups contain higher amounts. Many soups are now specially processed to be low fat or fat free and low-sodium or reduced-sodium. Criteria were designed to distinguish those soups that are lower in total fat and saturated fat from their higher-fat alternatives. Soups that contain 480 milligrams sodium or more per serving (20% or greater of the Daily Value) are considered high in sodium and are indicated with a ▲ symbol.

Criteria Key

▲ Best Choice: Fat Free or Low Fat

Products listed in this category meet the FDA's definition for "Fat Free," (less than
1/2 gram fat per serving, or "Low Fat" (3 grams or less fat per serving).

▲ Acceptable Choice: Contains Greater Than 3 Grams, but
                           Less Than or Equal to 5 Grams Total Fat

Products listed in this category **do not** meet the FDA's definition for "Low Fat."
They may also contain 5 or less grams of fat per serving. The 5 grams of total fat
cut-off was used in order to be consistent with the amount of fat equal to one
diabetes diet fat exchange and is also equivalent to 1 teaspoon of added fat.[75]
These products contribute a greater amount of fat to the overall daily diet.

▲ Occasional Choice: Contains Greater Than 5 Grams Total Fat

Those products that contain greater than 5 grams of total fat per serving are listed
in this category. These products can contribute a significant amount of fat to the
overall daily diet and should be consumed only on occasion.

BRAND	BEST CHOICE	ACCEPTABLE CHOICE	OCCASIONAL CHOICE
	Fat Free OR Low Fat	Contains Greater Than 3 Grams but Less Than or Equal to 5 Grams Total Fat	Contains Greater Than 5 Grams Total Fat
Baxters	▲☆ Chicken & Vegetable ▲☆ Country Garden ▲☆ Lentil & Vegetable ▲☆ Minestrone ▲☆ Onion ▲☆ Tomato, Bean & Vegetable		

Bearitos	Beans & Rice:
	  ▲★ Cajun Style
	  ▲★ Cuban Style
	  ▲☆ Mexican Style
	Fat Free Homestyle Naturals:
	  ▲☆ Mixed Bean
	  ▲☆ Navy Bean
	  ▲ Southwest Vegetable
	  ☆ Split Pea
	Homestyle Naturals:
	  ▲☆ Hearty Tex-Mex
	  ▲☆ Lentil
	  ▲ Minestrone		

Best of All	∇★ 3-Bean Chili Mix ∇★ Caribbean Black Bean Mix ∇★ New Orleans Red Beans & Rice Mix ▲★ Senate Soup Mix		

Borden	Soup Starter:
	  ▲ Beef Vegetable
	  ▲ Chicken Noodle
	  ▲ Hearty Chicken Vegetable		

Broccoli Time			▲ Cream of Broccoli Soup

Campbell's	▲ Chicken w/White & Wild Rice
	Chunky Soup:
	  ▲☆ Hearty Vegetable w/Pasta
	  ▲☆ Old Fashioned Chicken
	     w/Country Vegetables
	  ▲☆ Pepper Steak
	  ▲☆ Vegetable
		Chunky Soup:
		  ▲ Beef Pasta
		  ▲☆ Beef w/Country
		     Vegetables
		  ▲☆ Chicken Noodle
		     w/Mushrooms
		  ▲ Chicken Rice
		  ▲☆ Chicken Vegetable
		  ▲☆ Clam Chowder,
		     Manhattan Style
			▲☆ Chicken Mushroom
			     Chowder
			Chunky Soup:
			  ▲ Chicken Broccoli Cheese
			  ▲☆ Chicken Corn Chowder
			  ▲ New England Clam Chowder
			  ▲★ Old Fashioned Bean
			     and Ham
			  ▲☆ Sirloin Burger
			Condensed:
			  ▲ Broccoli Cheese

▲ High Sodium, 480 mg. or greater per serving.
∇ Low Sodium, 140 mg. or less per serving.
☆ Good Source of Fiber, between 2.5 g. and 5 g. per serving.
★ High Fiber, 5 g. or greater per serving.

BRAND	BEST CHOICE	ACCEPTABLE CHOICE	OCCASIONAL CHOICE
	Fat Free OR Low Fat	Contains Greater Than 3 Grams but Less Than or Equal to 5 Grams Total Fat	Contains Greater Than 5 Grams Total Fat
Campbell's (Cont.)	Condensed: ▲ Beef Broth ▲ Beef Consomme ▲ Beef Noodle ▲ Beef w/Vegetables & Barley ▲ Beefy Mushroom ▲★ Black Bean ▲ Chicken & Stars ▲ Chicken 'n Dumplings ▲ Chicken Broth ▲ Chicken Gumbo ▲ Chicken Noodle ▲ Chicken Noodle O's ▲ Chicken Vegetable ▲ Chicken w/Rice ▲ Chicken Wonton ▲ Clam Chowder, Manhattan Style ▲ Clam Chowder, New England Style ▲ Cream of Potato ▲ Double Noodle ▲ Fiesta Tomato ▲ French Onion ▲ Golden Mushroom ▲★ Green Pea ▲ Hearty Vegetable w/ Pasta ▲ Homestyle Chicken Noodle ▲ Italian Tomato ▲☆ Minestrone ▲ Old Fashioned Tomato Rice ▲ Old Fashioned Vegetable ▲ Scotch Broth ▲ Tomato ▲ Turkey Noodle ▲☆ Vegetable ▲ Vegetable Beef ▲ Vegetarian Vegetable Healthy Request: ▲ Chicken Noodle ▲ Chicken w/Rice ▲ Cream of Chicken	Chunky Soup: ▲ Classic Chicken Noodle ▲ Minestrone ▲☆ Old Fashioned Vegetable Beef ▲★ Split Pea and Ham ▲☆ Steak & Potato Condensed: ▲★ Bean w/Bacon ▲ Golden Corn ▲ Noodles & Ground Beef ▲ Pepper Pot ▲★ Split Pea w/Ham & Bacon Home Cookin' Soup: ▲ Chicken Noodle ▲☆ Chicken Vegetable ▲ Italian Vegetable	Condensed: ▲ Cheddar Cheese ▲ Cream of Asparagus ▲ Cream of Broccoli ▲ Cream of Celery ▲ Cream of Chicken ▲ Cream of Mushroom ▲ Cream of Shrimp ▲ Creamy Chicken Mushroom ▲ Creamy Chicken Noodle ▲ Creamy Onion ▲ Fiesta Nacho Cheese ▲ Nacho Cheese ▲ Oyster Stew Home Cookin' Soup: ▲☆ Cream of Mushroom ▲ New England Clam Chowder ▲★ Tuscany-Style Minestrone Ready to Serve, Low Sodium: ▽☆ Cream of Mushroom

▲ High Sodium, 480 mg. or greater per serving.
▽ Low Sodium, 140 mg. or less per serving.
☆ Good Source of Fiber, between 2.5 g. and 5 g. per serving.
★ High Fiber, 5 g. or greater per serving.

BRAND	BEST CHOICE	ACCEPTABLE CHOICE	OCCASIONAL CHOICE
	Fat Free OR Low Fat	Contains Greater Than 3 Grams but Less Than or Equal to 5 Grams Total Fat	Contains Greater Than 5 Grams Total Fat
Campbell's (Cont.)	Healthy Request: ▲ Cream of Mushroom ▲★ Split Pea w/Ham Tomato ▲ Turkey Vegetable w/ White & Wild Rice ▲ Vegetable ▲ Vegetable Beef Healthy Request Ready to Serve: ▲ Chicken Broth ▲ Hearty Chicken Noodle ▲ Hearty Chicken Rice Hearty Chicken Vegetable ▲☆ Hearty Minestrone Hearty Vegetable ▲ New England Clam Chowder Home Cookin' Soup: ▲★ Bean and Ham ▲ Chicken Rice ▲ Country Vegetable ▲☆ Fiesta ▲☆ Minestrone ▲★ Split Pea w/Ham ▲☆ Tomato Garden ▲☆ Vegetable Beef Low Fat Ramen Noodle Soup: ▲ Beef ▲ Chicken ▲ Oriental Microwavable Campbell's Cup: ▲ Chicken w/Rice Quality Soup Mix: ▲ Noodle Ready to Serve, Low Sodium: ▽ Chicken Broth Soup & Recipe Mix: ▲ Onion ▲ Onion Soup w/Chicken Broth		
Casbah	▲ Jambalaya Moroccan Stew	▲ Thai Yum	
College Inn	▲ Beef Broth ▲ Lower Sodium Beef Broth ▲ Lower Sodium Chicken Broth	▲ Chicken Broth	

▲ High Sodium, 480 mg. or greater per serving.
▽ Low Sodium, 140 mg. or less per serving.
☆ Good Source of Fiber, between 2.5 g. and 5 g. per serving.
★ High Fiber, 5 g. or greater per serving.

BRAND	BEST CHOICE	ACCEPTABLE CHOICE	OCCASIONAL CHOICE
	Fat Free OR Low Fat	Contains Greater Than 3 Grams but Less Than or Equal to 5 Grams Total Fat	Contains Greater Than 5 Grams Total Fat

Fantastic Foods	★ Black Bean Salsa Couscous
	★ Low Fat Cha-Cha Chili
	▲★ Country Lentil Soup
	▲★ Couscous w/Lentils
	▲ Creamy Corn & Potato Chowder
	▲ Low Fat Creamy Mushroom
	▲ Low Fat Creamy Tomato Rice Parmesano
	★ Five Bean Soup
	★ Jumpin' Black Bean Soup
	▲☆ Low Fat Creamy Broccoli in Cheddar Soup
	▲☆ Minestrone Soup
	Only A Pinch:
	   ∇★ Couscous w/Lentils
	   ∇★ Spanish Rice & Beans
	Ramen Noodles:
	   ▲☆ Vegetable Curry
	   ▲☆ Vegetable Miso
	   ▲☆ Vegetable Tomato
	   ▲☆ Vegetarian Chicken
	Rice & Beans:
	   ★ Bombay Curry
	   ▲★ Cajun
	   ▲★ Caribbean
	   ▲★ Northern Italian
	   ▲☆ Szechuan
	   ▲★ Tex-Mex
	★ Split Pea Soup
	☆ Vegetarian Chili		

Habitant		▲★ French-Canadian Pea	

Hain	99% Fat Free Soup:
	   ▲★ Black Bean
	   ▲☆ Mushroom Barley
	   ▲ Vegetarian Lentil
	   ▲★ Vegetarian Split Pea		

HamBeens	∇★ 15 Bean Soup ★ Chicken 15 Bean Soup ★ Chili 15 Bean Soup		

▲ High Sodium, 480 mg. or greater per serving.
∇ Low Sodium, 140 mg. or less per serving.
☆ Good Source of Fiber, between 2.5 g. and 5 g. per serving.
★ High Fiber, 5 g. or greater per serving.

BRAND	BEST CHOICE	ACCEPTABLE CHOICE	OCCASIONAL CHOICE
	Fat Free OR Low Fat	Contains Greater Than 3 Grams but Less Than or Equal to 5 Grams Total Fat	Contains Greater Than 5 Grams Total Fat
Health Valley	★ Fat Free 3 Bean Chili Fat Free Beef Broth Fat Free Chicken Broth ★ Fat Free Mild Black Bean Chili ▽★ Fat Free Mild Vegetarian Chili ▽★ Fat Free Mild Vegetarian Chili w/Lentils ▽★ Fat Free Mild Vegetarian Chili w/Beans, No Salt Fat Free Soup: 　☆ 14 Garden Vegetable 　★ 5-Bean Vegetable 　★ Black Bean 　★ Black Bean Vegetable 　★ Carotene Vegetable Power 　▽★ Country Corn & Vegetable 　★ Italian Plus Carotene 　★ Lentil & Carrots 　★ Real Italian Minestrone 　☆ Split Pea & Carrot 　★ Tomato Vegetable 　☆ Vegetable Barley Fat Free Soup in a Cup: 　☆ Chicken Flavored Noodles w/Vegetables 　☆ Creamy Potato w/Broccoli 　Garden Split Pea w/Carrots 　★ Lentil w/Couscous 　☆ Pasta Italiano 　★ Spicy Black Bean w/ Couscous 　☆ Zesty Black Bean w/Rice ★ Fat Free Spicy Black Bean Chili Fat Free Spicy Vegetarian Chili w/Beans: 　▽★ No Salt 　▽★ Regular ★ Organic Lentil ★ Organic Minestrone ★ Organic Mushroom Barley ☆ Organic Potato Leek ★ Organic Split Pea		

▽ Low Sodium, 140 mg. or less per serving.
☆ Good Source of Fiber, between 2.5 g. and 5 g. per serving.
★ High Fiber, 5 g. or greater per serving.

BRAND	BEST CHOICE	ACCEPTABLE CHOICE	OCCASIONAL CHOICE
	Fat Free OR Low Fat	Contains Greater Than 3 Grams but Less Than or Equal to 5 Grams Total Fat	Contains Greater Than 5 Grams Total Fat
Health Valley (Cont.)	☆ Organic Tomato ★ Organic Vegetable ★ Super Broccoli Carotene		
Healthy Choice	★ Bean and Ham ★ Chicken Corn Chowder ☆ Chicken w/Rice ★ Country Vegetable ★ Garden Vegetable ▲☆ Hearty Chicken ▲★ New England Clam Chowder Old Fashioned Chicken Noodle ★ Split Pea and Ham ★ Vegetable Beef		
Hormel	▲ Beef Vegetable ▲ Chicken Noodle	▲★ Ham & Bean ▲ New England Clam Chowder	▲ Broccoli Cheese w/Ham ▲ Potato Cheese w/Ham
L. B. Jamison's	Flavored Soup Base: ▲ Chicken		
Lipton	Cup-a-Soup: ▲ Broccoli and Cheese ▲ Chicken Noodle w/White Meat ▲ Hearty Chicken Spring Vegetable ▲ Tomato Kettle Creations: ▲☆ Bean Medley w/Pasta ▲ Chicken 'n Onion ▲☆ Chicken w/Pasta & Beans ▲☆ Minestrone Recipe Secrets: ▲ Beefy Onion ▲ Golden Onion ▲ Onion ▲ Onion Mushroom		
Manischewitz	Condensed: ▲☆ Barley and Mushroom Soup ▲ Chicken Soup		

▲ High Sodium, 480 mg. or greater per serving.
☆ Good Source of Fiber, between 2.5 g. and 5 g. per serving.
★ High Fiber, 5 g. or greater per serving.

BRAND	BEST CHOICE	ACCEPTABLE CHOICE	OCCASIONAL CHOICE
	Fat Free OR Low Fat	Contains Greater Than 3 Grams but Less Than or Equal to 5 Grams Total Fat	Contains Greater Than 5 Grams Total Fat
Manischewitz (Cont.)	Passover Gold Soup Cup: ▲ Hearty Potato ▲ Vegetarian Tomato		
Mayacamas	Just Enough: Alfredo Pasta ▲ Chicken-Style Rice w/ Broccoli ▲ Chicken-Style Vermicelli Mushroom & Pea Pasta Tomato Basil Pasta ▲ Tomato Vermicelli		
Mrs. Grass	Soup Mix: ▲ Homestyle Chicken Flavored Noodle ▲ Noodle Soup		
Nile Spice	▲ Black Bean ▲ Carrot Dill Soup ▲ Chicken Flavored Vegetable Soup ▲★ Chili & Corn Soup Chili 'n Beans: ▲★ Vegetarian ▲ Country Mushroom Soup ▲ Couscous Almondine ▲ Couscous Garbanzo ▲☆ Couscous Lentil Curry Soup ▲ Couscous Minestrone ▲ Couscous Parmesan ▲☆ Curry Lentil & Rice Soup ▲☆ Lentil Soup Mediterranean Pasta ▲☆ Minestrone Parmesan Pasta ▲☆ Potato Leek Soup ☆ Primavera Pasta ▲☆ Red Beans & Rice Soup ▲☆ Split Pea Sweet Corn Chowder ▲ Tomato & Rice Soup		
Pepperidge Farm	▲ Gazpacho Soup	▲ Chicken w/Wild Rice Soup	

▲ High Sodium, 480 mg. or greater per serving.
☆ Good Source of Fiber, between 2.5 g. and 5 g. per serving.
★ High Fiber, 5 g. or greater per serving.

Brand	Best Choice	Acceptable Choice	Occasional Choice
	Fat Free OR Low Fat	Contains Greater Than 3 Grams but Less Than or Equal to 5 Grams Total Fat	Contains Greater Than 5 Grams Total Fat
Pritikin	Chicken & Rice Chicken Broth Chicken Pasta Soup ☆ Hearty Vegetable ★ Lentil Soup ☆ Minestrone ★ Split Pea ★ Three Bean Chili Vegetable Broth Vegetarian: ☆ Vegetable		

Progresso	▲★ Bean & Ham
	▲ Chicken Noodle Soup
	▲ Chicken Rice w/Vegetables
	▲★ Green Split Pea
	Healthy Classics:
	  ▲☆ Beef Barley Soup
	  ▲ Chicken Noodle Soup
	  Chicken Rice Soup
	  ☆ Garlic & Pasta Soup
	  ▲ Minestrone
	  ▲ New England Clam
	    Chowder
	  Vegetable Soup
	▲★ Hearty Black Bean
	▲ Homestyle Chicken w/
	    Vegetables & Macaroni
	    Pearls
	▲★ Lentil
	Minestrone:
	  ▲★ Original Recipe
	Pasta Soups:
	  ▲☆ Broccoli & Shells
	  ▲☆ Chicken Vegetable &
	    Penne
	  ▲☆ Hearty Minestrone &
	    Shells
	  ▲ Hearty Penne in Chicken
	    Broth
	  ▲☆ Hearty Vegetable and
	    Rotini
	▲ Tortellini in Chicken Broth
	▲☆ Vegetable
		▲☆ Beef Barley
		▲★ Macaroni & Bean Soup
		Pasta Soups:
		  ▲ Spicy Chicken & Penne
			▲ New England Clam Chowder
			Pasta Soups:
			  ▲ Clam & Rotini Chowder
			  ▲ Meatballs & Pasta Pearls

▲ High Sodium, 480 mg. or greater per serving.
☆ Good Source of Fiber, between 2.5 g. and 5 g. per serving.
★ High Fiber, 5 g. or greater per serving.

BRAND	BEST CHOICE	ACCEPTABLE CHOICE	OCCASIONAL CHOICE
	Fat Free OR Low Fat	Contains Greater Than 3 Grams but Less Than or Equal to 5 Grams Total Fat	Contains Greater Than 5 Grams Total Fat
Sanwa			Ramen Pride: ▲ Beef ▲ Chicken ▲ French Onion ▲ Oriental ▲ Pork
Shari's Bistro	☆ Indian Black Bean & Rice ▲☆ Italian White Bean w/ Herb Soup ★ Mexican Bean Burrito Spicy French Green Lentil		
Spice Islands	Quick Meal: ▲ Chicken Rice Pilaf ☆ Curry Rice ▲ Garlic & Herb Pasta ▲★ Oriental Rice & Vegetables ★ Pasta Primavera ▲ Rice & Country Vegetables ★ Rice & Spicy Black Beans ★ Vegetarian Chili ★ Wild Rice & Vegetables		
Swanson	▲ Beef Broth ▲ Clear Chicken Broth ▲ Clear Vegetable Broth Natural Goodness with ⅓ Less Salt: ▲ Clear Chicken Broth		
Sweet Sue	▲ Beef Broth Clear Chicken Broth: ▲ Regular ▲ Reduced Sodium		
Tabatchnick	▲★ Barley and Mushroom ▲ Chicken Broth with Noodles and Dumplings ▲★ Pea		
The Spice Hunter	Brown & Wild Rice Amandine ▲ Cantonese Noodle		

▲ High Sodium, 480 mg. or greater per serving.
☆ Good Source of Fiber, between 2.5 g. and 5 g. per serving.
★ High Fiber, 5 g. or greater per serving.

BRAND	BEST CHOICE	ACCEPTABLE CHOICE	OCCASIONAL CHOICE
	Fat Free OR Low Fat	Contains Greater Than 3 Grams but Less Than or Equal to 5 Grams Total Fat	Contains Greater Than 5 Grams Total Fat
The Spice Hunter (Cont.)	▲ French Country Lentil ▲ Hunan Noodle ▲ Kasba Curry ▲ Mandarin Noodle ▲ Mediterranean Minestrone ▲ Moroccan Couscous ▲ Savory Fettuccini w/Broccoli ▲ Szechwan Noodle		

Wyler's	Instant Broth:
	  ▲ Beef
	  ▲ Chicken
	Instant Broth Low Sodium:
	  ∇ Chicken		

YOUR FAVORITE SOUPS NOT LISTED IN THE *GUIDE*			

▲ High Sodium, 480 mg. or greater per serving.
∇ Low Sodium, 140 mg. or less per serving.

NUT AND SEED BUTTERS

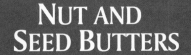

This category contains a selection of nut and seed butters. These products are all cholesterol- free, however, they are high in total fat. Although these products vary in the amount and type of fatty acids they contain, most nut and seed butters consist of predominately mono-unsaturated and polyunsaturated fatty acids.

The *Food Guide Pyramid* lists these products as part of the "Meat, Poultry, Fish, Dry Beans, Eggs, and Nut Group." Because many foods from other food groups also contain protein, most Americans can obtain adequate protein by consuming 2 to 3 servings from this group per day. Two and one-half to three ounces of cooked lean meat, poultry, or fish, count as one serving from this food group. Two tablespoons of peanut butter or other nut butters can be substituted for one ounce of lean meat (about 1/3 serving). Because nut and seed butters contain substantially more fat than lean meat, moderate use is usually appropriate. The FDA has established reference amounts or standardized serving sizes for use on the food label. The reference amount for nut and seed butters is 2 tablespoons. Be sure to read the *Nutrition Facts* label for the serving size information of your nut and seed butter choice. (See pages 51 and 52 for an explanation of reference amounts and the difference between serving sizes established by the FDA for food labeling and those recommended by the *Food Guide Pyramid*.)

The *Dietary Guidelines for Americans*[11] recommends a diet low in fat and saturated fat. The criteria were, therefore, designed to distinguish those products lower in total fat and saturated fat from their higher-fat alternatives.

Criteria Key

▲ **Best Choice:**   **Reduced Fat AND Less Than 4 Grams Saturated Fat**

The nut butters listed in this category meet the FDA's definition for "Reduced" (25% less fat than regular nut butters) and contain the lowest amounts of total fat per 2-tablespoon serving.

△ **Acceptable Choice:**   **"Regular Fat" AND Less Than 4 Grams Saturated Fat**

The nut butters listed in this category are the traditional butters that contain between 14 and 16 grams of total fat per 2-tablespoon serving. These butters also contain less than 4 grams of saturated fat per serving.

▲ **Occasional Choice:**   **High Saturated Fat**

The nut butters listed in this category are considered high in saturated fat because they contain 4 grams or more saturated fat per serving (20% or greater of the Daily Value). These products should be consumed only on occasion.

BRAND	BEST CHOICE	ACCEPTABLE CHOICE	OCCASIONAL CHOICE
	Reduced Fat and Contains Less Than 4 Grams Saturated Fat	Regular Fat and Contains Less Than 4 Grams Saturated Fat	High Saturated Fat
Arrowhead Mills		Peanut Butter: ∇ Creamy ∇ Creamy Sodium Free ∇ Crunchy Sodium Free	
Baron		Peanut Butter: ∇ Creamy ∇ Super Crunch	
Bozo		Peanut Butter	
Estee		∇ Peanut Butter	
Jif	Reduced Fat Peanut Spread: Creamy Crunchy	Peanut Butter: Creamy ∇ Extra Crunchy Simply Jif: ∇ Creamy ∇ Extra Crunchy	
Koeze's		Natural Peanut Butter: ∇ Crunchy	
Krema		Double Whipped: ∇ Peanut Butter Natural Peanut Butter: ∇ All Varieties	
Krinos		∇☆ Tahini	
Maranatha		∇ Cashew Butter ∇ Raw Almond Butter ∇ Roasted Almond Butter	∇ Macadamia Butter
Nutella		∇ Creamy Hazelnut Spread w/Milk Cocoa	
Peter Pan	Smart Choice: Creamy Crunchy	Peanut Butter: Creamy ∇ Extra Crunchy ∇ Sodium Free Whipped Peanut Butter: Creamy	
Reese's		Peanut Butter: ∇ Creamy ∇ Crunchy	

∇ Low Sodium, 140 mg. or less per serving.
☆ Good Source of Fiber, between 2.5 g. and 5 g. per serving.

BRAND	BEST CHOICE	ACCEPTABLE CHOICE	OCCASIONAL CHOICE
	Reduced Fat and Contains Less Than 4 Grams Saturated Fat	Regular Fat and Contains Less Than 4 Grams Saturated Fat	High Saturated Fat
Skippy	Peanut Butter: Reduced Fat	Peanut Butter: Creamy ∇ Super Chunk	
Smucker's		Goober Peanut Butter and Jelly Stripes: All Flavors Natural Peanut Butter: ∇ Creamy or Chunky Peanuts: Creamy Peanut Butter Crunchy Peanut Butter	
YOUR FAVORITE NUT AND SEED BUTTERS NOT LISTED IN THE *GUIDE*			

∇ Low Sodium, 140 mg. or less per serving.

BUTTER AND MARGARINE

This category contains a large variety of butter and margarines. They are available in liquid "squeeze," spray, tub, or stick forms. Some are advertised as "Fat Free," "Reduced Fat," "Low Saturated Fat," or "Low Sodium." Most margarines are made from vegetable oils, blends of vegetable oils, or vegetable oil/butter blends.

For the most part, all margarines are a mixture of liquid vegetable oils and hydrogenated vegetable oils. The process of hydrogenation increases the amount of saturated fat in a product. For this reason, the American Heart Association recommends selecting a margarine that lists "liquid" oil as the first ingredient, followed by hydrogenated oil. Margarine that has been reduced in fat should list water as its first ingredient, followed by liquid vegetable oil, then hydrogenated oil. Because ingredients are listed on the product label in order of predominance, this order will ensure that the product selected will be the lowest in saturated fat (Note: Many of these products may not be suitable for use in cooking or baking).

Butter and Margarine are included as part of the "Fats, Oils, and Sweets Group" at the tip of the *Food Guide Pyramid*. No recommendation has been established for intake from this group. Instead, the public is cautioned to use these foods sparingly. Because butter and margarine can contribute a substantial amount of fat and excess calories to the daily diet, limited use is recommended. The FDA has established reference amounts or standardized serving sizes for use on the food label. The reference amount for butter or margarine is 14 grams (1 Tablespoon). Be sure to read the *Nutrition Facts* label for the serving size information of your choice. (See pages 51 and 52 for an explanation of reference amounts and the difference between serving sizes established by the FDA for food labeling and those recommended by the *Food Guide Pyramid*.)

Although all vegetable-based margarines are cholesterol-free, some still contain saturated fat. Saturated fat is the key substance that contributes to elevated cholesterol, which increases one's risk for heart disease. Criteria were, therefore, designed to distinguish those products lower in total fat and saturated fat from their higher-fat alternatives.

Criteria Key

▲ **Best Choice:**   **Low Saturated Fat**

Products listed in this category meet the FDA's definition for "Low Saturated Fat," (1 gram or less saturated fat per serving).

△ **Acceptable Choice:**   **Contains Less than 2 Grams Saturated Fat**

Products listed in this category **do not** meet the FDA's definition for "Low Saturated Fat" but are lower in saturated fat content than those listed in the Occasional Choice category.

▲ **Occasional Choice:**   **Contains 2 Grams or Greater Saturated Fat**

Products listed in this category **do not** meet the FDA's definition for "Low Saturated Fat," and are higher in saturated fat content than those listed in the Acceptable Choice category, and, therefore, should be consumed only on occasion.

BRAND	BEST CHOICE	ACCEPTABLE CHOICE	OCCASIONAL CHOICE
	Low Saturated Fat	Contains Less Than 2 Grams Saturated Fat	Contains Greater Than or Equal to 2 Grams Saturated Fat
Blue Bonnet	∇ 48% Vegetable Oil Spread (Tub) Lower Fat Margarine (Tub): ∇ 34% Vegetable Oil	∇ 60% Pure Vegetable Oil Spread (Stick) ∇ 68% Pure Vegetable Oil Spread (Tub) Light Taste Spread: ∇ 52% Oil (Stick) ∇ 56% Vegetable Oil	
Brummel & Brown	Spread: ∇ Made w/Yogurt		
Butter Buds	∇ Spread		
Cole's			∇ Garlic Spread
Fleischmann's	Canola Choice: ∇ 56% Canola and Corn Oil Spread ∇ Fat Free Low Calorie Spread (Squeeze) Lower Fat Margarine Sticks: ∇ 40% Corn Oil Lower Fat Margarine Tubs: ∇ 31% Canola/Corn Oil	Light Taste Spread: ∇ 56% Corn Oil Move Over Butter Whipped Spread: ∇ 72% Vegetable Oil Soft Spread: ∇ 67% Corn Oil Squeeze Spread: ∇ 70% Corn Oil	Move Over Butter: ∇ 72% Vegetable Oil Spread Original Margarine: ∇ 80% Corn Oil Soft Spread: ∇ 75% Corn Oil ∇ Sweet Unsalted Margarine
Hain			∇ Safflower Oil Margarine
I Can't Believe It's Not Butter	Light: ∇ 40% Vegetable Oil Spread (Tub) ∇ Margarine Spray	Light: ∇ 52% Vegetable Oil Spread	∇ 70% Vegetable Oil Spread (Tub) 70% Vegetable Oils Spread: ∇ Sweet Cream Buttermilk (Quarters) ∇ Soft Margarine Squeezable 68% Vegetable Oil Spread: ∇ Sweet Cream Buttermilk
Imperial		Delight: ∇ 48% Vegetable Oil Spread (Tub) ∇ 52% Vegetable Oil Spread (Stick)	∇ 70% Vegetable Oil Spread (Stick) Soft: ∇ 68% Vegetable Oil Spread (Tub)
Kraft		Touch of Butter: ∇ 47% Vegetable Oil (Tub)	
Land O Lakes			Country Morning Blend Light: ∇ 40% Vegetable Oil & Butter Blend (Tub)

∇ Low Sodium, 140 mg. or less per serving.

BRAND	BEST CHOICE	ACCEPTABLE CHOICE	OCCASIONAL CHOICE
	Low Saturated Fat	Contains Less Than 2 Grams Saturated Fat	Contains Greater Than or Equal to 2 Grams Saturated Fat
Land O Lakes (Cont.)			Spread: ∇ 70% Vegetable Oil Spread (Stick) Spread w/Sweet Cream: ∇ 60% Vegetable Oil (Tub) ∇ 70% Vegetable Oil (Quarters) ∇ Stick Margarine ∇ Tub Margarine
Move Over Butter		∇ 72% Vegetable Oil Spread (Quarters) Whipped: ∇ 72% Vegetable Oil Spread (Tub)	
Parkay	Light: ∇ 40% Vegetable Oil Spread (Tub)	⅓ Less Fat: ∇ 53% Vegetable Oil Spread ∇ 50% Vegetable Oil Spread Squeeze: ∇ 64% Vegetable Oil Spread	∇ 70% Vegetable Oil Spread ∇ Soft Margarine
Promise	Extra: ∇ Light Margarine (Stick) ∇ Light Margarine (Tub) Ultra: ∇ 26% Vegetable Oil Spread ∇ Nonfat Margarine	∇ 68% Vegetable Oil Spread (Tub)	∇ 68% Vegetable Oil Spread (Stick)
Shedd's Spread		Country Crock: ∇ 48% Vegetable Oil ∇ 48% Vegetable Oil (Tub) Country Crock Churnstyle: ∇ 48% Vegetable Oil (Tub) Country Crock Spreadable Sticks: ∇ 64% Vegetable Oil Squeezable Country Crock: ∇ 64% Vegetable Oil	∇ Country Crock Churnstyle (Stick) Willow Run Soybean Margarine
Smart Beat	∇ Lower Fat Margarine		
Weight Watchers	∇ Light Margarine (Tub)		
BUTTER			
All Brands			∇ Butter
Land O Lakes			Country Morning Blend Margarine: ∇ Quarters

∇ Low Sodium, 140 mg. or less per serving.

296   **Butter and Margarine**

Brand	Best Choice	Acceptable Choice	Occasional Choice
	Low Saturated Fat	Contains Less Than 2 Grams Saturated Fat	Contains Greater Than or Equal to 2 Grams Saturated Fat

Land O Lakes (Cont.)			Light Butter:
			  ∇ Salted Quarters
			Sweet Cream Salted Butter:
			  ∇ Quarters
			Sweet Cream Whipped Butter:
			  ∇ Salted (Tub)
			Sweet Light Butter:
			  ∇ Unsalted Quarters
			Unsalted Sweet Butter:
			  ∇ Quarters
			Whipped Butter:
			  ∇ Unsalted

Purity Farms			Ghee: ∇ Clarified Butter
BUTTER SUBSTITUTES			
Butter Buds	∇ Butter Mix		
McCormick	Best O Butter: ∇ Original Butter		

Molly McButter	Natural Sprinkles:
	  Butter Flavor
	  ∇ Cheese Flavor
	  ∇ Garlic & Herb Flavor		

YOUR FAVORITE BUTTER AND MARGARINE NOT LISTED IN THE *GUIDE*			

∇ Low Sodium, 140 mg. or less per serving.

CREAM, CREAM SUBSTITUTES, AND TOPPINGS

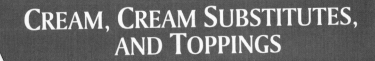

Products in this category have been divided into three sub-headings (fresh, frozen, and powders) for ease in locating these products. Brand-name products in this category range from fat-free creamers and toppings to full-fat versions that can contribute a significant amount of fat to the daily diet.

High-fat products listed in this category are included as part of the "Fats, Oils and Sweets Group" at the tip of the *Food Guide Pyramid*. There is no recommendation established for intake from this group. Instead, consumers are cautioned to use these foods sparingly. The FDA has established reference amounts or standardized serving sizes for use on the food label. The reference amount for these products varies depending on type. Reference amounts range from 2 grams (1 teaspoon) for powdered creamers to 30 milliliters (2 tablespoons) for Half & Half. Be sure to read the *Nutrition Facts* label for the serving size information of your cream product choice. (See pages 51 and 52 for an explanation of reference amounts and the difference between serving sizes established by the FDA for food labeling and those recommended by the *Food Guide Pyramid*.)

Products in this category range from those that are higher in fat and should be used in limited amounts, to those that contain little or no fat when used in their recommended serving size. The criteria were, therefore, designed to distinguish those products that are lower in total fat and saturated fat from their higher-fat alternatives.

Criteria Key

▲ **Best Choice:**   **Fat Free**

Products listed in this category meet the FDA's definition for "Fat Free" (less than $1/2$ gram fat per serving).

▲ **Acceptable Choice:**   **Low Fat AND Low Saturated Fat**

Products listed in this category meet the FDA's definition for "Low Fat" (3 grams or less fat per serving), and "Low Saturated Fat" (1 gram or less per serving).

▲ **Occasional Choice:**   **Contains Greater Than 3 grams Total Fat, or Greater Than 1 gram Saturated Fat**

Products listed in this category **do not** meet the FDA's definition for "Low Fat" or "Low Saturated Fat." Since excessive use of these products can significantly increase your intake of total fat and saturated fat, they should be consumed only on occasion.

BRAND	BEST CHOICE	ACCEPTABLE CHOICE	OCCASIONAL CHOICE
	Fat Free	Low Fat AND Low Saturated Fat	Contains Greater Than 3 Grams Total Fat OR Greater Than 1 Gram Saturated Fat
FRESH			
All Brands			Cream: ∇ Light ∇ Medium - 25% Fat ∇ Half & Half Sour Cream: ∇ Cultured Whipping Cream: ∇ Heavy ∇ Light
Berne'A	∇ Nonfat Sour Cream	∇ Lowfat Sour Cream	∇ Old Fashioned Sour Cream
Breakstone's	∇ Free Sour Cream		Sour Cream: ∇ Half & Half ∇ Regular
Broughton Foods			Real Cream: ∇ Whipped Light Cream
C.F. Burger			∇ Half & Half
Carnation	Fat Free Coffee-Mate ∇ All Flavors	Coffee-Mate: ∇ Amaretto ∇ Cinnamon Creme ∇ French Vanilla ∇ Hazelnut ∇ Irish Cream ∇ Liquid Non-Dairy Creamer ∇ Lite Liquid Non-Dairy Creamer	
Country Fresh	∇ Nonfat Sour Cream	∇ Lowfat Sour Cream	∇ Sour Cream
Dean Foods		∇ Light Sour Cream Ultra: ∇ Non-Dairy Creamer	∇ Cultured Sour Cream Ultra: ∇ Half & Half
Farm Rich	Non-Dairy Creamer: ∇ Fat Free	Non-Dairy Creamer: ∇ Light ∇ Original	
International Delight	No Fat Cappuccino Creamer: ∇ All Flavors No Fat Creamer: ∇ All Flavors	Non-Dairy Creamer: ∇ All Flavors	

∇ Low Sodium, 140 mg. or less per serving.

BRAND	BEST CHOICE	ACCEPTABLE CHOICE	OCCASIONAL CHOICE
	Fat Free	Low Fat AND Low Saturated Fat	Contains Greater Than 3 Grams Total Fat OR Greater Than 1 Gram Saturated Fat
Knudsen	∇ Fat Free Sour Cream		∇ Hampshire Sour Cream ∇ Light Sour Cream
Land O Lakes	∇ No Fat Sour Cream		∇ Light Sour Cream
Light N' Lively	Free: ∇ Nonfat Sour Cream Alternative	∇ Light Sour Cream	
Melody Farms		∇ Real Whip	∇ Coffee Cream ∇ Cultured Sour Cream ∇ Half and Half ∇ Heavy Whipping Cream ∇ Lite Sour Cream
Naturally Yours	∇ No Fat Sour Cream		
Parmalat			∇ Long Life Half & Half
Real Dairy	Sour Cream: ∇ No Fat		
Reddi Wip		Real Whipped Light Cream: ∇ Instant ∇ Whipped Topping	∇ Deluxe Real Heavy Whipped Cream
Rich's		Coffee Rich: ∇ Light Non-Dairy Creamer ∇ Non-Dairy Creamer Coffee Rich Cholesterol & Lactose Free: ∇ Non-Dairy Creamer Rich Whip: ∇ Whip Topping	
Sante			Creme Fraiche: ∇ Cooking and Topping Cream
Sealtest	∇ Fat Free Sour Cream		∇ Light Sour Cream ∇ Sour Cream
Stonyfield Farm			∇ Light Sour Cream ∇ Sour Cream
Yoder's	∇ Fat Free Sour Cream		∇ Light Sour Cream ∇ Old Fashioned Sour Cream

∇ Low Sodium, 140 mg. or less per serving.

302   **Cream, Cream Substitutes and Toppings**

BRAND	BEST CHOICE	ACCEPTABLE CHOICE	OCCASIONAL CHOICE
	Fat Free	Low Fat AND Low Saturated Fat	Contains Greater Than 3 Grams Total Fat OR Greater Than 1 Gram Saturated Fat
FROZEN			
Cool Whip		∇ Lite Whipped Topping	∇ Extra Creamy Whipped Topping ∇ Non-Dairy Whipped Topping ∇ Regular Whipped Topping
Reddi Wip		∇ Lite Whipped Topping	
POWDERS			
Borden	Cremora Lite: ∇ Non-Dairy Creamer	Cremora: ∇ Non-Dairy Creamer	
Carnation	Coffee-Mate: ∇ Fat Free Non Dairy Creamer ∇ Lite Non-Dairy Creamer	Coffee-Mate: ∇ Regular	Powdered Coffee-Mate: ∇ All Flavors
D-Zerta		∇ Reduced Calorie Whipped Topping Mix	
Dream Whip		∇ Whipped Topping Mix	
YOUR FAVORITE CREAM AND TOPPINGS NOT LISTED IN THE *GUIDE*			

∇ Low Sodium, 140 mg. or less per serving.

FATS AND OILS

This category contains selections of fats and oils. These products range from liquid vegetable oils or sprays to solid animal fats such as lard. All products in this section, whether from a vegetable source or an animal source, provide 100% of calories from fat!

Although fat is an essential nutrient, it is needed in only small amounts. Fats in food carry some vitamins into the body and are necessary for skin health and some nervous system tissue.

Fat is very dense in calories. In fact, the caloric content of one gram of fat is greater than two times the caloric content of one gram of carbohydrate or protein. Hence, for adults who are concerned about weight control, it is recommended to limit all fats in the diet so that no more than 30% of total calories comes from fat.

Fats and oils are included as part of the "Fats, Oils, and Sweets Group" at the tip of the *Food Guide Pyramid.* There is no recommendation established for intake from this group. Instead, the public is cautioned to use these foods sparingly. The FDA has established reference amounts or standardized serving sizes for use on the food label. The reference amount for oils is 1 tablespoon (14 grams). Be sure to read the *Nutrition Facts* label for the serving size information of your vegetable oil choice. (See pages 51 and 52 for an explanation of reference amounts and the difference between serving sizes established by the FDA for food labeling and those recommended by the Food Guide Pyramid.)

Choosing appropriate types of fat is just as important as monitoring the amount of fat you eat. Although all vegetable fats are cholesterol-free, it is important to keep in mind that they all provide 100% of their calories from fat and still may contain some saturated fat, which is the key substance that contributes to elevated blood cholesterol. Another key concept for the consumer to consider is the amount of fat that is eaten. A small serving of a food product that contains saturated fat can be part of a heart-healthy diet. Conversely, eating large amounts of a low-saturated-fat food may provide more saturated fat and calories than is recommended for a heart-healthy diet.

Diets high in monounsaturated fatty acids have been shown to lower LDL-cholesterol, without lowering the protective HDL-cholesterol, when substituted in the diet for saturated fatty acids. On the other hand, diets high in

polyunsaturated fatty acids have been shown to lower the protective HDL-cholesterol as well as lowering the LDL-cholesterol. Without a doubt, the most significant dietary factor contributing to elevated cholesterol levels is a high intake of saturated fat. Use Table 8 on page 42 to help guide you in your fat selections.

As previously mentioned in the introduction of this book, fats and oils do not consist of only one type of fatty acid, but instead are a mixture of saturated, polyunsaturated, and monounsaturated fatty acids. Therefore, for the purpose of evaluating these products, fats and oils are classified according to their predominant fatty acid. For example, olive oil contains significantly more monounsaturated fat (77% by weight) than saturated (14% by weight) or polyunsaturated (9% by weight). Olive oil is therefore classified as a monounsaturated fat source.

Criteria were therefore designed to distinguish those fats and oils that consist of predominantly monounsaturated, polyunsaturated, or saturated fatty acids.

Criteria Key

▲ **Best Choice:**   **Predominantly Monounsaturated Fatty Acids**

Fats and Oils listed in this category are the richest sources of monounsaturated fat, which is a type of fat known to lower LDL-cholesterol levels. Guidelines set by the National Cholesterol Education Program (NCEP II), see pages 34 and 35, recommend that the greatest proportion of fat in the diet come from monounsaturated sources.[35]

▲ **Acceptable Choice:**   **Predominantly Polyunsaturated Fatty Acids**

Fats and Oils listed in this category are the richest sources of polyunsaturated fat. Polyunsaturated fat is known to lower LDL-cholesterol levels, but may also lower HDL-cholesterol. Although small amounts of these fats are important for health, it is recommended that they be limited to no more than 10% of total calories.

▲ **Occasional Choice:**   **Predominantly Saturated Fatty Acids**

Conclusive scientific evidence exists that the most significant dietary factor contributing to elevated blood cholesterol levels is a high intake of saturated fat. For this reason products listed in this category should be consumed only on occasion.

BRAND	BEST CHOICE	ACCEPTABLE CHOICE	OCCASIONAL CHOICE
	Predominantly Monounsaturated Fat	Predominantly Polyunsaturated Fat	Predominantly Saturated Fat
OILS			
Alessi	∇ Extra Vergine Di Oliva		
All Brands	∇ Avocado Oil ∇ Canola Oil ∇ High Oleic Safflower ∇ High Oleic Sunflower ∇ Olive Oil ∇ Peanut Oil	∇ Corn Oil ∇ Safflower Oil ∇ Sesame Oil ∇ Soybean Oil ∇ Sunflower Oil	∇ Coconut Oil
Arrowhead Mills		∇ Flax Seed Oil	
Bella	∇ Olive Oil		
Bellino	Olive Oil: ∇ Extra Virgin		
Bertolli	Olive Oil: ∇ Classico ∇ Extra Light		
Calavo	∇ Avocado Oil		
California Naturals	∇ Fra Diavalo Hot Oil ∇ Pesto Pasta Oil		
Colavita	∇ Extra Virgin Olive Oil ∇ Limonolio ∇ Olive Oil ∇ Pepperolio		
Crisco	∇ Corn and Canola Oil Blend ∇ Natural Blend Oil ∇ Pure Vegetable Oil ∇ Puritan Canola Oil		
DaVinci	∇ 100% Pure Olive Oil ∇ Extra Virgin Olive Oil		
Delallo	∇ Olive Oil		
Dell' Alpe	∇ Extra Virgin Olive Oil ∇ Olive Oil		
Ferrara	∇ 100% Extra Virgin Olive Oil		
Filippo Berio	Olive Oil: ∇ Extra Mild ∇ Extra Virgin ∇ Regular		

∇ Low Sodium, 140 mg. or less per serving.

BRAND	BEST CHOICE	ACCEPTABLE CHOICE	OCCASIONAL CHOICE
	Predominantly Monounsaturated Fat	Predominantly Polyunsaturated Fat	Predominantly Saturated Fat
Giralda	∇ Olive Oil		
Hain	∇ Canola Oil ∇ High Oleic Sunflower Oil ∇ Olive Oil ∇ Peanut Oil	∇ All Blend Oil ∇ Garlic Oil ∇ Safflower Oil ∇ Sesame Oil ∇ Soy Oil ∇ Sunflower Oil	
Hollywood	∇ Canola Oil ∇ Peanut Oil	∇ Safflower Oil	
International Bazaar	Olive Oil: ∇ Extra Virgin		
Italica	∇ Olive Oil		
La Preferida	∇ Extra Virgin Olive Oil		
Little Crow		∇ Popcorn Oil	

Loriva	∇100% Canola Oil
	∇ Basil Flavored Oil
	Canolive Supreme:
	   ∇ Canola and Olive Oil
	   Blend
	∇ Garlic Flavored Oil
	∇ Peanut Oil
	∇ Rice Bran Oil
		∇ Safflower Oil
		∇ Extra Virgin Sesame Oil
		∇ Walnut Oil	

Mazola	∇ Right Blend	∇ 100% Pure Corn Oil	
Old Monk	∇ Extra Virgin Olive Oil		
Olio Sasso	∇ Extra Virgin Olive Oil		
Orville Redenbacher		Popping & Topping Popcorn Oil: ∇ Buttery Flavor	
Planters	∇ 100% Pure Peanut Oil		
Pompeian	∇ Extra Virgin Olive Oil		

Progresso	Olive Oil:
	   ∇ Extra Mild
	   ∇ Extra Virgin
	   ∇ Regular		

Racconto	∇ 100% Italian Olive Oil ∇ Extra Virgin Olive Oil		
RS	∇ Extra Virgin Olive Oil		

∇ Low Sodium, 140 mg. or less per serving.

308   **Fats and Oils**

BRAND	BEST CHOICE	ACCEPTABLE CHOICE	OCCASIONAL CHOICE
	Predominantly Monounsaturated Fat	Predominantly Polyunsaturated Fat	Predominantly Saturated Fat
Spectrum Naturals	▽ Almond Oil ▽ Apricot Kernel Oil ▽ Avocado Oil ▽ Canola & Olive Oil ▽ Canola Oil ▽ Extra Virgin Olive Oil ▽ Peanut Oil	▽ Corn Oil ▽ Safflower Oil ▽ Sesame Oil ▽ Soy Oil ▽ Toasted Sesame Oil ▽ Walnut Oil	
Tirreno	Olive Oil: ▽ All Types		
Vigo	▽ Olive Oil		

Wesson	▽ Best Blend
	▽ Canola Oil
	▽ Pure Olive Oil
	▽ Stir Fry Oil
		▽ Corn Oil
		Vegetable Oil:
		  ▽ Kosher for Passover
		  ▽ Light Tasting
		  ▽ Original	

SPRAYS			
Bake Eez	Canola Oil Pan Coating: ▽ Butter Flavor		
Baker's Joy		▽ Baking Spray	
Mazola		No Stick: ▽ Corn Oil Cooking Spray	
Naturally Lite	▽ Butter Flavored Spray ▽ Canola Cooking Spray ▽ Real Garlic Flavored Spray		

Pam	No Stick Cooking Spray:
	  ▽ "All Natural Butter Flavor"
	  ▽ "All Natural Original"
	▽ Non-Aerosol Pump Spray		

Tryson House		▽ Buttery Delight ▽ Garlic Mist	
Weight Watchers	▽ Canola Cooking Spray	▽ Buttery Spray	
Wesson	▽ No Stick Cooking Spray		
LARDS			
All Brands			▽ Lard
Armour			▽ Armour Lard

▽ Low Sodium, 140 mg. or less per serving.

BRAND	BEST CHOICE	ACCEPTABLE CHOICE	OCCASIONAL CHOICE
	Predominantly Monounsaturated Fat	Predominantly Polyunsaturated Fat	Predominantly Saturated Fat
Oscar Mayer			∇ Lard
YOUR FAVORITE FATS AND OILS NOT LISTED IN THE *GUIDE*			

∇ Low Sodium, 140 mg. or less per serving.

SALAD DRESSING

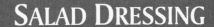

Salad dressings add zest to healthy salads. Unfortunately, many of these can provide a lot of fat, even if consumed in the small reference serving size of 2 tablespoons. The good news is that food manufacturers have responded to consumer demands for lower-fat foods by developing reduced-fat or fat-free versions of our favorites.

Salad dressings are included as part of the "Fats, Oils, and Sweets Group" at the tip of the *Food Guide Pyramid*. There is no recommendation established for intake from this group. Instead, the public is cautioned to use these foods sparingly. Serving sizes and the number of servings that you eat can make a big difference in this category. The higher-fat choices may be part of a heart-healthy diet, in particular, if the amount eaten is small and they are consumed occasionally.

The FDA has established reference amounts or standardized serving sizes for use on the food label. The reference amount for salad dressings is 30 grams (2 tablespoons). Be sure to read the *Nutrition Facts* label for the serving size information of your salad dressing choice. (See pages 51 and 52 for an explanation of reference amounts and the difference between serving sizes established by the FDA for food labeling and those recommended by the *Food Guide Pyramid*.)

Products in the Salad Dressing category range from fat-free to those that are higher in fat. Some also contain higher levels of saturated fat, particularly the creamy variety; yet others are a source of unsaturated fat, such as the vinaigrettes. Criteria are, therefore, designed to distinguish those products lower in total fat and saturated fat from their higher-fat alternatives.

Criteria Key

▲ **Best Choice:**   **Fat Free or Low Fat, AND Low Saturated Fat**

Products listed in this category meet the FDA's definition for "Fat Free" (less than $1/2$ gram fat per serving) or "Low Fat" (3 grams or less fat per serving) and "Low Saturated Fat" (1 gram or less saturated fat per serving).

△ **Acceptable Choice:**   **Contains Greater Than or Equal to 3 Grams but Less Than 13 Grams Total Fat, AND Low Saturated Fat**

Products listed in this category **do not** meet the FDA's definition for "Low Fat" but **do** meet the definition for "Low Saturated Fat."

▲ **Occasional Choice:**   **High Fat or Contains Greater Than 1 Gram Saturated Fat**

Products listed in this category contain 13 grams or more total fat per serving (20% or greater of the Daily Value) and are, therefore, considered high in total fat. These products also **do not** meet the FDA's definition for "Low Saturated Fat." Because these products can contribute a greater amount of total fat and saturated fat to the overall daily diet, they should be consumed only on occasion.

BRAND	BEST CHOICE	ACCEPTABLE CHOICE	OCCASIONAL CHOICE
	Fat Free or Low Fat AND Low Saturated Fat	Contains Greater Than 3 Grams But Less Than 13 Grams Total Fat AND Low Saturated Fat	High Fat OR Contains Greater Than 1 Gram Saturated Fat
Annie's	Organic Yogurt Dressing w/Dill: No Fat	∇ Balsamic Vinaigrette ∇ Cilantro & Lime Vinaigrette Gingerly Vinaigrette Goddess Dressing ∇ Raspberry Vinaigrette Roasted Red Pepper Vinaigrette	Cowgirl Ranch Dressing Shiitake & Sesame Vinaigrette

Arnie's	Fat Free:
	    Raspberry Vinaigrette
	    ∇ Riviera
			Riviera Dressing
			Raspberry Vinaigrette

Bernstein's		Light Fantastic: Parmesan Garlic Ranch	
Blanchard & Blanchard	Spa Dressing: All Flavors		

Cardini's			Dressing:
			    The Original Caesar
			Dressing & Marinade:
			    Italian
			    Lemon Herb
			    Pesto Pasta
			    Zesty Garlic

Christie's		Greek Dressing	

Estee	Low Calorie Dressing:
	    ∇ Creamy French
	    ∇ Thousand Island		

Girard's	Fat Free Salad Dressing:
	    Balsamic Vinaigrette
	    Raspberry
	    Red Wine Vinaigrette
		Light Caesar	Caesar
			Champagne
			▲ Old Venice Italian
			∇ Raspberry
			Romano Cheese
			Spinach Salad Dressing

Henri's	Fat Free:
	    Honey Mustard
	    Italian
	    Ranch
	Light Original French
	Light Ranch
	Light Tas-Tee
	Light Thousand Island
		Tangy Dijon Honey Mustard	Bacon and Tomato
			Caesar Ranch
			Original French
			Ranch
			Tas-Tee
			Thousand Island
			▲ Traditional Italian

▲ High Sodium, 480 mg. or greater per serving.
∇ Low Sodium, 140 mg. or less per serving.

BRAND	BEST CHOICE	ACCEPTABLE CHOICE	OCCASIONAL CHOICE
	Fat Free or Low Fat AND Low Saturated Fat	Contains Greater Than 3 Grams But Less Than 13 Grams Total Fat AND Low Saturated Fat	High Fat OR Contains Greater Than 1 Gram Saturated Fat
Herb Magic	Fat Free Dressing: All Flavors		
Hidden Valley Ranch	Fat Free: Blue Cheese Coleslaw Dressing Creamy Parmesan Honey Dijon Ranch Italian Parmesan Low Fat Original Ranch	Light Original Ranch	Cole Slaw Dressing ▲ Creamy Parmesan Fiesta Ranch For Kids: Nacho Cheese Ranch Pizza Ranch Super Cheese Ranch Super Creamy Ranch Taco Ranch Honey Dijon Ranch Original Ranch Original Ranch w/Bacon
Ken's		▲ Lite Caesar Lite Creamy Parmesan w/ Cracked Peppercorn Lite Ranch ▽ Raspberry Walnut Vinaigrette	Balsamic & Basil Vinaigrette Caesar Dressing Country French w/Vermont Honey Italian w/Aged Romano Ranch Spicy Italian
Knott's Berry Farm		▽ Fruit Salad Dressing	Ground Peppercorn ▽ Honey Mustard Poppyseed Sun-Dried Tomato Vinaigrette Dressing
Kraft	Deliciously Right: French Free: Blue Cheese Catalina French Honey Dijon Italian Peppercorn Ranch Ranch Thousand Island	Deliciously Right: Catalina Cucumber Ranch Italian Thousand Island Salsa Zesty Garden	Bacon and Tomato Buttermilk Ranch Caesar Caesar Ranch Catalina French Catalina w/Honey Cucumber Ranch Deliciously Right: Ranch French Honey Dijon House Italian w/Olive Oil Presto Italian Ranch Roka Blue Cheese Salsa Ranch

▲ High Sodium, 480 mg. or greater per serving.
▽ Low Sodium, 140 mg. or less per serving.

BRAND	BEST CHOICE	ACCEPTABLE CHOICE	OCCASIONAL CHOICE
	Fat Free or Low Fat AND Low Saturated Fat	Contains Greater Than 3 Grams But Less Than 13 Grams Total Fat AND Low Saturated Fat	High Fat OR Contains Greater Than 1 Gram Saturated Fat
Kraft (Cont.)			Sour Cream & Onion Ranch Thousand Island ▲ Zesty Italian
La Martinique	Nonfat Dressing: Red Wine Vinegar		∇ A True French Vinaigrette Blue Cheese Vinaigrette
Lawry's		▲ Red Wine Vinaigrette	Caesar Dressing w/Imported Anchovies Creamy Caesar w/Cracked Black Pepper Italian w/Aged Parmesan Cheese ▲ Italian w/Bleu Cheese Lemon Pepper w/Lemon Juice ▲ San Francisco w/Romano Cheese
Manischewitz	Passover Gold: Fat Free Italian		
Maple Grove Farms		Lite Dressing: Caesar Honey Mustard Honey Ranch & Cracked Pepper Italian Wine & Cheese Lemon 'n Dill Pesto Parmesan Vermont: Sweet 'n Sour	Vermont: ∇ Honey 'n Lemon Poppyseed Honey Mustard
Marie's	Luscious Low Fat: Zesty Ranch Zesty Fat Free: ∇ Raspberry Vinaigrette Red Wine Vinaigrette		Chunky Blue Cheese Honey Mustard
Marzetti	Fat Free: Slaw Dressing	Light California French Slaw Dressing: Light	Light Ranch Potato Salad Dressing Ranch Slaw Dressing: Southern Recipe The Original Sweet & Saucy Thousand Island
Nayonaise	∇ Vegi Dressing & Spread		

▲ High Sodium, 480 mg. or greater per serving.
∇ Low Sodium, 140 mg. or less per serving.

BRAND	BEST CHOICE	ACCEPTABLE CHOICE	OCCASIONAL CHOICE
	Fat Free or Low Fat AND Low Saturated Fat	Contains Greater Than 3 Grams But Less Than 13 Grams Total Fat AND Low Saturated Fat	High Fat OR Contains Greater Than 1 Gram Saturated Fat
Newman's Own	Light Italian Dressing		Caesar Dressing Olive Oil and Vinegar Dressing Ranch Dressing
Old Dutch	▲ Sweet & Sour Dressing		
Old Family Recipe			Caesar Dill & Lemon Gourmet Blue Cheese House Vinaigrette Lite Parmesan Pepper Parmesan Pepper
Pritikin	Fat Free Salad Dressing: ∇ All Flavors		
Robb Ross		▲ Red Wine Vinegar Oil	
S & W	Vintage Lites Oil Free Dressing: All Flavors		
Seven Seas	Fat Free: Ranch Red Wine Vinegar	Reduced Calorie: Viva Italian Two Cheese Italian	▲ Creamy Italian Honey Mustard Ranch Dressing ▲ Red Wine Vinegar & Oil ▲ Viva Italian
Smart Temptations	Nonfat Salad Dressing: All Flavors		

T. Marzetti's	Fat Free:
	Honey French
	Italian
	Peppercorn Ranch
	∇ Raspberry
		Lite Honey French
		Lite Slaw Dressing
			Buttermilk Vegetable Dip and
			    Dressing
			Classic Caesar Ranch
			∇ Creamy Garlic Italian
			Dijon Honey Mustard Dip and
			    Dressing
			Fresh Buttermilk Bacon Ranch
			Fresh Buttermilk Ranch
			Homestyle Thousand Island
			Lite Buttermilk Ranch
			Lite Chunky Blue Cheese
			Old Fashioned Poppyseed
			Olde World Caesar
			Original Slaw Dressing
			∇ Wilde Raspberry Dressing

▲ High Sodium, 480 mg. or greater per serving.
∇ Low Sodium, 140 mg. or less per serving.

316   **Salad Dressing**

BRAND	BEST CHOICE	ACCEPTABLE CHOICE	OCCASIONAL CHOICE
	Fat Free or Low Fat AND Low Saturated Fat	Contains Greater Than 3 Grams But Less Than 13 Grams Total Fat AND Low Saturated Fat	High Fat OR Contains Greater Than 1 Gram Saturated Fat
Thomson Berry Farms			∇ Susan's Sweet Raspberry Dressing
Waldon Farms	Fat Free Salad Dressing: All Varieties		
Weight Watchers	Salad Celebrations: Fat Free Caesar Fat Free Creamy Italian Fat Free French Style Fat Free Honey Dijon Fat Free Italian Fat Free Ranch Low Fat Thousand Island Low Fat Three Cheese Caesar		
Western	Fat Free French Lite French		Bacon Dressing French
Wish-Bone	Healthy Sensation: Fat Free Honey Dijon Fat Free Italian Fat Free Ranch ▲ Lite Italian Dressing	Lite Olive Oil Caesar Olive Oil Italian Olive Oil Vinaigrette Russian	Chunky Blue Cheese ▲ Italian Lite Ranch Ranch ▲ Robusto Italian Dressing Sweet and Spicy French Thousand Island Dressing
SANDWICH SPREADS: 1 TABLESPOON SERVING			
Hain			∇ Eggless Mayonnaise
Hellman's	∇ Low Fat Mayonnaise Dressing Low Fat Tartar Sauce ∇ Reduced Fat Mayonnaise	∇ Light Mayonnaise	∇ Real Mayonnaise
Kraft	Free: ∇ Mayonnaise Dressing Tartar Sauce Miracle Whip: ∇ Light Salad Dressing Miracle Whip Free: ∇ Nonfat Dressing ∇ Reduced Fat Sandwich Spread	∇ Light Mayonnaise Miracle Whip: ∇ Coleslaw Dressing ∇ Salad Dressing ∇ Sandwich Spread & Burger Sauce	∇ Real Mayonnaise Sauceworks: Tartar Sauce

▲ High Sodium, 480 mg. or greater per serving.
∇ Low Sodium, 140 mg. or less per serving.

BRAND	BEST CHOICE	ACCEPTABLE CHOICE	OCCASIONAL CHOICE
	Fat Free or Low Fat AND Low Saturated Fat	Contains Greater Than 3 Grams But Less Than 13 Grams Total Fat AND Low Saturated Fat	High Fat OR Contains Greater Than 1 Gram Saturated Fat
Smart Beat	∇ Nonfat Mayonnaise Dressing		
Spectrum Naturals		∇ Canola Mayonnaise	
Weight Watchers	∇ Fat Free Whipped Dressing ∇ Light Mayonnaise		
Westbrae Natural			∇ Mayonnaise
YOUR FAVORITE SALAD DRESSINGS NOT LISTED IN THE *GUIDE*			

∇ Low Sodium, 140 mg. or less per serving.

DESSERTS

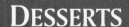

This category contains a large variety of dessert products, such as frozen dairy and non-dairy desserts, prepared cakes and pies, puddings and gelatins. These dessert products range in fat and sugar content from those that are fat-free and sugar-free to the more traditional high-fat, high-sugar desserts.

The *Food Guide Pyramid* includes some dessert-type foods as part of the "Bread, Cereal, Rice, and Pasta Group," while others are included as part of the "Milk, Yogurt, and Cheese Group," and yet others are included as part of the "Fats, Oils, and Sweets Group." It is generally recommended that dessert-type products, regardless of what food group they are identified with in the *Food Guide Pyramid*, be chosen less often in order to limit intake of excess calories, fat, and saturated fat, especially by those persons who need to reduce their body weight or those with medical conditions such as heart disease or diabetes. The FDA has established reference amounts or standardized serving sizes for use on the food label. The reference amounts for these foods vary greatly depending on type of product. Be sure to read the *Nutrition Facts* label for the serving size information of your dessert choice. (See pages 51 and 52 for an explanation of reference amounts and the difference between serving sizes established by the FDA for food labeling and those recommended by the *Food Guide Pyramid*.)

The criteria were designed to distinguish those dessert products lower in total fat and saturated fat from their higher-fat alternatives.

Criteria Key

▲ **Best Choice:**   **Fat Free or Low Fat**

Products listed in this category meet the FDA's definition for "Fat Free" (less than 1/2 gram fat per serving) or "Low Fat" (3 grams or less fat per serving).

▲ **Acceptable Choice:**   **Contains Greater Than 3 Grams but Less Than 13 Grams Total Fat, AND Less Than 4 Grams Saturated Fat**

Products listed in this category **do not** meet the FDA's definition for "Low Fat." These products contain less than 20% of the Daily Value for total fat and saturated fat and are, therefore, not considered high in total fat or saturated fat.

▲ **Occasional Choice:**   **High Fat or High Saturated Fat**

Products listed in this category contain 13 grams or more total fat per serving (20% or greater of the Daily Value) or 4 grams or more saturated fat per serving (20% or greater of the Daily Value). These foods are, therefore, considered high in total fat or high in saturated fat and should be consumed only on occasion. If foods from this category were selected as part of a regular diet, it would be difficult to meet the *Dietary Guidelines for Americans*[11] for choosing a diet low in fat and saturated fat.

BRAND	BEST CHOICE	ACCEPTABLE CHOICE	OCCASIONAL CHOICE
	Fat Free OR Low Fat	Contains Greater Than 3 Grams but Less Than 13 Grams Total Fat AND Less Than 4 Grams Saturated Fat	High Fat OR High Saturated Fat
CAKES & PIES			
Amy's		Chocolate Fudge Cake Golden Honey Spice Cake	Strawberry Cheesecake
Awrey's Best		Almond Crunch Dunker Chocolate Dessert: French Butter Cream Strawberry Dessert Cake Pound Cake	

Banquet			Banana Cream Pie
			Chocolate Cream Pie
			Coconut Cream Pie
			Lemon Cream Pie
			Ready To Bake:
			   Apple Pie
			   Cherry Pie

Chez de Prez	Fat Free Cheesecake:
	   ∇ New York Style
	   ∇ Pumpkin Swirl
	   ∇ Raspberry Swirl
	   ∇ Strawberry Swirl
			Premium Cheesecake:
			   Amaretto
			   Black Forest
			   Chocolate Chip
			   Chocolate Swirl
			   Cookies n' Cream
			   Double Chocolate
			   Dutch Apple
			   Irish Cream Mint
			   Irish Mint
			   Margarita
			   New York
			   Pumpkin
			   Raspberry Swirl
			   Triple Chocolate Raspberry
			   White Chocolate Raspberry

Eli's			Original Cheesecake

Entenmann's	Fat Free:
	   Banana Crunch Cake
	   Cherry Beehive Pie
	   Chocolate Loaf Cake
	   Golden Loaf Cake
	   Marble Loaf Cake
	   Mocha Iced Chocolate Cake
	   Raisin Loaf Cake
		Banana Crunch Cake
		Raisin Loaf
			All Butter Pound Loaf
			Apple Strudel
			Banana Cake
			Carrot Cake
			Creme Filled Chocolate Cake
			Homestyle Apple Pie
			Lemon Pie
			Louisiana Crunch Cakes

∇ Low Sodium, 140 mg. or less per serving.

BRAND	BEST CHOICE	ACCEPTABLE CHOICE	OCCASIONAL CHOICE
	Fat Free OR Low Fat	Contains Greater Than 3 Grams but Less Than 13 Grams Total Fat AND Less Than 4 Grams Saturated Fat	High Fat OR High Saturated Fat
Entenmann's (Cont.)			Marshmallow Iced Devil's Food Cake Thick Fudge Golden Cake
Mountain Top			Apple Pie

Mrs. Smith's		Bake & Serve Pie:
		  Apple
		  Blueberry
		  Cherry
		  Peach
		  Pumpkin Custard
		  Red Raspberry
		  Strawberry Rhubarb
		Ready to Serve Dessert:
		  ∇ Boston Cream
		  Lemon Meringue
			Bake & Serve Pie:
			  Coconut Custard
			  Dutch Apple Crumb
			Ready to Serve Dessert:
			  French Silk Chocolate

Nabisco		SnackWell's Reduced Fat:
		  Apple Pie
		  Cherry Pie	

Oregon Farms			Carrot Cake

Pepperidge Farm		Apple Dumplings
		∇ Puff Pastry Bake It Fresh
		    Sheets
		Special Recipe:
		  ∇ Pineapple Cream
			Apple Turnovers
			Cake:
			  Chocolate Fudge
			  Coconut
			  German Chocolate
			  Vanilla
			∇ Puff Pastry Shells
			Special Recipe:
			  ∇ Chocolate Mousse Cake
			  Classic Carrot Cake
			  ∇ Lemon Mousse Cake

Pet-Ritz			Cream Pie: All Flavors

Sara Lee		Free & Light:
		  Pound Cake
		Homestyle:
		  Lemon Meringue
			All Butter Pound Cake
			Cake:
			  German Chocolate
			Cream Cheesecake:
			  Original
			  Original Strawberry

∇ Low Sodium, 140 mg. or less per serving.

BRAND	BEST CHOICE	ACCEPTABLE CHOICE	OCCASIONAL CHOICE
	Fat Free OR Low Fat	Contains Greater Than 3 Grams but Less Than 13 Grams Total Fat AND Less Than 4 Grams Saturated Fat	High Fat OR High Saturated Fat
Sara Lee (Cont.)			French Cheesecake: Strawberry Homestyle: Apple Pie Blueberry Pie Chocolate Cream Pie Coconut Cream Pie Dutch Apple Pie ▲ Pecan Pie
FROZEN			
All Brands	Frozen Yogurt: ∇ Non Fat ∇ Non Fat Soft Serve ∇ Fruit and Juice Bars ∇ Ice Milk ∇ Sherbet	Frozen Yogurt: ∇ Soft Serve	∇ Premium Ice Cream Ice Cream Bars: ∇ Vanilla w/Chocolate Coating
Ben & Jerry's	Frozen Yogurt: ∇ Apple Pie ∇ Banana Strawberry ∇ Blueberry Cheesecake ∇ Bluesberry ∇ Cherry Garcia No Fat Frozen Yogurt: ∇ All Flavors	Frozen Yogurt: ∇ Chocolate Fudge Brownie ∇ English Toffee Bar Crunch	Ice Cream: ∇ All Flavors Peace Pops: ∇ All Flavors Smooth Frozen Dessert: ∇ All Varieties
Bexley's		Ice Cream: ∇ Cherry Pie ∇ Mackinaw Fudge Brownie ∇ Pralines & Cream ∇ Rocky Road ∇ Vanilla	
Blue Bunny	∇ Bomb Pop Frozen Yogurt Bars: ∇ All Flavors ∇ Fudge Lites Lowfat Frozen Yogurt: ∇ All Flavors Nonfat Frozen Yogurt Cups: ∇ All Flavors Nonfat No Added Sugar Ice Cream Cups: ∇ All Flavors		Ice Cream Bars: ∇ Crunch Bar ∇ English Toffee Bar ∇ Peanut Sticks ∇ Premium Ice Cream Bar Ice Cream Cups: ∇ All Flavors

▲ High Sodium, 480 mg. or greater per serving.
∇ Low Sodium, 140 mg. or less per serving.

Brand	Best Choice	Acceptable Choice	Occasional Choice
	Fat Free OR Low Fat	Contains Greater Than 3 Grams but Less Than 13 Grams Total Fat AND Less Than 4 Grams Saturated Fat	High Fat OR High Saturated Fat
Blue Bunny (Cont.)	Reduced Fat Ice Cream: ∇ All Flavors Sherbet: ∇ All Flavors Sherbet Cups: ∇ All Flavors		
Borden	Fat Free Ice Cream: ∇ All Flavors Low Fat Ice Cream: ∇ Chocolate Chip Cookie Dough ∇ Chocolate Marshmallow Swirl ∇ Cookies 'n Cream Premium Frozen Yogurt: ∇ Chocolate ∇ Strawberry ∇ Vanilla	Ice Cream: ∇ All Flavors	
Breyers	Fat Free Frozen Yogurt: ∇ All Flavors Fat Free Ice Cream: ∇ All Flavors Lowfat Frozen Yogurt: ∇ Strawberry	Frozen Yogurt: ∇ Strawberry Cheesecake ∇ Vanilla Light Ice Cream: ∇ Chocolate ∇ Heavenly Hash ∇ Natural Strawberry Premium Light Ice Cream: ∇ All Flavors Reduced Fat Ice Cream: ∇ Mocha Almond Fudge ∇ Praline Almond Crunch ∇ Swiss Almond Fudge Twirl	Ice Cream: ∇ All Flavors Viennetta: ∇ Premium Chocolate Ice Cream Cake
Cascadian Farm	Frozen Yogurt: ∇ All Flavors Sorbet & Cream: ∇ All Flavors ∇ Strawberry Sorbet		∇ Dark Chocolate Cherry Bars ∇ Dark Chocolate Raspberry Bars ∇ Dark Chocolate Vanilla Bars
Columbo	Lowfat Frozen Yogurt: ∇ All Flavors Shoppe Style Lowfat Yogurt: ∇ All Flavors Slender Scoops Nonfat Frozen Yogurt: ∇ All Flavors	Shoppe Style Gourmet: ∇ Cappuccino Coffee Bean ∇ Caramel Pecan Chunk ∇ Chocolate Chip Cookie Dough ∇ Cookies & Cream ∇ Peanut Butter Cup	Shoppe Style Gourmet: ∇ Bavarian Chocolate Chunk ∇ White Chocolate Almond

∇ Low Sodium, 140 mg. or less per serving.

BRAND	BEST CHOICE	ACCEPTABLE CHOICE	OCCASIONAL CHOICE
	Fat Free OR Low Fat	Contains Greater Than 3 Grams but Less Than 13 Grams Total Fat AND Less Than 4 Grams Saturated Fat	High Fat OR High Saturated Fat
Columbo (Cont.)		Shoppe Style Gourmet: ∇ Toffee Bar Crunch	
Country Fresh	Assorted Pops: ∇ No Sugar Added ∇ Fudge Bar Frostbite Guilt Free, Nonfat Frozen Yogurt: ∇ All Flavors Guilt Free, Nonfat Ice Cream: ∇ All Flavors Lowfat Frozen Yogurt: ∇ All Flavors Lowfat Ice Cream: ∇ All Flavors Nonfat Frozen Yogurt: ∇ All Flavors Sherbet: ∇ All Flavors		Ice Cream: ∇ Butter Pecan ∇ Chocolate ∇ Chocolate Chip ∇ Chocolate Chip Cookie Dough ∇ Chocolate Marshmallow ∇ Cookies 'n Cream ∇ French Vanilla ∇ Golden Vanilla ∇ Heavenly Holstein ∇ Mint Chocolate Chip ∇ Neapolitan ∇ Ryba's Mackinac Island Fudge ∇ Tin Roof Sundae ∇ Vanilla ∇ Ice Cream Bar Ice Cream Limited Edition: ∇ Chocolate Polka-Dots ∇ Peppermint Stick Ice Cream Sandwich ∇ Pride Vanilla Ice Cream
Crowley	Frozen Yogurt: ∇ All Flavors		
Dean Foods	∇ Dreamsicles Fat Free Ice Cream: ∇ All Flavors Frozen Yogurt: ∇ Black Cherry ∇ Chocolate ∇ Peach ∇ Strawberry Banana ∇ Vanilla Guilt Free Nonfat Ice Cream: ∇ All Flavors Popsicles: ∇ Sugar Free ∇ Premium Stick-Em-Up Frozen Dessert Sherbet: ∇ All Flavors	Frozen Yogurt: ∇ Toffee Light Ice Cream: ∇ Cookies 'N Cream ∇ Heavenly Hash ∇ Strawberry Cheesecake ∇ Tin Roof Light Sandwich: Vanilla Flavored Sundae Cup: ∇ Strawberry Swirl Ice Cream	Bar: ∇ Toffee Flavored Ice Cream ∇ Vanilla Flavored Ice Cream ∇ Vanilla Flavored Light Ice Cream Country Charm Ice Cream: ∇ All Flavors ∇ Premium Toffee Bars Sundae Cup: ∇ Chocolate Swirl Ice Cream ∇ Vanilla Cups

∇ Low Sodium, 140 mg. or less per serving.

BRAND	BEST CHOICE	ACCEPTABLE CHOICE	OCCASIONAL CHOICE
	Fat Free OR Low Fat	Contains Greater Than 3 Grams but Less Than 13 Grams Total Fat AND Less Than 4 Grams Saturated Fat	High Fat OR High Saturated Fat
Dean Foods (Cont.)	Twin Pops: ∇ All Flavors		
Dole	Fruit 'N Juice Bars: ∇ All Flavors Fruit Sorbet: ∇ All Flavors		
Dove			Bite Size Ice Cream: ∇ Cherry Royale ∇ Classic Vanilla ∇ Double Chocolate ∇ French Vanilla Ice Cream Bars: ∇ All Flavors
Edy's	Fat Free Frozen Yogurt: ∇ All Flavors Frozen Yogurt: ∇ Chocolate ∇ Raspberry Vanilla Swirl ∇ Vanilla Grand Fat Free Ice Cream No Sugar Added: ∇ All Flavors ∇ Strawberry Kiwi Sherbet ∇ Swiss Orange Sherbet	Frozen Yogurt: ∇ Cookies 'n Cream ∇ Heath Bar Crunch ∇ Strawberry Chocolate Chip Grand Ice Cream No Sugar Added: ∇ All Flavors Grand Light: ∇ All Flavors	Grand Cones: ∇ All Flavors Grand Ice Cream: ∇ All Flavors Grand Ice Cream Bars: ∇ Cookies 'n Cream Grand Ice Cream Lactose Reduced: ∇ All Flavors
Eskimo Pie		Frozen Dairy Dessert: ∇ Fudge Ripple ∇ Vanilla	∇ Dark Chocolate Coating w/Vanilla Ice Cream Frozen Dairy Dessert: ∇ Butter Pecan
Espirit	Lowfat Frozen Yogurt: ∇ All Flavors		
Freezer Pleezer	∇ Assorted Pops ∇ Banana Pops ∇ Fruit Chillers ∇ Fudge Bars ∇ Juice Coolers ∇ Orange Creme Treats ∇ Root Beer Float Pops ∇ Sugar Free Fudge Treats ∇ Tropical Pops ∇ Twin Pops	∇ Ice Cream Sandwiches	∇ Chocolate Eclair Bars ∇ Crispy Bars ∇ Ice Cream Bars ∇ Ice Milk Bars ∇ Toffee Bars

∇ Low Sodium, 140 mg. or less per serving.

BRAND	BEST CHOICE	ACCEPTABLE CHOICE	OCCASIONAL CHOICE
	Fat Free OR Low Fat	Contains Greater Than 3 Grams but Less Than 13 Grams Total Fat AND Less Than 4 Grams Saturated Fat	High Fat OR High Saturated Fat
Frozen Fruitstick	Cherry Chill Lemon Chill Strawberry Chill		
Gold Mine	Bullets: 　All Flavors		
Good Humor	Creamsicle: 　∇ Original 　∇ Reduced Calorie Cream 　　Pops Fudgesicle: 　∇ Original 　∇ Reduced Calorie Popsicle: 　∇ Juice Jets 　∇ Twister Popsicle Ice Pops: 　∇ All Flavors 　∇ Low Calorie	∇ Chocolate Eclair	∇ Candy Center Crunch ∇ Chocolate Almond ∇ Original Ice Cream Bar ∇ Strawberry Shortcake ∇ Toasted Almond
Haagen Dazs	Frozen Yogurt: 　∇ Chocolate 　∇ Coffee 　∇ Raspberry Rendezvous 　∇ Strawberry Daiquiri Bar 　∇ Vanilla Frozen Yogurt & Sorbet: 　∇ Orange Tango 　∇ Pina Colada 　∇ Strawberry Duet Frozen Yogurt & Sorbet Bars: 　∇ All Flavors Sorbet: 　∇ Chocolate 　∇ Mango 　∇ Raspberry		Extraas: 　∇ Caramel Cone Explosion 　∇ Cookie Dough Dynamo 　　Peanut Butter Burst 　　Strawberry Cheesecake 　　Craze 　∇ Triple Brownie Overload Extraas - Frozen Yogurt: 　∇ Strawberry Cheesecake 　　Craze Frozen Yogurt & Sorbet: 　∇ Raspberry Ice Cream: 　∇ All Flavors Ice Cream Cordials: 　∇ Baileys Original Irish 　　Cream 　∇ Disaronno Amaretto ∇ Vanilla & Almonds Bar ∇ Vanilla & Dark Chocolate Bar ∇ Vanilla & Milk Chocolate Bar ∇ Vanilla Caramel & Peanut 　　Brittle Bars
Healthy Choice	Premium Low Fat Ice Cream: 　∇ All Flavors		

∇ Low Sodium, 140 mg. or less per serving.

BRAND	BEST CHOICE	ACCEPTABLE CHOICE	OCCASIONAL CHOICE
	Fat Free OR Low Fat	Contains Greater Than 3 Grams but Less Than 13 Grams Total Fat AND Less Than 4 Grams Saturated Fat	High Fat OR High Saturated Fat
Healthy Choice (Cont.)	Special Creations Frozen Dessert: ∇ All Varieties		
Homemade	Frozen Yogurt: ∇ All Flavors Premium Yogurt Singles: ∇ Vanilla	Premium Light Ice Cream: ∇ All Flavors Yogurt Sundaes: ∇ Vanilla Yogurt w/Chocolate Fudge Topping	Ice Cream: ∇ All Flavors Premium Ice Cream Singles: ∇ All Flavors
House of Flavors			Ice Cream: ∇ All Flavors
Kemps	Frozen Yogurt: ∇ Nonfat Chocolate Toffee Sundae ∇ Nonfat Fudge Marble ∇ Nonfat Vanilla ∇ Raspberry ∇ Strawberry ∇ Sugar Free Strawberry ∇ Vanilla	Frozen Yogurt: ∇ Chocolate Almond ∇ Chocolate Chip Cookie Dough ∇ Pralines N Caramel Kids' Ice Cream: ∇ All Varieties Sundae Toppers Frozen Yogurt: ∇ Heath Crunch	Ice Cream: ∇ Butter Pecan ∇ Chocolate Monster ∇ Natural Vanilla
Klondike			Ice Cream Bars: ∇ All Flavors ∇ Lite Original
Life Savers	Flavor Pops: ∇ Original ∇ Sugar Free		
London's	Nonfat Ice Cream: ∇ All Flavors Sherbet: ∇ All Flavors		
Luigi's	Real Italian Ice: ∇ All Flavors		
Mama Tish's	Original Italian Ices: ∇ All Flavors		
Marie Callender's			Peach Cobbler
Mars	Milky Way: ∇ Lowfat Milk Shake	Milky Way Dark: ∇ Reduced Fat Vanilla Ice Cream Bars	3-Musketeers Ice Cream Bars: ∇ All Flavors Milky Way Ice Cream Bars: ∇ All Flavors

∇ Low Sodium, 140 mg. or less per serving.

BRAND	BEST CHOICE	ACCEPTABLE CHOICE	OCCASIONAL CHOICE
	Fat Free OR Low Fat	Contains Greater Than 3 Grams but Less Than 13 Grams Total Fat AND Less Than 4 Grams Saturated Fat	High Fat OR High Saturated Fat
McArthur	Lowfat Frozen Yogurt: ▽ All Flavors TG Lee Fat Free Non-Dairy Desserts: ▽ All Flavors		
Melody Farms	▽ Fudge Bars ▽ Melody Mini Pops ▽ Orange Cream Bars Sherbet: ▽ All Flavors ▽ Twin Pops	▽ Ice Cream Sandwiches	Ice Cream: ▽ All Flavors ▽ Ice Cream Bars Ice Cream Sundaes: ▽ All Flavors
Merritt Foods Company	▽ Bomb Pop Jr.		
Micro Shake			▽ Vanilla Milkshake Yogurt: Chocolate Milkshake
Mike's Original			Cheesecake Ice Cream Bar: ▽ Graham Cracker Crunch ▽ Strawberry Sorbet
Mocha Mix		Non Dairy Dessert: ▽ Dutch Chocolate ▽ Neopolitan ▽ Vanilla	
Nestle	Cool Cream Push-Ups: ▽ Sherbet Treats Cool Creations: ▽ Ice Pops ▽ Surprise Ice Pops Flintstones Push-Up: ▽ Orange ▽ Sherbet Treats	Cool Creations: ▽ Mickey Mouse Ice Cream Bars ▽ Mini Ice Cream Sandwiches	▽ Butterfinger Ice Cream Bar Crunch: ▽ Vanilla Drumstick: ▽ All Flavors ▽ Heath Ice Cream Bar Pebbles Push-Up: ▽ Ice Cream Treats
Nutty Buddy			▽ Chocolate Nut Sundae Cones
R W Frookie	▽ Cool Fruit Freezers		
Reese's			▽ Peanut Butter Ice Cups
Rice Dream		Non-Dairy Dessert: ▽ Vanilla	Frozen Pies: Chocolate Dream

▽ Low Sodium, 140 mg. or less per serving.

BRAND	BEST CHOICE	ACCEPTABLE CHOICE	OCCASIONAL CHOICE
	Fat Free OR Low Fat	Contains Greater Than 3 Grams but Less Than 13 Grams Total Fat AND Less Than 4 Grams Saturated Fat	High Fat OR High Saturated Fat
Savino	Sorbet: 　▽ All Flavors		
Sealtest	Fat Free Frozen Desserts: 　▽ Chocolate Lowfat Frozen Yogurt: 　▽ All Flavors		
Snickers			▽ Ice Cream Bars
Starburst	Lowfat Frozen Yogurt Snacks: 　▽ All Flavors		
Stonyfield Farm	Frozen Yogurt: 　▽ Dutch Chocolate 　▽ Mocha Almond Fudge 　▽ Very Vanilla		
Stroh's		Reduced Fat Ice Cream: 　▽ All Flavors	1919 Brand Ice Cream: 　▽ All Flavors Premium Ice Cream: 　▽ All Flavors
Superior Dairy	Free Supreme Nonfat Ice Cream: 　▽ All Flavors		
Sweet Nothings	Fat-Free Non-Dairy Frozen Desserts: 　▽ All Flavors		
TCBY	Frozen Yogurt: 　▽ All Flavors		
Tofutti	Better Than Yogurt Frozen Dessert: 　▽ All Flavors ▽ Chocolate Fudge Treats Frutti: 　▽ All Flavors ▽ Teddy Fudge Bars	Cuties Frozen Dessert: 　▽ Chocolate Sandwiches 　▽ Vanilla Sandwiches Premium Frozen Dessert: 　▽ Chocolate Cookies 　Supreme 　Chocolate Supreme Vanilla 　▽ Vanilla Almond Bark 　▽ Vanilla Fudge 　Wildberry Supreme	Premium Frozen Dessert: 　Better Pecan
Trix	▽ Pops		

▽ Low Sodium, 140 mg. or less per serving.

BRAND	BEST CHOICE	ACCEPTABLE CHOICE	OCCASIONAL CHOICE
	Fat Free OR Low Fat	Contains Greater Than 3 Grams but Less Than 13 Grams Total Fat AND Less Than 4 Grams Saturated Fat	High Fat OR High Saturated Fat
United Dairy Farmers	Quality Sherbet: ▽ All Flavors		Quality Ice Cream: ▽ All Flavors
Valet		Ice Cream: ▽ All Flavors	

Weight Watchers	▽ Chocolate Mousse Bars
	Oh! So Very Vanilla:
	  ▽ Light Ice Cream
	▽ Orange Vanilla Treat
	Sweet Celebrations:
	  Caramel Fudge a La Mode
	  ▽☆ Chocolate Frosted
	    Brownie
	  Double Fudge Brownie
	    Parfait
	  ▽☆ Peanut Butter Fudge
	    Brownie
	  ▽ Praline Toffee Crunch
	    Parfait
	  Strawberry Shortcake a La
	    Mode
		▽ Arctic D'Lites
		▽ English Toffee Crunch Bars
		Sweet Celebrations:
		  ☆ Brownie a la Mode
		  ☆ Brownie Cheesecake
		  ▽ Chocolate Chip Cookie
		    Dough Sundae
		  Chocolate Eclairs
		  ▽ Chocolate Mocha Pie
		  ☆ Chocolate Mousse
		  Double Fudge Cake
		  ▽ Mississippi Mud Pie
		  ▽ Praline Pecan Mousse
		  Strawberry Cheesecake
		  ☆ Toasted Almond
		    Amaretto Cheesecake
		  ▽ Triple Chocolate Caramel
		    Mousse
		  Triple Chocolate Cheesecake
		Triple Chocolate Tornado:
		  ▽ Light Ice Cream
		Vanilla Sandwich Bars
			▽ Caramel Nut Bars

Welch's	Fruit Juice Bars: ▽ Light ▽ Variety Pack		
Wunderbar			Cherry Dipped in Dark Chocolate
Yoplait	▽ Double Fruit Low Fat Frozen Yogurt Bars		
PUDDING, GELATIN & PIE FILLING			
Axelrod	Mini-Desserts: ▽ Rice Pudding		
Betty Crocker	Gelooze: ▽ All Flavors		

▽ Low Sodium, 140 mg. or less per serving.
☆ Good Source of Fiber, between 2.5 g. and 5 g. per serving.

BRAND	BEST CHOICE	ACCEPTABLE CHOICE	OCCASIONAL CHOICE
	Fat Free OR Low Fat	Contains Greater Than 3 Grams but Less Than 13 Grams Total Fat AND Less Than 4 Grams Saturated Fat	High Fat OR High Saturated Fat
Borden	None Such Mincemeat		
Comstock	∇ Red Ruby Cherry Pie Filling ∇ Royal Blueberry Pie Filling		
Crosse & Blackwell	Pie Filling: ∇ All Flavors		

D-Zerta	Low Calorie Gelatin:
	  ∇ All Flavors
	Reduced Calorie Pudding:
	  ∇ All Flavors		

Del Monte	Gel Snack Cups:
	  ∇ All Flavors
	Lite Pudding Cups:
	  ∇ All Flavors
		Pudding:
		  Butterscotch
		Pudding Cups:
		  ∇ Chocolate
		  Chocolate Fudge
		  ∇ Chocolate Marshmallow
		  ∇ Tapioca	

Hershey	Free Pudding Packs:
	  Hershey's Chocolate & Vanilla
	    Pudding Variety Pack
	  Hershey's Kisses Chocolate
	    & Vanilla Pudding
	  Tapioca		

Hunt's	Snack Pack:
	  ∇ Lemon
	Snack Pack Light:
	  ∇ All Flavors
	Snack Pack, Fat Free:
	  All Flavors
		Snack Pack:
		  Banana
		  Butterscotch
		  Chocolate
		  Chocolate Fudge
		  ∇ Chocolate Marshmallow
		  ∇ Tapioca
		  ∇ Vanilla
		Snack Pack Swirl:
		  Chocolate Caramel
		  ∇ S'Mores	

Jell-O	∇ 1-2-3
	Americana:
	  ∇ Custard Dessert
	  ∇ Rice Pudding
	  ∇ Tapioca
	Cook N' Serve Pudding:
	  Banana Cream
		Pudding Packs:
		  Banana & Vanilla
		  Chocolate Pudding
		  Chocolate-Vanilla Swirls
		  Swirls-Variety Pack
		  Vanilla & Chocolate	

∇ Low Sodium, 140 mg. or less per serving.

BRAND	BEST CHOICE	ACCEPTABLE CHOICE	OCCASIONAL CHOICE
	Fat Free OR Low Fat	Contains Greater Than 3 Grams but Less Than 13 Grams Total Fat AND Less Than 4 Grams Saturated Fat	High Fat OR High Saturated Fat

Jell-O (Cont.)	Cook N' Serve Pudding:
	  ∇ Butterscotch
	  ∇ Chocolate
	  Coconut Cream
	  ∇ Lemon
	  ∇ Vanilla
	Free Pudding Snacks:
	  Chocolate
	  Swirls Variety Pack
	Gelatin Dessert:
	  ∇ All Flavors
	Gelatin Jigglers:
	  ∇ All Flavors
	Instant Pudding and Pie Filling:
	  Butterscotch
	  Chocolate
	  Chocolate Fudge
	  Coconut Cream
	  Lemon
	  Milk Chocolate
	  Pistachio
	  Vanilla
	Sugar Free Cook N' Serve Pudding and Pie Filling:
	  ∇ Chocolate
	  ∇ Vanilla
	Sugar Free Gelatin:
	  ∇ All Flavors
	Sugar Free Instant Pudding and Pie Filling:
	  Banana
	  Butterscotch
	  Chocolate
	  Chocolate Fudge
	  Pistachio
	  Vanilla		

Knox	∇ Unflavored Gelatin		
Kozy Shack	∇ Flan w/Creme Caramel ∇ Rice Pudding		
Kraft	Handi Snacks Gels: ∇ All Flavors		
Libby's	∇ Solid Pack Pumpkin		

∇ Low Sodium, 140 mg. or less per serving.

BRAND	BEST CHOICE	ACCEPTABLE CHOICE	OCCASIONAL CHOICE
	Fat Free OR Low Fat	Contains Greater Than 3 Grams but Less Than 13 Grams Total Fat AND Less Than 4 Grams Saturated Fat	High Fat OR High Saturated Fat
Lundberg	Elegant Rice Pudding: ∇ Honey Almond		
Minute	∇ Tapioca		
Nabisco Royal	Sugar Free Gelatin Dessert: ∇ All Flavors Sugar Free Instant Pudding and Pie Filling: Butterscotch		
Reese	Tapioca: ∇ Small Pearl		
Thank You	Cream Filling or Topping: Chocolate Filling or Topping: ∇ Berry Patch Strawberry ∇ Blueberry ∇ Country Peach ∇ Dark Sweet Cherry ∇ Lemon ∇ More Fruit Apple ∇ More Fruit Peach ∇ Ruby Red Cherry Light Filling or Topping: ∇ Cherry Premium More Fruit: ∇ Blueberry ∇ Pure Pumpkin The Ultimate Pudding: Rice The Ultimate Pudding & Pie Filling: Lemon	The Ulitmate Pudding & Pie Filling: Banana Butterscotch The Ultimate Pudding: Chocolate Chocolate Fudge Tapioca Vanilla	
YOUR FAVORITE DESSERTS NOT LISTED IN THE *GUIDE*			

∇ Low Sodium, 140 mg. or less per serving.

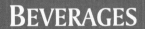

BEVERAGES

This category contains a large variety of beverages that are grouped into six different headings for ease of locating products. The headings are: carbonated, fruit, non-carbonated, powders/syrups, sport, and vegetable. Beverages supply the body's major source of water. Although not considered a nutrient *per se*, water is more essential to life than food itself. The average person can survive for weeks without food but only a few days without water. To ensure adequate fluid intake, adults need a minimum of six to eight cups of water or other beverages daily.

The *Food Guide Pyramid* does not have a specific food group for beverages. However, sweetened soft drinks are included as part of the "Fats, Oils, and Sweets Group" at the tip of the *Food Guide Pyramid*, and fruit and vegetable juices are included as part of the "Fruit Group" and "Vegetable Group" respectively. The recommended serving sizes will vary depending on their food group classification.

The FDA has established reference amounts or standardized serving sizes for use on the food label. The reference amount for beverages is 240 milliliters (8 fluid ounces). Be sure to read the *Nutrition Facts* label for the serving size information of your beverage choice. (See pages 51 and 52 for an explanation of reference amounts and the difference between serving sizes established by the FDA for food labeling and those recommended by the *Food Guide Pyramid*.)

Beverages in this category range from those that are fat-free, sugar-free, and low-sodium, such as sparkling waters and diet soft drinks, to those that contain significant amounts of sugar, fat, saturated fat, and sodium, such as regular soft drinks, chocolate milk beverages, and some vegetable juices.

Criteria were, therefore, designed to distinguish those products lower in total fat, saturated fat, and sugar from their higher-fat, higher-sugar alternatives. Although sodium was not used as a criteria for assessing acceptability of products, those

beverages that contain 480 milligrams sodium or more per serving (20% of the Daily Value) are considered high in sodium and are are marked with a ▲ symbol. Products meeting the FDA's definition for "Low Sodium" (less than 140 milligrams sodium) are likewise marked with a ∇ symbol.

Criteria Key

▲ **Best Choice:**   **Fat Free AND Without Added Sugars (May Contain Sugar Substitutes)**

Beverages listed in this category meet the FDA's definition for "Fat Free" (less than 1/2 gram fat per serving) and do not contain added sugars.

△ **Acceptable Choice:**   **Fat Free or Low Fat AND Low Saturated Fat AND With Added Sugars**

Beverages listed in this category meet the FDA's definition for "Fat Free" or "Low Fat" (3 grams fat or less per serving) and "Low Saturated Fat" (1 gram or less saturated fat per serving) and contain added sugars. According to FDA's ruling, "added sugar" is defined as any sweeteners added during processing such as: fruit juices, fructose, honey, molasses, maltose, sucrose, corn syrups, or high-fructose corn syrup.

▲ **Occasional Choice:**   **Contains Greater Than 3 Grams Total Fat or Greater Than 1 Gram Saturated Fat**

Products listed in this category **do not** meet the FDA's definition for "Low Fat" or "Low Saturated Fat." Since excessive use of these products may significantly increase your intake of total fat and saturated fat, they should be consumed only on occasion.

BRAND	BEST CHOICE	ACCEPTABLE CHOICE	OCCASIONAL CHOICE
	Fat Free AND Without Added Sugars (May Contain Sugar Substitutes)	Fat Free or Low Fat AND Low Saturated Fat AND With Added Sugars	Contains Greater Than 3 Grams Total Fat OR Greater Than 1 Gram Saturated Fat
CARBONATED			
7-Up	∇ Diet 7-Up ∇ Diet Cherry 7-Up	∇ 7-Up ∇ Cherry 7-Up	
A&W	∇ Diet Cream Soda ∇ Diet Root Beer	∇ Cream Soda ∇ Root Beer	
Barq's	∇ Diet Root Beer	∇ Root Beer	
Big Red		∇ Big Red Cola	

Canada Dry	∇ Club Soda
	Diet:
	  ∇ Cranberry Gingerale
	  ∇ Gingerale
	  ∇ Tonic Water
		Gingerale:
		  ∇ Cranberry
		  ∇ Regular
		  ∇ Tahitian Treat
		Tonic Water:
		  ∇ All Flavors	

Canfield's	Diet Sodas:
	  ∇ All Flavors
	Seltzer Water:
	  ∇ All Flavors
		50/50:
		  ∇ Grapefruit/Lime
		Clear:
		  ∇ All Flavors
		∇ Cola
		∇ Tonic Water	

Cap 10	Natural Mineral Water: ∇ All Flavors		
Cascadia	Carbonated Beverage: ∇ All Flavors		

Chaos	Diet Beverage:
	  ∇ All Flavors
		Beverage:
		  ∇ All Flavors	

Clearly Canadian	Clearly 2:
	  ∇ All Flavors
		Sparkling Waters:
		  ∇ All Flavors	

Coca-Cola	∇ Caffeine Free Diet Coke ∇ Diet Cherry Coke ∇ Diet Coke ∇ Sugar Free Tab	∇ Cherry Coke ∇ Classic ∇ Mello Yello	
Country Springs		∇ Sparkling Water Beverage	

Crystal Bay		Flavored Sparkling Water:
		  ∇ Blackberry
		  ∇ Cherry	

∇ Low Sodium, 140 mg. or less per serving.

BRAND	BEST CHOICE	ACCEPTABLE CHOICE	OCCASIONAL CHOICE
	Fat Free AND Without Added Sugars (May Contain Sugar Substitutes)	Fat Free or Low Fat AND Low Saturated Fat AND With Added Sugars	Contains Greater Than 3 Grams Total Fat OR Greater Than 1 Gram Saturated Fat
Crystal Bay (Cont.)		Flavored Sparkling Water: ∇ Raspberry	
Crystal Clear	Sparkling Water Diet Beverage: ∇ All Flavors		
Culligan	Sparkling Water: ∇ All Flavors		
Dad's	∇ Diet Old Fashioned Root Beer	∇ Red Creme Soda Rouge ∇ Root Beer	
Diet Rite	Diet Rite Soda: ∇ All Flavors		
Dr. Brown's	Diet Flavored Soda: ∇ All Flavors	∇ Flavored Sodas	
Dr. Pepper	∇ Diet Dr. Pepper	∇ Dr. Pepper	
Equator		Naturally Flavored Cocktail: ∇ All Flavors	
Faygo	∇ Club Soda Diet Soda: ∇ All Flavors ∇ Diet Tonic Water Sparkling Water: ∇ All Flavors	Sodas: ∇ All Flavors ∇ Tonic Water	
Fresca	∇ Fresca		
Hires	∇ Diet Root Beer	∇ Root Beer	
IBC Root Beer Co.	∇ Diet Root Beer	∇ Root Beer	
Jamaican		Flavored Soda: ∇ All Flavors	
Koala		Flavored Fruit Juice Beverage: ∇ All Flavors	
La Croix	Sparkling Mineral Water: ∇ All Flavors		
Marquée	∇ Diet Cola Sparkling Water Beverage: ∇ All Flavors	Soda: ∇ All Flavors	

∇ Low Sodium, 140 mg. or less per serving.

BRAND	BEST CHOICE	ACCEPTABLE CHOICE	OCCASIONAL CHOICE
	Fat Free AND Without Added Sugars (May Contain Sugar Substitutes)	Fat Free or Low Fat AND Low Saturated Fat AND With Added Sugars	Contains Greater Than 3 Grams Total Fat OR Greater Than 1 Gram Saturated Fat
Minute Maid		∇ Orange Soda	
Mistic		Sparkling Water Beverage: ∇ All Flavors	
Mountain Dew	∇ Caffeine-Free Diet Mountain Dew ∇ Diet Mountain Dew	∇ Caffeine-Free Mountain Dew ∇ Mountain Dew	
Moxie	Diet Soda: ∇ All Flavors	Soda: ∇ All Flavors	
Naturale 90	Diet Natural Soda: ∇ All Flavors	Natural Soda: ∇ All Flavors	
Old Tyme		∇ Cola Champagne ∇ Jamaican Style Ginger Brew ∇ Park Avenue Punch	
Pepsi	∇ Caffeine Free Diet Pepsi ∇ Diet Crystal Pepsi ∇ Diet Mandarin Orange Slice ∇ Diet Pepsi ∇ Diet Slice	∇ Caffeine Free Pepsi ∇ Crystal Pepsi ∇ Pepsi Slice: ∇ All Flavors	
Perrier	Mineral Water: ∇ All Flavors		
Poland Spring	Sparkling Spring Water: ∇ All Flavors		
Quest	2 Calorie Quest: ∇ All Flavors		
Quibell	Sparkling Spring Water: ∇ All Flavors		
Royal Crown Cola	∇ Diet Rite Cola	∇ RC Cola	
RW Knudsen	Fruit TeaZer: ∇ All Flavors		
Schweppes	∇ Club Soda ∇ Diet Raspberry Gingerale ∇ Diet Tonic Water Seltzer Water: ∇ All Varieties	Ginger Ale ∇ Raspberry Gingerale ∇ Tonic Water	

∇ Low Sodium, 140 mg. or less per serving.

BRAND	BEST CHOICE	ACCEPTABLE CHOICE	OCCASIONAL CHOICE
	Fat Free AND Without Added Sugars (May Contain Sugar Substitutes)	Fat Free or Low Fat AND Low Saturated Fat AND With Added Sugars	Contains Greater Than 3 Grams Total Fat OR Greater Than 1 Gram Saturated Fat
Seagrams	∇ Club Soda ∇ Diet Gingerale	∇ Gingerale ∇ Tonic Water	

Shasta	A Sante Sparkling Waters:
	  ∇ All Flavors
	Diet Soda:
	  ∇ All Flavors
		Soft Drinks:
		  ∇ All Flavors
		Spree All Natural Soda:
		  ∇ All Flavors	

SoHo		Soda: ∇ All Flavors	
Sprite	∇ Diet Sprite	∇ Sprite	
Squirt	∇ Diet Squirt	∇ Ruby Red ∇ Squirt	
Stewart's		∇ Diet Rootbeer ∇ Rootbeer	

Sunkist	Diet Sunkist:
	  ∇ Lemonade
		Sunkist:
		  ∇ Grape
		  ∇ Orange Soda
		  ∇ Sparkling Lemonade	

Vernors	∇ Diet Vernors	∇ Vernors	
Virgil's		∇ Root Beer	
Welch's		Sparkling Soda: ∇ All Flavors	
West End		All Natural Soda Brew: ∇ All Flavors	
FRUIT			
After the Fall	Fruit Juices: ∇ All Flavors		

All Brands	100% Fruit Juice:
	  ∇ No Added Sugars
		Fruit Drinks:
		  ∇ with Added Sugars	

Arizona		Fruit Beverages: ∇ All Flavors	
Awake		∇ Frozen Orange Beverage	

∇ Low Sodium, 140 mg. or less per serving.

340   **Beverages**

BRAND	BEST CHOICE	ACCEPTABLE CHOICE	OCCASIONAL CHOICE
	Fat Free AND Without Added Sugars (May Contain Sugar Substitutes)	Fat Free or Low Fat AND Low Saturated Fat AND With Added Sugars	Contains Greater Than 3 Grams Total Fat OR Greater Than 1 Gram Saturated Fat
Betty Crocker	Squeezit 100: ∇ All Flavors	Squeezit Fruit Drink: ∇ All Flavors	
Bluebird	∇ 100% Pink Grapefruit Juice		
Boku		Fruit Juice Cooler: ∇ All Flavors Fruit Juice Cooler Boxes: ∇ All Flavors	
Borden	ReaLemon: ∇ Premium Lemon Juice ReaLime: ∇ Lime Juice From Concentrate		
Capri Sun		100% Natural Fruit Drinks: ∇ All Flavors	
Chief Lake	∇ Apple Juice		
Chiquita	100% Fruit Juice Blends: ∇ All Flavors 100% Juice Frozen Concentrate: ∇ All Flavors		
Citrus Valley	∇ 100% Orange Juice Concentrate Mini Juice Boxes: All Flavors		
Crystal Geyser	Juice Squeeze: ∇ Mountain Raspberry ∇ Passion Fruit & Mango ∇ Pink Lemonade ∇ Ruby Grapefruit ∇ Wild Berry		
Daily's		Harvest Best Fruit Drinks: ∇ All Flavors	
Dean Foods	∇ 100% Grapefruit Juice ∇ 100% Pure Orange Juice From Concentrate	Pink Grapefruit Juice ∇ Pink Grapefruit Juice Cocktail	
Dole	100% Juice: ∇ All Flavors	∇ Fruit Fiesta Juice Drink ∇ Pacific Pink Grapefruit Juice Drink	

∇ Low Sodium, 140 mg. or less per serving.

BRAND	BEST CHOICE	ACCEPTABLE CHOICE	OCCASIONAL CHOICE
	Fat Free AND Without Added Sugars (May Contain Sugar Substitutes)	Fat Free or Low Fat AND Low Saturated Fat AND With Added Sugars	Contains Greater Than 3 Grams Total Fat OR Greater Than 1 Gram Saturated Fat
Dole (Cont.)	100% Juice Frozen Concentrate: ∇ All Flavors Pure and Light: ∇ All Flavors ∇ Sun Ripe Grapefruit Juice ∇ Tropical Fruit Juice Unsweetened Juice: ∇ All Flavors		
Everfresh		Refreshers: ∇ All Flavors	
Faygo		Bottled Lemonade: ∇ All Flavors	
Five Alive		Frozen Concentrate Citrus Beverages: ∇ All Flavors	
Florida Gold	∇ Pure 100% Valencia Orange Juice		
Hawaiian Punch		Diet Hawaiian Punch ∇ Fruit Juicy Red Fruit Juicy: ∇ All Flavors Fruit Punch: ∇ All Flavors Typhoon Blasters: ∇ All Flavors	
HI-C		Fruit Drink: ∇ All Flavors	
Indian Summer	100% Apple Juice: ∇ From Concentrate	Cosmic Cooler Fruit Drink: ∇ All Flavors	
Juicyful	∇ 100% Apple Juice	Drink Boxes: ∇ Fruit Punch ∇ Grape ∇ Orange	
Kool-Aid		Bursts: ∇ All Flavors Koolers: ∇ All Flavors	
Libby's	Juicy Juice: ∇ All Flavors	∇ Apricot Nectar ∇ Peach Nectar ∇ Pear Nectar	

∇ Low Sodium, 140 mg. or less per serving.

BRAND	BEST CHOICE	ACCEPTABLE CHOICE	OCCASIONAL CHOICE
	Fat Free AND Without Added Sugars (May Contain Sugar Substitutes)	Fat Free or Low Fat AND Low Saturated Fat AND With Added Sugars	Contains Greater Than 3 Grams Total Fat OR Greater Than 1 Gram Saturated Fat
Liberty Gold	∇ Pineapple Juice		
London's	∇ 100% Pure Orange Juice		
Martinelli's	∇ 100% Apple Cider ∇ 100% Apple Juice		
McCain	Junior Juice: ∇ All Flavors		
Melody Farms	100% Pure: ∇ Orange Juice	∇ Grape Drink ∇ Orange Drink	

Minute Maid	100% Orange Juice from Concentrate:
	  ∇ Calcium Fortified
	∇ 100% Pure Apple Juice
	100% Pure Orange Juice:
	  ∇ All Varieties
	Frozen Concentrate:
	  ∇ Apple Juice
	  ∇ Country Style Orange Juice
	  ∇ Grapefruit Juice
	  ∇ Orange Juice
	  ∇ Pulp Free Orange Juice
	Premium Choice Orange Juice:
	  ∇ Country Style, Regular
		All Natural Drink Boxes:
		  ∇ All Flavors
		Frozen Concentrate:
		  ∇ Berry Punch
		  ∇ Country Style Lemonade
		  ∇ Fruit Punch
		  ∇ Limeade
		  ∇ Pink Lemonade
		  ∇ Raspberry Lemonade
		  ∇ Regular Lemonade
		Fruit Punch:
		  ∇ All Flavors
		Fruitopia:
		  ∇ All Flavors
		Lemonade:
		  ∇ All Flavors
		Naturals:
		  ∇ All Flavors	

Mondo		Fruit Squeezers: ∇ All Flavors	
Mott's	∇ 100% Juice Boxes ∇ 100% Pure Apple Juice ∇ Prune Juice		
Musselman's	∇ 100% Apple Juice ∇ Apple Juice Box ∇ Natural Apple Juice ∇ Premium Apple Juice		
Ocean Spray	∇ 100% Grapefruit Juice	Cran-Raspberry: ∇ Reduced Calorie	

∇ Low Sodium, 140 mg. or less per serving.

Brand	Best Choice	Acceptable Choice	Occasional Choice
	Fat Free AND Without Added Sugars (May Contain Sugar Substitutes)	**Fat Free or Low Fat AND Low Saturated Fat AND With Added Sugars**	**Contains Greater Than 3 Grams Total Fat OR Greater Than 1 Gram Saturated Fat**

Ocean Spray (Cont.)		Cranapple:
		    ∇ Reduced Calorie
		Cranberry Juice Cocktail:
		    ∇ Reduced Calorie
		Drink Boxes:
		    ∇ All Flavors
		Juice Drinks:
		    ∇ All Flavors
		Lemonade:
		    ∇ All Flavors
		Mauna Lai Fruit Drink:
		    ∇ All Flavors
		    ∇ Pink Grapefruit Juice
		        Cocktail
		Reduced Calorie Drinks:
		    ∇ Cranberry Juice Cocktail
		Refreshers:
		    ∇ All Flavors
		    ∇ Ruby Red
		    ∇ Ruby Red and Tangerine
		    ∇ Ruby Red Grapefruit Juice	

Old Orchard	Frozen Concentrate:
	    ∇ Apple Juice
	    ∇ Orange Juice
		Four Seasons from Concentrate:
		    ∇ All Flavors
		Frozen Concentrate:
		    ∇ Cranberry Juice Cocktail
		    ∇ Pink Lemonade	

Rich N' Ready		California Citrus Punch:
		    ∇ Orange
		    ∇ Raspberry Orange
		    ∇ Citrus Punch
		    ∇ Fruit Punch	

Royal Select	∇ Apple Juice		

RW Knudsen	∇ Apple Raspberry
	Fruit Floats:
	    ∇ All Flavors
	    ∇ Guava Strawberry
	    ∇ Natural Apple
	Nectar:
	    ∇ All Flavors
	    ∇ Orange Mango
	    ∇ Vita Juice		

Santa Cruz Natural		Organic Orangeade	

∇ Low Sodium, 140 mg. or less per serving.

BRAND	BEST CHOICE	ACCEPTABLE CHOICE	OCCASIONAL CHOICE
	Fat Free AND Without Added Sugars (May Contain Sugar Substitutes)	Fat Free or Low Fat AND Low Saturated Fat AND With Added Sugars	Contains Greater Than 3 Grams Total Fat OR Greater Than 1 Gram Saturated Fat
Seneca	Frozen Concentrate: ∇ Granny Smith Apple Juice	Frozen Concentrate: ∇ Cranberry Juice Cocktail Frozen Concentrate: ∇ White Grape Juice Cocktail	
Shasta		Plus - 10% Juice Beverage: ∇ All Flavors	
Snapple		Bottled Drinks: ∇ All Varieties	
Speas Farm	∇ Apple Juice		
Summer Song	100% Fruit Juice Blends: ∇ All Flavors		
Sunkist	Frozen Concentrate: ∇ Grapefruit Juice ∇ Orange Juice		
Sunny Delight		∇ Enriched Citrus Beverage w/Calcium Enriched Citrus Beverage: ∇ All Flavors Florida Citrus Punch	
Sunsweet	∇ Prune Juice		
Tampico		∇ Citrus Punch	
Texsun	∇ Pink Grapefruit Juice		
TreeSweet	∇ 100% Orange Juice ∇ 100% Pure Pink Grapefruit Juice		
TreeTop	∇ 100% Apple Juice		
Tropicana	∇ 100% Pure Grapefruit Juice 100% Pure Orange Juice From Concentrate: ∇ All Varieties ∇ Grovestand Orange Juice Pure Premium: ∇ 100% Pure Orange Juice, All Varieties	∇ Lemon Citrus Fruit Tea Twister Fruit Beverage: ∇ All Flavors	

∇ Low Sodium, 140 mg. or less per serving.

BRAND	BEST CHOICE	ACCEPTABLE CHOICE	OCCASIONAL CHOICE
	Fat Free AND Without Added Sugars (May Contain Sugar Substitutes)	Fat Free or Low Fat AND Low Saturated Fat AND With Added Sugars	Contains Greater Than 3 Grams Total Fat OR Greater Than 1 Gram Saturated Fat
Tropicana (Cont.)	Pure Premium: ∇ Ruby Red Grapefruit Juice ∇ Ruby Red Orange Season's Best: ∇ All Flavors Twister Light Fruit Beverage: ∇ All Flavors		
Veryfine	∇ Apple Juice ∇ Grape Juice ∇ Grapefruit Juice ∇ Orange Juice ∇ Orange Juice Blend ∇ Pineapple Juice	Apple Quenchers Cocktail: ∇ All Varieties	
Vrüit	∇ All Flavors		
Welch's	100% Grape Juice: ∇ from Concentrate (can) ∇ 100% White Grape Juice Frozen Concentrate: ∇ 100% Grape Juice ∇ Light Cranberry Juice Cocktail	Frozen Concentrate: ∇ Cranberry Juice Cocktail ∇ Cranberry Orange Juice Cocktail ∇ Cranberry Raspberry Juice Cocktail ∇ Grape Juice ∇ Grape Juice Cocktail ∇ White Grape Juice Fruit Juice Cocktail: ∇ Apple, Grape, Raspberry ∇ Orange, Pineapple, Apple ∇ Grape Juice Beverage Orchard Drink Boxes: ∇ All Flavors Orchard Frozen Concentrate: ∇ Harvest Blend	
Wilderness	∇ Apple Juice		
NON-CARBONATED			
All Brands	∇ Pure Spring Water		
Aqua Vie		Spring Water Beverage: ∇ All Flavors	
Arizona	∇ Diet Iced Tea	Iced Tea: ∇ All Flavors	
Aspire		Iced Cafe: ∇ Amaretto	

∇ Low Sodium, 140 mg. or less per serving.

BRAND	BEST CHOICE	ACCEPTABLE CHOICE	OCCASIONAL CHOICE
	Fat Free AND Without Added Sugars (May Contain Sugar Substitutes)	Fat Free or Low Fat AND Low Saturated Fat AND With Added Sugars	Contains Greater Than 3 Grams Total Fat OR Greater Than 1 Gram Saturated Fat
Aspire (Cont.)		Iced Cafe: ∇ Cappucino ∇ Decaffeinated ∇ Regular ∇ Vanilla	
Caffe Fantastico		Iced Cappuccino Drink Box: ∇ Skim Milk	
Carnation		Instant Breakfast (cans): Cafe Mocha	Instant Breakfast (cans): Creamy Milk Chocolate
Celestial Seasonings		Tea Drinks: ∇ All Flavors	
Dean Foods		Chocolate Drink	∇ Vitamite
Faygo	Bottled Diet Iced Tea: ∇ All Flavors Bottled Unsweeted Iced Tea: ∇ All Flavors	Bottled Iced Tea: ∇ All Flavors	
Gatorade		∇ Iced Tea Cooler	
Hershey		Drink Boxes: ∇ Genuine Chocolate Hershey's Bottle Chocolate Drink	
Ice Mountain	Spring Water		
Lipton	Brisk Iced Tea: ∇ Diet Originals Brewed Tea: ∇ Unsweetened Originals Diet: ∇ Natural Lemon Flavor	Brisk Iced Tea: ∇ All Flavors Originals Brewed Tea: ∇ Mountain Berry Apple ∇ Sweetened Originals Iced Tea: ∇ Sweetened-Natural Lemon	
Maxwell House			Cappio: ∇ Mocha ∇ Vanilla Iced Cappuccino: ∇ Coffee ∇ Mocha ∇ Vanilla
Mistic		Spring Water Iced Tea: ∇ w/Lemon	

∇ Low Sodium, 140 mg. or less per serving.

BRAND	BEST CHOICE	ACCEPTABLE CHOICE	OCCASIONAL CHOICE
	Fat Free AND Without Added Sugars (May Contain Sugar Substitutes)	Fat Free or Low Fat AND Low Saturated Fat AND With Added Sugars	Contains Greater Than 3 Grams Total Fat OR Greater Than 1 Gram Saturated Fat

Nestea		Cool:
		  ∇ Lemon Iced Tea
		Ice Tea, Bottled:
		  ∇ Lemon	

Snapple	Bottled Drinks:
	  ∇ Diet Iced Tea-Lemon
		Bottled Drinks:
		  ∇ Lemon Flavored Iced Tea	

Tradewinds	Tea:
	  ∇ Unsweetened
		Iced Tea:
		  ∇ All Flavors	

YooHoo		Chocolate Flavored Drink	
POWDERS / SYRUPS			

Alba	Reduced Calorie Shake Mix:
	  ∇ All Flavors
	Sugar Free Hot Cocoa Mix:
	  ∇ Chocolate and
	    Marshmallow
	  ∇ Milk Chocolate		

Alba '77	Reduced Calorie Dairy Shake Mix		

All Brands	Instant Coffee:
	  ∇ Decaffeinated
	  ∇ Regular
	Instant Tea:
	  ∇ Decaffeinated
	  ∇ Herbal
	  ∇ Regular		

Bosco		∇ Real Chocolate Flavored Syrup	

Carnation	Diet Hot Cocoa Mix:
	  Rich Chocolate
	Fat Free Hot Cocoa Mix:
	  w/NutraSweet
	Instant Breakfast No Sugar
	  Added Powders:
	  ∇ All Flavors
	Sugar Free Hot Cocoa:
	  Rich Chocolate
		Hot Cocoa Mix:
		  ∇ Milk Chocolate
		  ∇ Rich Chocolate
		  ∇ w/Marshmallows
		Instant Breakfast Powders:
		  ∇ All Flavors
		Malted Milk:
		  ∇ Chocolate
		  ∇ Original	

Country Time	Sugar Free Drink Mix:
	  ∇ All Flavors
		Drink Mix:
		  ∇ Lemonade
		  ∇ Pink Lemonade	

∇ Low Sodium, 140 mg. or less per serving.

BRAND	BEST CHOICE	ACCEPTABLE CHOICE	OCCASIONAL CHOICE
	Fat Free AND Without Added Sugars (May Contain Sugar Substitutes)	Fat Free or Low Fat AND Low Saturated Fat AND With Added Sugars	Contains Greater Than 3 Grams Total Fat OR Greater Than 1 Gram Saturated Fat
Crystal Light	Low Calorie Soft Drink Mix: ∇ All Flavors		
Dr. Cool		∇ Soft Drink Mix	
Fountain Shake		∇ Fat Free Strawberry Supreme ∇ Fat Free Vanilla Dream ∇ Imperial Chocolate	
General Foods		International Coffee: ∇ Cafe Amaretto ∇ Cafe Vienna ∇ French Vanilla Cafe ∇ Hazelnut Belgian Cafe ∇ Italian Cappucino ∇ Kahlua Cafe ∇ Orange Cappucino ∇ Suisse Mocha ∇ Viennese Chocolate Cafe Sugar Free International Coffee: ∇ Cafe Vienna ∇ French Vanilla Cafe ∇ Orange Cappuccino ∇ Suisse Mocha ∇ Suisse Mocha-Decaf	International Coffee: ∇ Cafe Francais
Ghirardelli		Hot Chocolate: ∇ All Flavors	
Hershey		Hershey's: ∇ Chocolate Malt Syrup ∇ Chocolate Syrup ∇ Strawberry Syrup ∇ Hershey's Syrup Hot Cocoa Collection: ∇ All Flavors	
Kool-Aid	Sugar Free Drink Mixes: ∇ All Flavors Unsweetened Soft Drink Mix: ∇ All Flavors	Sweetened Soft Drink Mix: ∇ All Flavors	
Land O Lakes			Cocoa Classics: All Flavors

∇ Low Sodium, 140 mg. or less per serving.

BRAND	BEST CHOICE	ACCEPTABLE CHOICE	OCCASIONAL CHOICE
	Fat Free AND Without Added Sugars (May Contain Sugar Substitutes)	Fat Free or Low Fat AND Low Saturated Fat AND With Added Sugars	Contains Greater Than 3 Grams Total Fat OR Greater Than 1 Gram Saturated Fat
Lipton	Iced Tea Mix: ∇ 100% Instant (Unsweetened) ∇ Decaffeinated (Unsweetened) Low Calorie Iced Tea: ∇ Natural Lemon Sugar Free Iced Tea Mix: ∇ All Flavors	Iced Tea Mix: ∇ Lemon Flavor Sweet Tea: ∇ Sugar, No Lemon	
Maxwell House		Cappuccino: ∇ Cinnamon ∇ Coffee ∇ Mocha ∇ Mocha Decaffeinated ∇ Vanilla ∇ Vanilla Decaffeinated	
Nescafe		Cappuccino: ∇ Authentic ∇ Authentic Mocha ∇ Authentic Sweetened	
Nestea	Instant Herb Tea: ∇ Orange Spice ∇ Lemon Splash ∇ Sugar Free Iced Tea Mix	100% Iced Tea Mix: w/Sweetener	
Nestle		European Hot Chocolate: ∇ Chocolate Irish Creme ∇ French Chocolate Creme ∇ Suisse Chocolate Truffle ∇ Nescafe Cappuccino Quik: ∇ Chocolate Flavored Syrup ∇ Chocolate Powder ∇ No Sugar Added Chocolate Powder ∇ Strawberry Powder	
Old Fashioned		∇ Instant Egg Nog Mix	
Ovaltine		∇ Original Malt Flavor ∇ Traditional Chocolate Malt Flavor	
Postum		Postum Instant Hot Beverage: ∇ Coffee Flavor ∇ Original	

∇ Low Sodium, 140 mg. or less per serving.

BRAND	BEST CHOICE	ACCEPTABLE CHOICE	OCCASIONAL CHOICE
	Fat Free AND Without Added Sugars (May Contain Sugar Substitutes)	Fat Free or Low Fat AND Low Saturated Fat AND With Added Sugars	Contains Greater Than 3 Grams Total Fat OR Greater Than 1 Gram Saturated Fat
Stephen's		Fat-Free Sipping Hot Wassail: ∇ All Flavors	Sipping Hot Cocoa Mix: All Flavors
Swiss Miss	Hot Cocoa Mix: Fat Free ∇ Sugar Free ∇ Sugar Free w/ Marshmallows	Hot Cocoa Mix: Lite Marshmallow Lovers ∇ Milk Chocolate Milk Chocolate w/Mini-Marshmallows Rich Chocolate Premiere Cocoas: Chocolate English Toffee Swisse Chocolate Truffle ∇ Spiced Apple Cider	Premiere Cocoas: Chocolate Raspberry Truffle
Tang	∇ Sugar Free Tang	Drink Mix: ∇ Orange	
Weight Watchers	Hot Cocoa Mix: Chocolate Marshmallow Milk Chocolate	Shake Mix: Chocolate Fudge Orange Sherbet	
SPORT			
All Sport		Thirst Quencher: ∇ All Flavors	
Gatorade		Gatorade Thirst Quencher: ∇ All Flavors	
Jogging in a Jug	∇ Jogging in a Jug		
Powerade		Thirst Quencher: ∇ All Flavors	
RW Knudsen	Recharge: ∇ Lemon Thirst Quencher		
Shasta		Body Works Sports Drink: All Flavors	
Twinlab		Ultra Fuel: ∇ All Flavors	

∇ Low Sodium, 140 mg. or less per serving.

BRAND	BEST CHOICE	ACCEPTABLE CHOICE	OCCASIONAL CHOICE
	Fat Free AND Without Added Sugars (May Contain Sugar Substitutes)	Fat Free or Low Fat AND Low Saturated Fat AND With Added Sugars	Contains Greater Than 3 Grams Total Fat OR Greater Than 1 Gram Saturated Fat
VEGETABLE			
Campbell's	Tomato Juice: ▽ Low Sodium ▲ Regular		
Del Monte	▲ Tomato Juice		
Frank's	▲ Kraut Juice		
Heinz	▲ Fancy Tomato Juice		
Hollywood	▽ 100% Natural Carrot Juice		
Hunt's	Tomato Juice: ▽ No Salt Added		
Mott's		▲ Clamato	
Red Gold	▲ Tomato Juice		
RW Knudsen	Organic Tomato Juice Very Veggie: ▽ Low Sodium ▲ Original ▲ Spicy		
Sacramento	Vegetable Cocktail		
V8	100% Vegetable Juice: ▲ All Flavors ▽ Low Sodium Vegetable Juice Picante Juice: ▲ Mild Flavor		
YOUR FAVORITE BEVERAGES NOT LISTED IN THE *GUIDE*			

▲ High Sodium, 480 mg. or greater per serving.
▽ Low Sodium, 140 mg. or less per serving.

352 **Beverages**

DIPS AND SALSAS

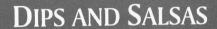

This category contains a large variety of dips and salsas that help add zest and enhance the flavor of many dishes. Many dips are tomato-based or chili pepper-based and are a nice complement to the many brands of reduced-fat and fat-free chips currently available. The higher-fat sour cream-based dips have the potential of adding many calories from fat and saturated fat to the daily diet.

Depending on the primary ingredient of the dip or salsa, the *Food Guide Pyramid* may consider these products part of either the "Fats, Oils, and Sweets Group," "Vegetable Group," or "Milk, Yogurt, and Cheese Group." The recommended serving sizes will vary depending on their food group classification. The FDA has established reference amounts or standardized serving sizes for use on the food label. The reference amount for dips and salsas is 2 tablespoons. Be sure to read the *Nutrition Facts* label for the serving size information of your product choice. (See pages 51 and 52 for an explanation of reference amounts and the difference between serving sizes established by the FDA for food labeling and those recommended by the *Food Guide Pyramid*.)

Dips and salsas range from those that are fat-free, low-fat and low saturated fat, to those that contain substantial amounts of fat and saturated fat. Criteria were therefore designed to distinguish those products lower in total fat and saturated fat from their higher-fat alternatives.

Criteria Key

▲ **Best Choice:**   **Fat Free**

Products listed in this category meet the FDA's definition for "Fat Free" (less than $1/2$ gram fat per serving).

▲ **Acceptable Choice:**   **Low Fat AND Low Saturated Fat**

Products listed in this category meet the FDA's definition for "Low Fat" (3 grams or less fat per serving), and "Low Saturated Fat" (1 gram or less per serving).

▲ **Occasional Choice:**   **Contains Greater Than 3 grams Total Fat, or Greater Than 1 gram Saturated Fat**

Products listed in this category **do not** meet the FDA's definition for "Low Fat" or "Low Saturated Fat." Since excessive use of these products can significantly increase your intake of total fat and saturated fat, they should be consumed only on occasion.

BRAND	BEST CHOICE	ACCEPTABLE CHOICE	OCCASIONAL CHOICE
	Fat Free	Low Fat AND Low Saturated Fat	Contains Greater Than 3 Grams Total Fat OR Greater Than 1 Gram Saturated Fat
Avo-King			Guacamole: ∇ Southwestern
Bearitos		∇ Bean Dip	
Bonavita		Vegetarian Pate: ∇ All Flavors	
Breakstone's			Sour Cream Dip: Bacon & Onion Chesapeake Clam Jalapeno Cheddar Toasted Onion
Bruno & Luigi's	Fat Free Chip Dip: ∇ All Varieties		
Calavo		Avocado Guacamole Lite	
Casbah			Hummus Mix
Cheese Shoppe	Mexican Salsa: ∇ Spicy ∇ w/Cheese		
Chi Chi's	Chunky Restaurante Salsa: Hot ∇ Medium Mild Picante Sauce: All Varieties Pico de Gallo Salsa: All Flavors Taco Sauce: ∇ Thick & Chunky		
Dairy Fresh		∇ French Onion Party Dip	
Dean Foods	No Fat French Onion Dip Veggie No Fat Dip	Light French Onion Dip Light Green Onion Dip	French Onion Dip: Non-Dairy French Onion Dip ∇ Ranch Dip ∇ Salsa Dip
Eagle	Salsa: All Flavors	Bean Dip: Mild Black Bean Dip: ∇ Mild	

∇ Low Sodium, 140 mg. or less per serving.

BRAND	BEST CHOICE	ACCEPTABLE CHOICE	OCCASIONAL CHOICE
	Fat Free	Low Fat AND Low Saturated Fat	Contains Greater Than 3 Grams Total Fat OR Greater Than 1 Gram Saturated Fat
Enrico's	Black Bean Dip: 　Mild 　Spicy Chunky Style Salsa: 　∇ Hot 　∇ Mild 　∇ Mild, No Salt Added Fat Free Nacho Cheese Dip: 　Mild		
Fantastic Foods		Hummus	
Festida	Thick 'n' Chunky Salsa: 　∇ All Varieties		
Frito Lay	Tostitos Black Bean Dip: 　Fat Free Tostitos Restaurant Style Salsa: 　All Varieties Tostitos Restaurant Style Black 　Bean Dip: 　All Varieties Tostitos Salsa: 　All Flavors	Cheese Dip: 　Jalapeno and Cheddar 　Mild Cheddar Fritos Bean Dip: 　∇ Original Tostitos Restaurant Style Salsa 　Con Queso: 　▲ All Varieties	French Onion Dip Ruffles Dip: 　Ranch
Gourmet Jose	Salsa: 　All Flavors		
Guiltless Gourmet	Black Bean Dip: 　∇ All Flavors Nacho Dip: 　All Flavors Pinto Bean Dip: 　∇ All Flavors Salsa: 　∇ All Flavors		
Hickory Farms			Nacho Cheese Sauce: 　Cheddar & Jalapeno
Hidden Valley Ranch	Party Dip: 　∇ French Onion 　∇ Garden Vegetable 　Original Ranch		
Hunt's	Homestyle Alfresco Salsa: 　All Flavors		

▲ High Sodium, 480 mg. or greater per serving.
∇ Low Sodium, 140 mg. or less per serving.

356　**Dips and Salsas**

BRAND	BEST CHOICE	ACCEPTABLE CHOICE	OCCASIONAL CHOICE
	Fat Free	Low Fat AND Low Saturated Fat	Contains Greater Than 3 Grams Total Fat OR Greater Than 1 Gram Saturated Fat

Hunt's (Cont.)	Homestyle Picante Sauce:
	  All Varieties
	Homestyle Salsa:
	  All Varieties		

Kaukauna	Mexican Salsa:
	  All Flavors
	Picante Sauce
		Pretzel Dip:
		  Sweet Hot Mustard	

Keebler			Salsa Verde

Knudsen			Premium Real Sour Cream Dip:
			  Bacon & Onion
			  French Onion
			  Nacho Cheese

Kraft			Avocado Dip Bacon & Horseradish Dip Clam Dip French Onion Dip Jalapeno Cheese Dip Jalapeno Dip Nacho Cheese Dip

La Famous	Thick 'n Chunky Salsa:
	  All Flavors
		Nacho Cheese Dip:
		  Mild
		  Spicy	

La Victoria	Salsa:
	  ∇ All Flavors
	Taco Sauce:
	  ∇ Green
	  ∇ Red		

Marie's			∇ Caramel Dip for Apples
			Dip:
			  Bacon Ranch
			  ∇ Parmesan Garlic
			  ∇ Sun Dried Tomato

Marzetti			∇ French Onion Dip
Mexican	Salsa Chunky Style: All Flavors		
Napa Valley	Gourmet Salsa: All Varieties		

∇ Low Sodium, 140 mg. or less per serving.

Dips and Salsas 357

BRAND	BEST CHOICE	ACCEPTABLE CHOICE	OCCASIONAL CHOICE
	Fat Free	Low Fat AND Low Saturated Fat	Contains Greater Than 3 Grams Total Fat OR Greater Than 1 Gram Saturated Fat
Newman's Own	Salsa: All Varieties		

Old El Paso	Homestyle Chunky Salsa:
	  ∇ All Flavors
	Salsa:
	  Medium Picante
	Salsa Thick & Chunky:
	  ∇ All Flavors
	  ∇ Picante, All Flavors
	Taco Sauce:
	  ∇ All Flavors
		Cheese-n-Salsa Dip:
		  All Flavors	

Ortega	Garden Style Salsa:
	  All Flavors
	Thick & Chunky Salsa:
	  All Varieties
	Thick & Smooth Taco Sauce:
	  ∇ All Varieties		

Pablo's	Medium Salsa Mild Salsa		▲ Jalapeno Cheese Sauce ▲ Nacho Cheese Sauce

Pace	Picante Sauce:
	  All Flavors
	Salsa Dip:
	  All Varieties
	Thick & Chunky Salsa:
	  All Varieties		

Ranger Luke's	7J Ranch Texasalsa: ∇ All Varieties		
Rojo's	∇ Salsa Ranchero		

Sargento	Salsa:
	  All Varieties
	Sonora Valley:
	  Chunky Salsa
	  Thick 'n Chunky Picante
		Beans w/Cheese Dip	Nacho Cheese Dip
			Sonora Valley:
			  ▲ Nacho Cheese Sauce
			  ▲ Salsa Con Queso

Sealtest			French Onion Dip
Shotgun Willie's	Picante Sauce: ∇ Hotter 'N Hell		
Smart Temptations	Fat Free Salsa: ∇ All Varieties		

▲ High Sodium, 480 mg. or greater per serving.
∇ Low Sodium, 140 mg. or less per serving.

358 **Dips and Salsas**

Brand	Best Choice	Acceptable Choice	Occasional Choice
	Fat Free	Low Fat AND Low Saturated Fat	Contains Greater Than 3 Grams Total Fat OR Greater Than 1 Gram Saturated Fat
Smart Temptations (Cont.)	∇ Mild Pinto Bean Dip		
Smucker's	Fat Free Apple Dip: ∇ Caramel		

T. Marzetti's			∇ Chocolate Fruit Dip
			∇ Old Fashioned Caramel Apple Dip
			∇ Peanut Butter Caramel Apple Dip
			∇ Reduced Fat Caramel Apple Dip
			Veggie Dip:
			  Blue Cheese
			  Ranch
			  Salsa Con Queso
			  Southwestern Ranch
			  Spinach

Taco Bell	Fat Free Black Bean Dip:
	  All Varieties
	Picante Sauce:
	  All Varieties
	Thick 'n Chunky Salsa:
	  All Varieties
		Salsa Con Queso:
		  All Varieties	

Thank You			Creamy French Onion Dip Creamy Ranch Dip
YOUR FAVORITE DIPS AND SALSAS NOT LISTED IN THE *GUIDE*			

∇ Low Sodium, 140 mg. or less per serving.

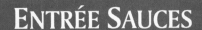

This category contains a large variety of entrée sauces, ranging from the fat-free or low-fat tomato-based sauces to the higher-fat pesto and Alfredo sauces. The higher-fat cream-based sauces have the potential of adding many calories from fat and saturated fat to the daily diet. To add variety and enhance nutrient density of pasta dinners, fresh cut-up vegetables can be added to tomato-based pasta sauces. Depending on the primary ingredient of the entrée sauces, the *Food Guide Pyramid* may consider these products part of either the "Fats, Oils, and Sweets Group," "Vegetable Group," or "Milk, Yogurt, and Cheese Group." The recommended serving sizes will vary depending on their food group classification. The FDA has established reference amounts or standardized serving sizes for use on the food label. The reference amount entrée sauces range from 1/4 cup for "minor" entrée sauces such as pizza sauce, pesto sauce, gravy, or white sauce to 125 grams (1/2 cup) for "major" entrée sauces such as spaghetti sauces. Be sure to read the *Nutrition Facts* label for the serving size information of your product choice. (See pages 51 and 52 for an explanation of reference amounts and the difference between serving sizes established by the FDA for food labeling and those recommended by the *Food Guide Pyramid*.)

Entrée sauces range from those that are fat-free, low-fat and low saturated fat, to those that contain substantial amounts of fat and saturated fat. Criteria were, therefore, designed to distinguish those products lower in total fat and saturated fat from their higher-fat alternatives. Entrée Sauces that contain 480 milligrams sodium or more per serving (20% of the Daily Value) are considered high in sodium and are indicated with a ▲ symbol.

Criteria Key

△ Best Choice: **Fat Free or Low Fat, AND Low Saturated Fat**

Products listed in this category meet the FDA's definition for "Fat Free" (less than
$1/2$ gram fat per serving), or "Low Fat" (3 grams or less fat per serving), and "Low
Saturated Fat" (1 gram or less saturated fat per serving).

△ Acceptable Choice: **Contains Greater Than 3 Grams, but
Less Than or Equal to 5 Grams Total Fat,
AND Low Saturated Fat**

Products listed in this category **do not** meet the FDA's definition for "Low Fat,"
but **do** meet the criteria for "Low Saturated Fat." The 5 grams of total fat cut-off
was used in order to be consistent with the amount of fat equal to one diabetes
diet fat exchange and is also equivalent to 1 teaspoon of added fat.[75] Although
these products contribute a greater amount of fat to the overall daily diet, they
are acceptable if consumed in moderation.

▲ Occasional Choice: **Contains Greater Than 5 Grams Total Fat,
or Greater Than 1 Gram Saturated Fat**

Products listed in this category **do not** meet the FDA's definition for either "Low
Fat," or "Low Saturated Fat." These products can contribute a significant amount
of fat to the overall daily diet and should be consumed only on occasion.

BRAND	BEST CHOICE	ACCEPTABLE CHOICE	OCCASIONAL CHOICE
	Fat Free or Low Fat AND Low Saturated Fat	Contains Greater Than 3 Grams but Less Than or Equal to 5 Grams Total Fat AND Low Saturated Fat	Contains Greater Than 5 Grams Total Fat OR Greater Than 1 Gram Saturated Fat
Balsamic	Pasta Sauce: ▲ Tomato Basil ▲ Traditional		
Boboli	Pizza Sauce		
Campbell's	Simmer Chef Cooking Sauce: Golden Honey Mustard ▲ Hearty Onion & Mushroom Oriental Sweet & Sour Zesty Tomato Mexicali Spaghetti Sauce: Extra Garlic & Onion ▲☆ Ground Beef Homestyle Italian Style ▲☆ Mushroom & Garlic ▲ Traditional		Simmer Chef Cooking Sauce: ▲ Creamy Broccoli ▲ Creamy Mushroom & Herb ▲ Family-Style Stroganoff
Chef Boyardee	Pizza Sauce w/Cheese		
Christopher Ranch			☆ Pesto Sauce
Ci'Bella	Pasta Sauce: ▲ w/Garden Vegetables		
Classico	Pasta Sauce: ▲ Mushrooms & Ripe Olives Spicy Red Pepper Tomato & Basil	Pasta Sauce: ▲ Beef & Pork ▲ Four Cheese Onion and Garlic Sun-Dried Tomato Sweet Peppers & Onions	
Colavita	Tomato Sauce: Classic Hot Marinara		
Contadina	Chunky Pizza Sauce: All Varieties Light Chunky Tomato Sauce ▲☆ Light Garden Vegetable Sauce	Marinara Sauce ▲☆ Spicy Italian Sausage & Bell Pepper Sauce	Alfredo Sauce: ▲ Light ▲ Regular ▲ Four Cheese Sauce w/White Wine & Shallots

▲ High Sodium, 480 mg. or greater per serving.
☆ Good Source of Fiber, between 2.5 g. and 5 g. per serving.

BRAND	BEST CHOICE	ACCEPTABLE CHOICE	OCCASIONAL CHOICE
	Fat Free or Low Fat AND Low Saturated Fat	Contains Greater Than 3 Grams but Less Than or Equal to 5 Grams Total Fat AND Low Saturated Fat	Contains Greater Than 5 Grams Total Fat OR Greater Than 1 Gram Saturated Fat
Contadina (Cont.)	Pasta Ready Tomato Sauce: ▲ Crushed Red Pepper ▲ Mushroom Pizza Sauce: Original Regular Pizza Squeeze Pizza Sauce: Italian Cheeses ☆ Plum Tomato w/Basil		Pesto w/Basil Sauce ▲☆ Pesto w/Sun Dried Tomato Sauce ▲ Red Bell Pepper Cream Sauce
Dei Fratelli	Marinara Sauce Tomato Sauce		
Del Monte	Spaghetti Sauce: Traditional w/Garlic and Onion ▲ w/Mushrooms		
Di Giorno	Light Pasta Sauce: Chunky Tomato w/Basil Pasta Sauce: Plum Tomato & Mushroom	Pasta Sauce: ▲ Marinara	Light Pasta Sauce: ▲ Reduced Fat Alfredo Pasta Sauce: ▲ Alfredo Four Cheese ▲ Olive Oil & Garlic w/ Grated Cheese ▲ Traditional Meat ▲ Pesto Sauce
Enrico's	Pasta Sauce: ▲ Garlic Marinara Hot & Spicy Arabiati ∇ Italian Style No Salt Added Traditional Fat Free ∇ Traditional Fat Free No Salt Spaghetti Sauce: All Natural All Natural w/Mushrooms ∇ No Salt Added		
Healthy Choice	Pasta Sauce: Chunky Mushrooms Extra Chunky Garlic & Onions		

▲ High Sodium, 480 mg. or greater per serving.
∇ Low Sodium, 140 mg. or less per serving.
☆ Good Source of Fiber, between 2.5 g. and 5 g. per serving.

BRAND	BEST CHOICE	ACCEPTABLE CHOICE	OCCASIONAL CHOICE
	Fat Free or Low Fat AND Low Saturated Fat	Contains Greater Than 3 Grams but Less Than or Equal to 5 Grams Total Fat AND Low Saturated Fat	Contains Greater Than 5 Grams Total Fat OR Greater Than 1 Gram Saturated Fat
Healthy Choice (Cont.)	Pasta Sauce: 　Extra Chunky Italian Style 　　Vegetables 　Garlic & Herbs 　Mushrooms 　Super Chunky Mushrooms 　　& Sweet Peppers 　Super Chunky Vegetable 　Primavera 　Traditional		
Heinz	Homestyle Gravy: 　All Varieties		
Hunt's	Chunky Spaghetti Sauce: 　▲ Italian Style Vegetables 　▲ Marinara 　▲ Tomato, Garlic & Onion 　　w/Tomato Chunks Homestyle Spaghetti Sauce: 　▲ Traditional 　▲ w/Mushrooms Original Spaghetti Sauce: 　▲ Traditional 　▲ w/Meat 　▲ w/Mushrooms Ready Tomato Sauce: 　Chunky Garlic & Herb 　Chunky Italian 　Chunky Mexican 　Chunky Salsa 　▽ Chunky Special 　Original Country Herb Spaghetti Sauce: 　▲ Classic Italian w/Garlic 　　and Herb 　▲ Classic Italian w/ 　　Parmesan		
Libby's		Country Gravy: 　Chicken	Country Gravy: 　Sausage
Mamma Rizzo's	▲ Marinara Italian Sauce		
Muir Glen	Organic Fat Free Pasta Sauce: 　☆ Garlic and Onion	Chef Sauce: 　Italian	

▲ High Sodium, 480 mg. or greater per serving.

▽ Low Sodium, 140 mg. or less per serving.

☆ Good Source of Fiber, between 2.5 g. and 5 g. per serving.

BRAND	BEST CHOICE	ACCEPTABLE CHOICE	OCCASIONAL CHOICE
	Fat Free or Low Fat AND Low Saturated Fat	Contains Greater Than 3 Grams but Less Than or Equal to 5 Grams Total Fat AND Low Saturated Fat	Contains Greater Than 5 Grams Total Fat OR Greater Than 1 Gram Saturated Fat
Muir Glen (Cont.)	Organic Fat Free Pasta Sauce: ☆ Sweet Pepper & Onion ☆ Tomato Basil Organic Pasta Sauce: ☆ Chunky Style ☆ Mushrooms and Green Peppers ☆ Romano Cheese		
Newman's Own	Sockarooni: ▲ Spaghetti Sauce ▲ Spicy Simmer Sauce for Chicken & Seafood Venetian Spaghetti Sauce: ▲ All Natural Marinara Style ▲ Marinara w/Mushrooms		
Pastorelli	Italian-Chef Pizza Sauce		
Pepperidge Farm	Gravy: ∇ All Flavors		
Prego	Extra Chunky Spaghetti Sauce: ▲ Garden Combination ▲ Zesty Oregano w/ Mushrooms Pizza Sauce: Traditional w/Sliced Mushrooms Spaghetti Sauce: ▲ Three Cheese X-tra Chunky: ▲ Garden Sauce	Extra Chunky Spaghetti Sauce: ▲ Mushroom and Diced Tomato Mushroom and Green Pepper ▲ Mushroom w/Extra Spice ▲ Zesty Garlic & Cheese	Extra Chunky Spaghetti Sauce: ▲ Mushroom and Diced Onion ▲ Tomato Onion Garlic ▲ Zesty Basil Spaghetti Sauce: ▲ Fresh Mushrooms ∇ Low Sodium ▲ Traditional ▲ With Meat
Pritikin	Marinara Sauce Spaghetti Sauce: ∇ Chunky Garden Style ∇ Original		
Progresso	Pizza Sauce: ∇ Italian Style	Spaghetti Sauce: ▲ Marinara ▲ Meat ▲ Mushroom	White Clam Sauce

▲ High Sodium, 480 mg. or greater per serving.
∇ Low Sodium, 140 mg. or less per serving.
☆ Good Source of Fiber, between 2.5 g. and 5 g. per serving.

BRAND	BEST CHOICE	ACCEPTABLE CHOICE	OCCASIONAL CHOICE
	Fat Free or Low Fat AND Low Saturated Fat	Contains Greater Than 3 Grams but Less Than or Equal to 5 Grams Total Fat AND Low Saturated Fat	Contains Greater Than 5 Grams Total Fat OR Greater Than 1 Gram Saturated Fat
Progresso (Cont.)		Spaghetti Sauce: ▲ Regular	
Ragu	100% Natural Pizza Sauce Chicken Tonight: 　▲ Chicken Cacciatore 　Sweet & Sour Chicken Chicken Tonight Light: 　Honey Mustard 　▲ Italian Primavera 100% Natural Pasta Sauce: 　☆ Hearty Italian Tomato Light Pasta Sauce: 　Chunky Mushroom 　Tomato & Herb Pizza Quick Sauce: 　Chunky Mushroom	Chunky Gardenstyle: 　▲ Mushroom & Green Pepper 　▲ Super Mushroom 100% Natural Pasta Sauce: 　▲☆ Flavored w/Sauteed Beef 　▲ Parmesan 　▲☆ Sauteed Onion & Garlic 　▲☆ Sauteed Onion & Mushroom Homestyle 100% Natural Spaghetti Sauce: 　▲ Flavored w/Meat 　▲ Mushroom Old World Style: 　▲ Meat 　▲ Mushroom 　▲ Traditional	Chicken Tonight: 　▲ Country French Chicken 　▲ Creamy Mushroom
Romance	☆ Marinara Sauce		▲ Alfredo Sauce Pesto Sauce
Santa Barbara Olive Co.		▲ Chunky Olive Pasta Sauce	
Sinatra's	Sugo Da Tavola: 　▲ Tomato Basil w/Parmesan		Alfredo Sauce Cooking Sauce: 　Marsala 　Scampi Pesto Sauce
Stokely's	Tomato Sauce		
Stouffer's			Welsh Rarebit: 　Cheddar Cheese Sauce
Sutter Home		▲ Italian Style Pasta Sauce ▲ Marinara Sauce ▲ Sicilian Style Pasta Sauce	▲ Spicy Mediterranean Style Pasta Sauce
Tasty Tomato	Premium Spaghetti Sauce: 　All Varieties		

▲ High Sodium, 480 mg. or greater per serving.
☆ Good Source of Fiber, between 2.5 g. and 5 g. per serving.

BRAND	BEST CHOICE	ACCEPTABLE CHOICE	OCCASIONAL CHOICE
	Fat Free or Low Fat AND Low Saturated Fat	Contains Greater Than 3 Grams but Less Than or Equal to 5 Grams Total Fat AND Low Saturated Fat	Contains Greater Than 5 Grams Total Fat OR Greater Than 1 Gram Saturated Fat

Uncle Dave's	Excellent Marinara:
	  Chunky Tomato
	  Chunky Tomato & Mushroom
	Pasta Sauce:
	  Sundried Tomato Basil
			Pasta Sauce:
			  ▲ Spicy Peanut

Weight Watchers	Smart Options Pasta Sauce: Mushroom		
YOUR FAVORITE ENTREE SAUCES NOT LISTED IN THE *GUIDE*			

▲ High Sodium, 480 mg. or greater per serving.

APPENDIX A

BODY MASS INDEX

The Body Mass Index (BMI) is a method used to determine degree of overweight. This method is used by many researchers to define overweight because it is closely related to the amount of body fat a person has.[72] BMI tends to be high in persons who have a large proportion of body fat. BMI is a ratio of weight to height which is calculated as follows:

$$\textbf{BMI} = \frac{\text{weight in kilograms}}{(\text{height in meters})^2}$$

To convert pounds to kilograms, divide by 2.2; to convert inches to meters, multiply by 0.0254.

The BMI for a 170 pound (77 kilogram) man, who is 6 feet (1.83 meters) tall is:

$$\textbf{BMI} = \frac{77 \text{ kilograms}}{(1.83 \text{ meters})^2} = \textbf{23}$$

Recent health survey data defines overweight as having a BMI greater than or equal to 27.8 for men and 27.3 for women, and severe overweight as having a BMI greater than or equal to 31.1 for men and 32.3 for women.[18,73] According to these definitions, the man in the example above is not overweight.

APPENDIX B

WAIST-TO-HIP RATIO

Determining your body shape can be done with two simple measurements used to measure waist-to-hip ratio. This ratio indicates which of these two areas (waist or hips) contains relatively more fat. Here is how you do it:

1. Measure around your waist near your navel while you stand relaxed, not pulling in your stomach.

2. Measure around your hips, over the buttocks, where they are largest.

3. Divide the waist measurement by the hips measurement to get your waist-to-hip ratio.

EXAMPLE

Waist	=	42 inches
Hips	=	36 inches
Waist-to-Hip Ratio	=	42 ÷ 36 = 1.166

A value greater than 1.0 means the measure for the waist is larger than the hips (an "apple" body shape). In general, a value greater than 1.0 means that too much fat is carried in the abdomen. More specifically, values above 0.80 for women and above 0.95 for men have been linked to greater risk for several chronic diseases such as cardiovascular disease, hypertension, and gallbladder disease.[13] However, ratios have not been defined for all populations or age groups.

If your weight is within the ranges in Table 2, page 25, if your waist-to-hip ratio is below 1.0 for men and 0.8 for women, and if you have no medical problem for which your doctor advises you to gain or lose weight, there appears to be no health advantage to changing your weight. If you do not meet all of these conditions, or if you are not sure, you may want to talk to your doctor about how your weight might affect your health and what you might do about it.

APPENDIX C

NUTRIENT CONTENT CLAIMS AND DEFINITIONS

Nutrient Content Claim	Definition
"Free"	A serving contains no or an inconsequential amount: <5 calories, <5 mg of sodium, <0.5 g fat, <0.5 g saturated fat, <2 mg cholesterol, or <0.5 g of sugar
"No Added Sugar"	• No sugars or ingredients containing functional sugars added during processing • Substitutes for food that contains sugars • No ingredients containing added sugars • Not processed to increase sugars content
"Low"	A serving contains no more than 40 calories; 140 mg of sodium; 3 g fat, 1 g (and 15% or less calories) from saturated fat; or 20 mg cholesterol; not defined for sugar; for "very low sodium": no more than 35 mg of sodium
"Unsalted"	• No salt added during processing; and • Substitutes for a food that contains salt
"Lean"	A 3 oz serving (and 100 g) of meat, poultry, seafood, and game meats contains <10 g fat, ≤4.5 g saturated fat, and <95 mg cholesterol
"Extra Lean"	A 3 oz serving (and 100 g) of meat, poultry, seafood, and game meats contains <5 g of fat, <2 g of saturated fat, and <95 mg of cholesterol
"High"	A serving contains 20% or more of the Daily Value (DV) for a particular nutrient
"Good Source"	A serving contains 10-19% of the DV for a particular nutrient
"Reduced" or "Less"	Sodium, sugar, fat, saturated fat, calories, or cholesterol has been reduced by at least 25% from an appropriate reference food

Table continues on next page.

NUTRIENT CONTENT CLAIMS AND DEFINITIONS (Continued)

Nutrient Content Claim	Definition
"Light"	• An altered-product contains $1/3$ fewer calories or 50% of the fat in a reference food, OR • The sodium content of a low-calorie, low-fat food has been reduced by 50%, OR • The term describes such properties as texture and color, as long as the label explains the intent (e.g., "light brown sugar")
"More"	A serving contains at least 10% of the DV of a nutrient more than a reference food
"% Fat Free"	A product must be low-fat or fat-free, and the percentage must accurately reflect the amount of fat in 100 g of food
"Healthy"	A food is low in fat and saturated fat, and a serving contains no more than 480 mg of sodium and no more than 60 mg of cholesterol; also must contain at least 10% of the recommended Daily Value for one of six nutrients: Vitamin A, Vitamin C, calcium, fiber, iron, protein
"Fresh"	• A food is raw, has never been frozen or heated, and contains no preservatives (irradiation at low levels is allowed), OR • The term accurately describes the product (e.g., "fresh milk" or "freshly baked bread")
"Fresh Frozen"	The food has been quickly frozen while still fresh; blanching is allowed before freezing to prevent nutrient breakdown

APPENDIX D

FAT SUBSTITUTIONS SUGGESTIONS

Original Ingredient	Substitution Option	Fat Grams Saved
1 C sour cream	1 C fat free sour cream 1 C non fat plain yogurt 1 C fat free cottage cheese (pureed) 1 C low-fat sour cream	40 40 40 24
1 C whole milk	1 C skim milk 1 C 1 % milk 1 C 2 % milk	9 6 4
1 whole egg	1/4 C egg substitute 2 egg whites	6 6
1 stick butter/ margarine	1/2 C applesauce + 3 Tbs. canola oil	56
1 C heavy cream	1 C evaporated skim milk 1 C evaporated whole milk 1 C half & half	90 71 61
1/4 C oil	2 Tbs. pureed prunes, bananas, applesauce or pumpkin + 2 Tbs. canola oil	84
1 C walnuts	1/2 C walnuts, lightly dry roasted to bring out the flavor	21

REFERENCES

1. American Heart Association. Heart and stroke facts: 1994 statistical supplement. Dallas: American Heart Association, 1993 [55 0515(COM).]

2. Stamler J, Wentworth D, Neaton JD. Is the relationship between serum cholesterol and risk of premature death from coronary heart disease continuous and graded: findings in 356,222 primary screenees of the Multiple Risk Factor Intervention Trial (MRFIT). JAMA 1986;256:2823-28.

3. Goldman L, Cook EF. The decline in ischemic heart disease mortality rates: An analysis of the comparative effects of medical interventions and changes in lifestyle. Ann Int Med 1984;101:825-36.

4. Carleton RA, Dwyer J, Finberg, Flora J, Goodman DS, Grundy SM et al. Report of the expert panel on population strategies for blood cholesterol reduction. Circulation 1991;83:2154-2232.

5. deLorgeril M, Renaud S, Mamelle N, Salen P et al. Mediterranean alpha-linolenic acid-rich diet in secondary prevention of coronary heart disease. Lancet 1994;343:1454-59.

6. Watts GF, Jackson P, Mandalia S, Brunt JN, Lewis E et al. Nutrient intake and progression of coronary artery disease. Am J Cardiol 1994;73:328-32.

7. Blankenhorn DH, Johnson RL, Mack W, Zein H, Vailas L. The influence of diet on appearance of new lesions in human coronary arteries. JAMA 1990;263:1646-52.

8. US Surgeon General. The Surgeon General's report on nutrition and health. Washington, DC: US Department of Health and Human Services; 1988. [DHHS publication (PHS) 88 50210.]

9. Connor WE, Connor SL. The key role of nutritional factors in the prevention of coronary heart disease. Prev Med I 1972;1:49-83.

10. Federal Register. Nutrition Labeling and Education Act of 1990. PL 101-535. 104 Stat 2353.
11. US Department of Agriculture and US Department of Health and Human Service. Report of the dietary guidelines advisory committee on the dietary guidelines for Americans, 1995. Washington DC: US Department of Agriculture.

12. US Department of Agriculture, Human Nutrition Information Services. Report of the dietary guidelines, advisory committee on the dietary guidelines for Americans 1990. Hyattsville, MD, 1990.

13. National Research Council. Diet and health: implications for reducing chronic disease risk. Washington, DC: National Academy Press, 1989.

14. National Research Council. Recommended dietary allowances. 10th ed. Washington, DC: National Academy Press, 1989.

15. US Department of Health and Human Services. Healthy people 2000: national health promotion and disease prevention objectives. Washington, DC: National Academy Press, 1991. [DHHS publication (PHS) 91 50213.]

16. Saltos E, Davis C, Welsh S, Guthrie J, Tamaki J. Using food labels to follow the dietary guidelines for Americans: a reference. Washington, DC: US Department of Agriculture, Agriculture Information Bulletin 704, 1994.

17. US Department of Agriculture. The food guide pyramid. Washington DC: US Government Printing Office, 1992. [Home and Garden Bulletin 252.]

18. Kuczmarski RJ, Flegal KM, Campbell SM, Johnson CL. Increasing prevalence of overweight among US adults: the National Health and Nutrition Examination Surveys, 1960-1991. JAMA 1994;272:205-211.

19. Larsson B. Regional obesity as a health hazard in men: prospective studies. Acta Med Scand 1988;723:45-51.

20. Lapidus L, Bengtsson C, Larsson B, Pennert K, Rybo E, Sjostrom L. Distribution of adipose tissue and risk of cardiovascular disease and death: a 12 year follow-up of participants in the population study of women in Gothenburg, Sweden. Br Med J 1984;289:1257-61.

21. Tremblay A, Plourede G, Despres JP, Bouchard C. Impact of dietary fat content and fat oxidation on energy intake in humans. Am J Clin Nutr. 1989;49:799-805.

22. Weinhouse S, Bal D, Adamson R, Dwyer J, Kleinman R, Kritchevsky D, et al. American Cancer Society guidelines on diet, nutrition, and cancer. Can J Clin 1991;41:334-38.

23. La Vecchia C, Harris RE, Wynder EL. Comparative epidemiology of cancer between the United States and Italy. Can Res 1988;48:7285-93.

24. Colditz GA, Branch LG, Lipnick RJ, Willett WC, Rosner B, Posner BM, et al. Increased green and yellow vegetable intake and lowered cancer deaths in an elderly population. Am J Clin Nutr 1985;41:32-6.

25. LeMarchand L, Yoshizawa CN, Kolonel LN, Hankin JH, Goodman MT. Vegetable consumption and lung cancer risk: a population-based case control study in Hawaii. JNCI 1989;81:1158-64.

26. Bell LP, Hectorn KJ, Reynolds H, Hunninghake DB. Cholesterol-lowering effects of soluble-fiber cereals as part of a prudent diet for patients with mild to moderate hypercholesterolemia. Am J Clin Nutr 1990;52:1020-26.

27. Anderson JW, Garrity TF, Wood CL, Whitis SE, Smith BM, Oeltgen PR. Prospective, randomized, controlled comparison of the effects of low-fat and low-fat plus high-fiber diets on serum lipid concentrations. Am J Clin Nutr 1992;56:887-94.

28. Anderson JW. High fibre diets for diabetic and hypertriglyceridemic patients. J Can Med Assoc 1980;123:975-79.

29. Karlstrom B, Vessby B, Asp NG, Boberg M, Gustafsson IB, Lithell H, et al. Effects of an increased content of cereal fiber in the diet of Type-II (non-insulin dependent) diabetic patients. Diabetologia 1984;26:272-77.

30. Tippett K, Goldman J. Diets more healthful, but still fall short of dietary guidelines. Food Rev 1994;17:8-14.

31. Butrum RR, Clifford CK, Lanza E. NCI dietary guidelines: rationale. Am J Clin Nutr 1988;48:888-95 (supplement).

32a. US Department of Agriculture. Agriculture handbook number 8-9: composition of foods: fruits and fruit juices - raw, processed, prepared. Washington, DC: US Government Printing Office, 1982.

32b. US Department of Agriculture. Agriculture handbook number 8-11: composition of foods: vegetables and vegetable products - raw, processed, prepared. Washington, DC: US Government Printing Office, 1984.

32c. US Department of Agriculture. Agriculture handbook number 8-15: composition of foods: finfish and shellfish products - raw, processed, prepared. Washington, DC: US Government Printing Office, 1987.

32d. US Department of Agriculture. Agriculture handbook number 8-13: composition of foods: beef products - raw, processed, prepared. Washington, DC: US Government Printing Office, 1986.

32e. US Department of Agriculture. Agriculture handbook number 8-10: composition of foods: pork products - raw, processed, prepared. Washington, DC: US Government Printing Office, 1983.

32f. US Department of Agriculture. Agriculture handbook number 8-5: composition of foods: poultry products - raw, processed, prepared. Washington, DC: US Government Printing Office, 1979.

32g. US Department of Agriculture. Agriculture handbook number 8-17: composition of foods: lamb, veal, and game products - raw, processed, prepared. Washington, DC: US Government Printing Office, 1989.

32h. US Department of Agriculture. Agriculture handbook number 8-7: composition of foods: sausages and luncheon meats - raw, processed, prepared. Washington, DC: US Government Printing Office, 1980.

32i. US Department of Agriculture. Agriculture handbook number 8-1: composition of foods: dairy products - raw, processed, prepared. Washington, DC: US Government Printing Office, 1980.

32j. US Department of Agriculture. Agriculture handbook number 8-4: composition of foods: fats and oils - raw, processed, prepared. Washington, DC: US Government Printing Office, 1979.

33. Anderson JW. Plant fiber in foods. Lexington, KY: HCF Nutrition Research Foundation, Inc., 1990.

34. Pennington JAT (ed). Bowes and Church's food values of portions commonly used. 16th ed. Philadelphia, PA: J.B. Lippincott Company, 1994.

35. National Institutes of Health, National Cholesterol Education Program. Second report of the expert panel on detection, evaluation, and treatment of high blood cholesterol in adults. Washington DC, 1993. [NIH publication 93 3095.]

36. American Heart Association in Cooperation with National Heart, Lung, and Blood Institute. Dietary treatment of hypercholesterolemia: a manual for patients. Dallas: American Heart Association National Center printing office, 1988. [64 9545 (SA).]

37. Kannel W. Cholesterol in the prediction of atherosclerotic disease. Ann Int Med 1979;90:85-91.

38. Halgrer, Levin, Rossner, Vessby, Ledo. Diet and prevention of coronary heart disease and cancer: 4th international Bergelius symposium. New York, NY: Raven Press, 1986.

39. Grundy SM, Denke MA. Dietary influences on serum lipids and lipoproteins. J Lipid Res 1990;31:1149-72.

40. Pooling Project Research Group. Relationship of blood pressure, serum cholesterol, smoking habits, relative weight, and ECG abnormalities to incidence of major coronary events: final report of the pooling project. J Chron Dis 1978;31:201-12.

41. Johnson CL, Rifkind BM, Sempos CT, et al. Declining serum total cholesterol levels among US adults. JAMA 1993;269:3002-08.

42. Lipid Research Clinics Program. The lipid research clinics coronary primary prevention trial results: II, the relationship of reduction in incidence of coronary heart disease to cholesterol lowering. JAMA 1984;251:365-74.

43. Castelli WP, Garrison RJ, Wilson PW, et. al. Incidence of coronary heart disease and lipoprotein cholesterol levels: the Framingham study. JAMA 1986;256:2835-38.

44. Gordon DJ, Probstfield JL, Garrison RJ, et al. High-density lipoprotein cholesterol and cardiovascular disease: four prospective American studies. Circulation 1989;79:8-15.

45. Freeman, DJ, Griffin BA, Murray E, Lindsay GM, Gaffney D. Packard CJ, et al. Smoking and plasma lipoproteins in man: effects on low density lipoprotein cholesterol levels and high density lipoprotein subfraction distribution. Eur J Clin Inv 1993;23:630-40.

46. Brischetto CD, Connor WE, Conner SL, Matarazzo JD. Plasma lipid and lipoprotein profiles of cigarette smokers from randomly selected families: enhancement of hyperlipidemia and depression of high-density lipoproteins. Am J Cardiol 1983:52:675-680.

47. NIH Consensus Conference. Triglyceride, high-density lipoprotein, and coronary heart disease. JAMA 1993;269:505-10.

48. Cooper GR, Myers GL, Smith SJ, Schlant RC. Blood lipid measurements: variations and practical utility. JAMA 1992;267:1652-60.

49. Franz MJ, Horton ES, Bantle JP, Beebe CA, Brunzell JD, Coulston AM, et al. Nutrition principles for the management of diabetes and related complications. Diabetes Care 1994;17:490-518.

50. Keys A, Anderson JT, Grande F. Prediction of serum cholesterol responses of man to changes in fats in the diet. Lancet 1957;2:959-66.

51. Hestead DM, McGandy RB, Myers ML, Stare FJ. Quantitative effects of dietary fat on serum cholesterol in man. Am J Clin Nutr 1965;17:281-295.

52. Keys A. Coronary heart disease in seven countries. Circulation 1970;41(4 Suppl):I1-161.

53. Keys A, Menotti A, Karvonen MJ, Aravanis C, Blackburn H, Buzina R, et al. The diet and 15-year death rate in the seven countries study. Am J Epid 1986;124:903-15.

54. Grundy SM. Comparison of monounsaturated fatty acids and carbohydrates for lowering plasma cholesterol. N Eng J Med 1986;314:745-48.

55. Grundy SM, Florentin L, Nix D, et al. Comparison of monounsaturated fatty acids and carbohydrates for reducing raised levels of plasma cholesterol in man. Am J Clin Nutr 1988;47:965-69.

56. Grundy SM. Monounsaturated fatty acids, plasma cholesterol and coronary heart disease. Am J Clin Nutr 1987;45:1168-75.

57. Mattson FH, Grundy SM. Comparison of effects of dietary saturated, monounsaturated, and polyunsaturated fatty acids on plasma lipids and lipoproteins. J Lipid Res 1985;26:194-202.

58. Vega GL, Groszek E, Wolf R, Grundy SM. Influence of polyunsaturated fats on plasma lipoprotein composition and apolipoprotein. J Lipid Res 1982;23:811-22.

59. Shepherd J, Packard CJ, Grundy SM, et al. Effects of saturated and polyunsaturated fat diets on the chemical composition and metabolism of low-density lipoproteins in man. J Lipid Res 1980;2:91-99.

60. Nydahl M, Gustafsson IB, Vessby B. Lipid-lowering diets enriched with monounsaturated and polyunsaturated fatty acids but low in saturated fatty acids have similar effects on serum lipid concentrations in hyperlipidemic patients. Am J Clin Nutr 1994;59:115-22.

61. Parthasarathy S, Khoo JC, Miller E. et al. Low density lipoprotein rich in oleic acid is protected against oxidative modification: implications for dietary prevention of atherosclerosis. Proc Nat Acad Sci 1990;87:3894-98.

62. National Research Council. Diet, nutrition and cancer. Washington, DC: National Academy Press, 1982.

63. Denke MA, Grundy SM. Effects of fats high in stearic acid on lipid and lipoprotein concentrations in men. Am J Clin Nutr 1991;54:1036-40.

64. Derr J, Kris-Etherton PM, Pearson TA, Seligson FH. The role of fatty acid saturation on plasma lipids, lipoproteins, and apolipoproteins II: the plasma total and low-density lipoprotein cholesterol response of individual fatty acids. Metabolism 1993;42:130-34.

65. Mensink RP, Katan MB. Effect of dietary trans-fatty acids on high-density and low-density lipoprotein cholesterol levels in healthy subjects. N Eng J Med 1990;323:439-45.

66. Fifth Report of the Joint National Committee on Detection, Evaluation, and Treatment of High Blood Pressure. Arch Int Med 1993;153:154-83.

67. Stamler J. Blood pressure and high blood pressure: aspects of risk. Hypertension 1991;18:95-107 (supplement).

68. VanBrummelen P, Koolen MI. Difference in sodium sensitivity in human hypertensives. Clin Inv Med 1987;10:581-85.

69. Weinberger MH, Cohen SJ, Miller JZ, Luft FC, Grim CE, Finegerg NS. Dietary sodium restriction as adjunctive treatment of hypertension. JAMA 1988;259:2561-65.

70. Working Group Report on Primary Prevention of Hypertension. Archives of Internal Medicine 1993;153:186-208.

71. Opinion Research Corporation. Trends in the United States—consumer attitudes and the supermarket. Washington, DC: Food Marketing Institute; 1995.

72. Revicki DA, and Israel RG. Relationship between body mass indices and measure of body adiposity. Am J Pub Health 1986;76:992-94.

73. Najjar MF, Rowland M. Anthropometric reference data and prevalence of overweight, United States: 1976-80. Vit Health Stat 1987;238:1-73.

74. Block G, Dresser CM, Hartman AM, Carrol MD. Nutrient sources in the American diet: quantitative data from the NHANES II survey. Am J Epid 1985;122:13-26.

75. Exchange Lists for Meal Planning. American Diabetes Association, Inc. and The American Dietetic Association; Chicago, IL, 1995.

76. National Live Stock and Meat Board, Nutri-Facts. 444 North Michigan Ave., Chicago, IL 60611.

77. Kromhout D, Bosschieter EB, Coulander C. The relationship between fish consumption and 20-year mortality from coronary heart disease. N Eng J Med;1985;1205-09.

INDEX

3 DIAMONDS
Canned Fruit ... 182

7-UP
Soft Drinks ... 337

A TASTE OF THAI
Soft Jasmine Rice ... 151

A WHALE OF A SNACK
Fat Free Bars ... 123

A&W
Soft Drinks ... 337

ACT II
Microwave French Fries ... 170
Microwave Popcorn ... 105

AFTER THE FALL
Fruit Juices ... 340

AK-MAK
100% Stone Ground
Crackers ... 141

AL DENTE
Pasta ... 155
Pasta & Sauce ... 155

ALBA
Drink Mixes ... 348

ALDONS
Original Recipe
English Muffins ... 85

ALESSI
Olive Oil ... 307

ALL SPORT
Sport Drink ... 351

ALL STAR FOODS
Cookies ... 123

ALOUETTE
Cheese ... 189

ALPEN
Swiss Style Cereal ... 95

ALPINE LACE
Cheese ... 189

ALTA-DENA
Yogurt ... 205
Yogurt Beverage ... 200

AMAZAKE
Milk Alternative ... 200

AMERICAN BEAUTY
Pasta ... 155

AMERICAN GRAINS
Popsters ... 105

AMERICAN MEAL
Premium ... 73

AMERICAN PRAIRIE
Beans ... 247
Hot Creal ... 95

AMY'S
Burritos ... 262
California Veggie Burger ... 252

Cheese Ravioli ... 262
Desserts ... 321
Enchiladas ... 262
Macaroni & Cheese ... 262
Macaroni & Soy Cheeze ... 262
Mexican Tamale Pie ... 262
Pizza Pocket ... 262
Pot Pies ... 262
Shepherd's Pie ... 262
Vegetable Lasagne ... 262

ANCIENT HARVEST
Quinoa Pasta ... 155

ANDERSON
Pretzels ... 105

ANNIE'S
Cheddar Shells ... 155
Salad Dressings ... 313

ANTOINE'S
Pasta ... 155, 156

APPIAN WAY
Pizza ... 61

AQUA STAR
Cod Fillets ... 224

AQUA VIE
Spring Water Beverages ... 346

ARCHWAY
Cookies ... 123

ARIZONA
Fruit Beverages ... 340
Iced Teas ... 346

ARMOUR
Canadian Style Bacon ... 229
Chili ... 257
Homestyle Meatballs ... 209
Lard ... 309
Premium Pepperoni ... 229
Sliced Dried Beef ... 229
Treet Luncheon Loaf ... 229
Vienna Sausage ... 229

ARNIE'S
Salad Dressings ... 313

ARNOLD
Bran'Nola Muffins ... 85
Bread ... 73
Bread Crumbs ... 162
Croutons ... 162, 163
Rolls ... 73
Muffins ... 85
Pita ... 73
Stuffing Mixes ... 162, 163

ARROWHEAD MILLS
Biscuit Mix ... 61
Bread Mix ... 61
Cereal ... 95
Cornbread Mix ... 61
Dried Legumes ... 251
Flax Seed Oil ... 307
Griddle Lite Pancake Mix ... 61

Muffin Mixes ... 61
Pancake and Waffle Mix ... 61
Peanut Butters ... 291

ASPIRE
Iced Cafe ... 346, 347

ATHENS FOODS
Fillo Dough ... 85

AUBURN FARMS
98% Fat Free Spud Bakes ... 105
Fat Free 7-Grainers ... 141
Fat Free Brownies ... 123
Fat Free
Butterscotch Corn ... 105
Fat Free Caramel Corn ... 105
Fat Free Jammers ... 123
Fat Free Toast 'N Jammers ... 85
Fat Free Only Chips ... 105

AUNT FANNY'S
Fried Pies ... 123

AUNT GINNIE'S
Hot Bread ... 73

AUNT JEMIMA
Corn Meal Mix ... 61
French Toast ... 85
Original Pancake Batter ... 61
Pancake & Waffle Mix ... 61
Pancake Mix ... 61
Pancakes ... 85
Waffles ... 85

AUNT MILLIE'S
Bread ... 73, 74
Buns ... 73, 74
Donut Shoppe ... 85
Fat Free English Muffins ... 85
Peanutty Dunking Stix ... 85

AUNT NELLIE'S
Beans ... 247
Canned Vegetables ... 173

AUSTIN
Crackers ... 141

AUTUMN GRAIN
Bread ... 74

AVO-KING
Guacamole ... 355

AWAKE
Frozen Orange Beverage ... 340

AWREY'S BEST
Assorted Donuts ... 85
Desserts ... 321
Muffins ... 85
Pastry ... 123

AXELROD
Cheese ... 189
Rice Pudding ... 331
Yogurt ... 205

AZTECA
Salad Shells ... 85
Tortillas ... 85
AZUMAYA
Tofu ... 252
B & M
Baked Beans ... 247
Brown Bread ... 85
KC Masterpiece Beans ... 247
BAGEL BITES ... 262
BAGELS
All Brands ... 85
BAHLSEN
Cookies ... 123
BAKE EEZ
Cooking Spray ... 309
BAKER'S CHOICE
Breadsticks ... 74
BAKER'S JOY
Baking Spray ... 309
BAKERY WAGON
Cookies ... 124
BALSAMIC
Pasta Sauces ... 363
BANQUET
Desserts ... 321
Extra Helping Meals ... 262
Meals ... 262
BARBARA'S
Blue Corn Chips ... 105
Cereal ... 95
Cookies ... 124
Honeysweet Pretzels ... 124
Sweet Potato Chips ... 105
Wheatines ... 141
BARBER FOODS
Chicken Products ... 263
BARON
Peanut Butters ... 291
BARQ'S
Root Beer ... 337
BASCAM'S
Barley ... 151
Dried Legumes ... 251
BASIC COUNTRY GOODNESS
Shredded Hashbrowns ... 170
BAXTERS
Soups ... 279
BAYS
English Muffins ... 86
BEACH CLIFF
Kippered Snacks ... 237
BEAN CUISINE
Bean Mixes ... 257
Legumes ... 251
BEARITOS
Bean Dip ... 355
Beans ... 247
Crunchitos ... 105

Lite Cheddar Puffs ... 105
Microwave Popcorn ... 105
Popcorn ... 105, 106
Soups ... 279
Tortilla Chips ... 106
BEEF
All Cuts ... 209
BEEFALO
All Parts ... 209
BEEFSTEAK
Breads ... 74
BEL GIOIOSO
Cheese ... 190
BELLA
Olive Oil ... 307
BELLAVIE
Organic Pasta ... 156
BELLINO
Olive Oils ... 307
BEN & JERRY'S
Frozen Desserts ... 323
BERNE'A
Cheese ... 190
Sour Creams ... 301
BERNSTEIN'S
Salad Dressings ... 313
BERTOLLI
Olive Oils ... 307
BEST OF ALL
Soup Mixes ... 279
BEST'S KOSHER
Bagel Dog ... 229
Beef Frankfurters ... 229
Beef Knackwurst ... 229
Beef Polish Sausage ... 229
Cooked Corned Beef ... 229
Mini Bagel Dogs ... 229
BETTER MADE
Potato Chips ... 106
BETTER WAY
Bread ... 74
BETTY CROCKER
Angel Food Cake Mix ... 67
Bugles ... 106
Bugs Bunny Fruit Snacks ... 106
By Request
Microwave Popcorn ... 106
Coffee Cake & Muffin Mix ... 61
Creamy Chilled Desserts ... 67
Date Bar Mix ... 67
Dinner Sensations ... 151, 156
Dunkaroos ... 124
Easy Delicious Desserts ... 67
Fat Free Muffin Mix ... 67
Fruit By The Foot ... 106
Fruit Roll-Ups ... 106
Fruit Snacks ... 106
Fudge Brownie Mix ... 67
FundaMiddles ... 106
Gelooze ... 331

Gingerbread Cake
& Cookie Mix ... 67
Golden Pound Cake Mix ... 67
Gushers ... 106
Hamburger Helper ... 151, 156
Light Bugles ... 106
Muffin Mix ... 61, 67
Pineapple Upside
Down Cake ... 67
Pop Chips ... 106
Pop-Secret ... 106
Pop-Secret Popcorn Bars ... 124
Potatoes and
Potato Mixes ... 161
Squeezit 100 ... 341
Squeezit Fruit Drink ... 341
String Thing ... 106
Suddenly Salad ... 156
SuperMoist Cake Mix ... 67
Supreme Brownie Mix ... 67
Supreme Dessert Bar Mix ... 67
Swirl Angel Food Cake ... 67
Tuna Helper ... 156
BEXLEY'S
Ice Creams ... 323
BIG RED
Big Red Cola ... 337
BIG VALLEY
Frozen Fruits ... 182
BIRDSEYE
French Style Rice ... 151
Frozen Vegetables ... 170, 171
BISQUICK
All Purpose Baking Mix ... 61
Shake 'n Pour ... 61
BLACK DIAMOND
Cheese ... 190
BLACK JEWELL
Microwave Popcorn ... 106
Popcorn Kernels ... 106
BLANCHARD & BLANCHARD
Salad Dressings ... 313
BLUE BONNET
Margarine ... 295
BLUE BUNNY
Frozen Desserts ... 323, 324
BLUE DIAMOND
Nut-Crackers ... 141
BLUE RIBBON
Figs ... 186
BLUEBIRD
Juice ... 341
BOB EVANS
Burritos ... 261
Sausage ... 229
BOB'S RED MILL
Bread Mix ... 61
Brown Rice Farina ... 95
Cornbread Mix ... 61

Grande Whole Grains
  Cereal/Pilaf 95
Hot Cereal 95
Muffin Mix 61
Old Country Style Muesli 95
Wheat-Free Biscuit
  & Baking Mix 61

BOBOLI
  Pizza Crust 86
  Pizza Sauce 363

BOCA BURGER
  98% Fat Free Boca Burger 252
  Meatless Boca Burger 252

BOKU
  Fruit Juice Cooler 341
  Fruit Juice Cooler Boxes 341

BONAVITA
  Vegetarian Pâté 355

BORDEN
  Cheese 190
  Cottage Fries 171
  Cremora 303
  Eagle Brand
    Condensed Milk 200
  Egg Nog 199
  Frozen Desserts 324
  None Such Mincemeat 332
  Potato Chips 106
  ReaLemon 341
  ReaLime 341
  Red Cross Pasta 156
  Soup Starter 279

BOSCO
  Real Chocolate
    Flavored Syrup 348

BOX HILL
  Bread Mixes 61

BOZO
  Peanut Butters 291

BRAUN'S BAGELS
  Bagels 86

BREAD DU JOUR
  Bread Sticks 74
  French Loaves 74
  Rolls 74
  Soft Rye 74

BREADSHOP'S
  Cereal 95

BREAKSTONE'S
  Cheese 190
  Sour Cream Dips 355
  Sour Creams 301

BREAST O' CHICKEN
  Tuna 237

BREMNER
  Wafers 141

BREYERS
  Frozen Desserts 324
  Mix 'N Crunch Yogurt 205
  Yogurt 205

BROCCOLI TIME
  Pasta Mixes 257
  Soup 279

BROCK
  Fruit Snackers 106

BROOKS
  Beans 247
  Canned Tomatoes 174
  Chili Mix 247

BROUGHTON FOODS
  Real Cream 301

BROWN COW FARM
  Yogurt 205

BROWN RICE
  All Brands 151

BROWNBERRY
  Bran'nola 74
  Bread Cubes 163
  Breads 74, 75
  Hot Dog Rolls 75
  Sandwich Buns 75
  Stuffing Mixes 163

BRUMMEL & BROWN
  Yogurt Spread 295

BRUNO & LUIGI'S
  Fat Free Chip Dips 355
  Pasta Chips 106

BRUNSWICK
  Kippered Snacks 237

BUENA VITA
  Fat Free Flour Tortillas 86

BUFFALO
  All Cuts 215

BULLDOG
  Sardines 237

BUMBLE BEE
  Tuna 237
  Salmon 237

BURNS & RICKER
  Bagel Crips 107
  Pita Crisps 107

BURSTING WITH FRUIT
  Cookies 124

BUSH'S BEST
  Beans 247
  Canned Greens 174

BUTTER
  All Brands 296

BUTTER BUDS
  Butter Substitute 297
  Spread 295

BUTTER MOIST
  Turkey Roast 215

BUTTERBALL
  Fresh Turkey 230
  Lunchmeats 229, 230
  Turkey 215
  Turkey Bacon 230

BUTTERFIELD
  Shoestring Potato Sticks 107

BUTTERNUT
  Bread 75
  Old World Bagels 86

C.F. BURGER
  Egg Nog 199
  Half & Half 301
  Milk 199

CABANA
  Pork Rinds 107

CABANA
  Tostados 107

CAFFE FANTASTICO
  Iced Cappuccino
    Drink Box 347

CAIN'S
  Potato Chips 107

CALAVO
  Avocado Guacamole Lite 355
  Avocado Oil 307

CALHOUN BEND MILL
  Peach Cobbler Mix 68

CALIFORNIA NATURALS
  Oils 307

CAMACHO'S
  Nacho Corn Chips 107

CAMPBELL'S
  Beans 247
  Entrée Sauces 363
  Soup & Oyster Crackers 141
  Soups 279, 280, 281
  Tomato Juice 352

CANADA DRY
  Beverages 337

CANFIELD'S
  Beverages 337

CAP 10
  Natural Mineral Water 337

CAPE COD
  Popcorn 107
  Potato Chips 107

CAPRI SUN
  Fruit Drinks 341

CARDINI'S
  Salad Dressings 313

CARL BUDDIG
  Lunchmeats 230

CARLSON-ARBOGAST FARM
  Bean Appetit Beans 251

CARNATION
  Breakfast Bars 124
  Coffee Mate 301, 303
  Drink Mixes 348
  Evaporated Milk 200
  Instant Breakfast 347
  Nonfat Dry Milk Powder 199

CARR'S
Crackers 141
Home Wheat 124

CASA RICARDO
Tortilla Chips 107

CASBAH
Falafel Mix 252
Hummus Mix 355
Pilaf Mix 156
Soups 281

CASCADIA
Carbonated Beverage 337

CASCADIAN FARM
Frozen Desserts 324

CASTLEBERRY'S
Beef Stew 257

CAVENDISH
Hash Brown Patties 161

CEDAR LANE
Vegetable Stew 263

CELESTIAL SEASONINGS
Tea Drinks 347

CHADWICK FARMS
Vanilla Wafers 124

CHAMPION
Raisins 186

CHAOS
Beverage 337

CHATHAM VILLAGE
Croutons 163

CHEESE SHOPPE
Nacho Chips 107
Pretzels 107
Salsa 355
Tortilla Chips 107

CHEEZ WHIZ
Cheese Product 190

CHEF BOYARDEE
Italian Meals 258
Microwave Meals 258
Pasta and Sauce 257
Pizza Mix 258
Pizza Sauce 363

CHEZ DE PREZ
Cheesecakes 321

CHI CHI'S
Dips 355
Refried Beans 248
Shredded Cheese 190
Taco Shells 86
Tortilla Chips 107

CHICAGO HEARTH
Enriched Buns 75

CHICKEN
All Parts 215

CHICKEN OF THE SEA
Salmon 237
Tuna 237

CHICO SAN
Popcorn Cakes 107

CHIECKO
Tofu 252

CHIEF LAKE
Apple Juice 341

CHIFLES
Plantain Chips 107

CHILDERS
Fat Free Potato Chips 108

CHILLI MAN
Chili 258

CHIQUITA
100% Fruit Juice 341

CHRISTIE'S
Greek Dressing 313

CHRISTOPHER RANCH
Pesto Sauce 363

CHUNG'S
Beef & Broccoli 263
Chicken Fried Rice 263

CI'BELLA
Pasta Sauce 363

CITRUS VALLEY
Juice Concentrate 341
Mini Juice Boxes 341

CLASSICO
Pasta Sauce 363

CLASSIQUE FARE
Belgian Waffle Mix 62
Pancake Mix 62

CLEARLY CANADIAN
Clearly 2 337
Sparkling Waters 337

COCA-COLA
Beverages 337

COFFEE CAKES
All Brands 85

COLAVITA
Fats and Oils 307
Tomato Sauce 363

COLE'S
Breadsticks 75
Focaccia 86
Garlic Bread 75
Garlic Spread 295

COLEMAN NATURAL MEATS
Beef 209

COLLEGE INN
Soups 281

COLOMA
No Sugar Added
Frozen Fruit 182

COLONIAL
Cookies 124

COLUMBO
Frozen Desserts 324, 325
Light 100 205
Yogurt 205

COMBOS
Snacks 108

COMSTOCK
Pie Fillings 332

CONTADINA
Crushed Tomatoes 174
Entrée Sauces 363, 364

CONTESSA
Shrimp and Scallops 224

COOL CUPS
Yogurt 205

COOL WHIP
Whipped Toppings 303

CORNNUTS
Toasted Corn 108

CORTIELLA
Pasta 156

COUNTRY FRESH
Cottage Cheese 190
Frozen Desserts 325
Sour Creams 301

COUNTRY HEARTH
Bread 75, 76
English Muffins 86

COUNTRY SPRINGS
Sparkling Water Beverage 337

COUNTRY TIME
Drink Mixes 348

COUNTY FAIR
Enriched Buns 76

COUNTY LINE
Cheese 190

COUSIN WILLIE'S
Popcorn 108

CRACKER BARREL
Cheese 191

CRACKER JACK
Cracker Jack 108
Nutty Deluxe 108

CRACKLIN' GOOD
Toaster Pastries 86

CREAMETTE
Pasta 156

CREAMS
All Brands Fresh 301

CRISCO
Fats and Oils 307

CROISSANTS
All Brands 85

CROSSE & BLACKWELL
Pie Fillings 332

CROWLEY
Frozen Yogurt 325

CRUNCH 'N MUNCH
Popcorn 108

CRUSTACEANS
All Types 223

CRYSTAL BAY
Flavored Sparkling
Water 337, 338

CRYSTAL CLEAR
Beverage 338

CRYSTAL GEYSER
Juice Squeeze 341

CRYSTAL LIGHT
Drink Mixes 349

CULLIGAN
Sparkling Water 338

D'ITALIANO
Real Italian Bread 76

D-ZERTA
Pudding and Gelatin 332
Whipped Topping Mix 303

DA VINCI
Chick Peas 248

DAD'S
Red Creme Soda Rouge 338
Root Beer 338

DAILY BREAD COMPANY
Quick Loaf 62

DAILY'S
Harvest Best Fruit Drinks 341

DAIRY EASE
Lactose Reduced Milk 199

DAIRY FRESH
Cheese 191
French Onion Party Dip 355

DANNON
Yogurt 205

DARE
Harvest From the
Rainforest Cookies 124
Crackers 141

DAVINCI
Olive Oils 307
Pasta 157

DEAN FOODS
Buttermilk 199
Chocolate Drink 347
Cottage Cheese 191
Creams and
Cream Substitutes 301
Dairy Ease Lactose
Reduced Milk 199
Frozen Desserts 325, 326
Fruit Juices 341
Vitamite 347

DEBOLE'S
Pasta 157

DECECCO
Macaroni Products 157

DEI FRATELLI
Entrée Sauces 364

DEL MONTE
Canned Fruits 182, 183
Canned Vegetables 174, 175
Dessert Cups 332
Fruit Snacks 108
Spaghetti Sauces 364
Tomato Juice 352
Yogurt Raisins 108

DELALLO
Olive Oil 307

DELI
Cheese Sauce 191
Cheese Spread 191

DELICIOUS
Cookies 124, 125

DELL' ALPE
Artichoke Hearts 175
Fine Italian Foods 157
Olive Oils 307

DELTA-PRIDE
Catfish 224

DELVERDE
Pasta 157

DEMING'S
Salmon 237

DERBY
Beef Tamales 258

DEVONSHEER
Melba Round 142

DI GIORNO
Entrée Sauces 364
Parmesan Cheese 191
Romano Cheese 191

DIET RITE
Diet Rite Soda 338

DIMPFLMEIER
Bread 76

DINO & DAVID
Semolina Pasta 157

DINTY MOORE
American Classics 258
Beef Stew 259
Chicken & Dumplings 258
Chicken Stew 258
Corned Beef Hash 258
Hearty Burger Stew 258

DOLE
100% Juice 341
100% Juice Frozen
Concentrate 342
Canned Fruits 183
Dried Fruits 186
Fresh Salads 169
Frozen Desserts 326
Fruit Fiesta Juice Drink 341
Pacific Pink
Grapefruit Juice Drink 341
Pure and Light 342

Sun Ripe Grapefruit Juice 342
Tropical Fruit Juice 342
Unsweetened Juice 342

DOLLY MADISON BAKERY
Blueberry Muffins 86
Cinnamon Rolls 86
Cupcakes 125
Donut Gems 86

DON MARCOS
Tortillas 86

DORMAN'S
Light Cheda-Jack 191

DOUGHNUTS
All Brands 85

DOVE
Frozen Desserts 326

DOWNYFLAKE
Cinnamon Swirl
French Toast 86
Waffles 86

DOXSEE
Chopped Clams 238

DR. BROWN'S
Flavored Sodas 338

DR. COOL
Drink Mixes 349

DR. PEPPER
Soft Drinks 338

DREAM WHIP
Whipped Topping Mix 303

DROMEDARY BAKERY
Bread Machine Mix 62

DUCK
All Parts 215

DUNCAN HINES
Bar Mix 68
Brownie Mix 68
Cookie Mix 68
Moist Deluxe Cake Mix 68
Muffin Mix 62, 68

DUTCH TWINS
Assorted Creme Wafers 125
Fudge Sticks 125
Party Stix 125
Yes! Yes! 125

EAGLE
Bavarian Hard Pretzels 108

EAGLE
Dips and Salsas 355
El Grande Restaurant
Style Rounds 108
Nacho Thins 108
Potato Chips 108
Pretzel Sticks 108
Ranch Thins 108
Ripples 108
Snack Mix 109
Thins 109

EARTH BAR
Desert Delight Bar 125

EAGLE MILL'S
Best Loaf Bread
Machine Mix 62

EARTH BAR
Mountain Majesty Bar 125
Ocean Berry Bar 125
Rainforest Frost Bar 125
Tropical Splendor Bar 125

EARTHGRAINS
Garlic Rolls 76

ECKRICH
Franks 230
Lunchmeats 230, 231
Sausage 231
Smoky Links 230

EDEN
Beans 248

EDENSOY
Soy Beverage 200

EDENBLEND
Rice & Soy Beverage 200

EDENRICE
Rice Beverage 200

EDY'S
Frozen Desserts 326

EL MONTEREY
Burritos 263

EL RIO
Tortilla Chips 109

ELAM'S
Miller's Bran 95

ELI'S
Cheesecake 321

ELK
All Parts 215

EMPIRE
Chicken 215

EMPIRE KOSHER
Chicken Pie 263
Classics 263
Potato Onion Pierogies 263

EMPIRE
Lunchmeats 231

EMPRESS
Jack Mackerel 238

ENGLISH MUFFINS
All Brands 85

ENRICO'S
Dips and Salsas 356
Entrée Sauces 364

ENTENMANN'S
Coffee Cake 87
Cookies 125
Desserts 321, 322
Fat Free Products 86, 87
Muffins 87
Pastries 87

EQUATOR
Naturally Flavored Cocktail 338

EREWHON
Cereal 95, 96
Instant Oatmeal 95

ESKIMO PIE
Frozen Desserts 326

ESPIRIT
Frozen Yogurts 326

ESTEE
Caramel Popcorn 109
Cookies 125
Peanut Butter 291
Pretzels 109
Salad Dressings 313

EVERFRESH
Refreshers 342

FAMILIA
Cereal 96

FAMOUS AMOS
Cookies 125

FANTASTIC FOODS
Couscous 157
Falafel 252
Hummus 356
Instant Beans 252
Macaroni & Cheese 157
Nature's Burger 252
Soups 282
Tabouli Salad Mix 151
Tofu Classics 252

FARLEY'S
Fruit Snacks 109

FARM RICH
French Toast Sticks 87
Non-Dairy Creamers 301

FARMER PEET'S
Ham Steak 231

FARMLAND
Canned Ham 211
Salt Pork Belly 231

FAST SHAKE
Pancake Mix 62

FATHER SAM'S
Pocket Bread 76

FATS AND OILS
All Brands 307

FAYGO
Bottled Iced Tea 347
Bottled Lemonade 342
Sodas 338
Sparkling Water 338
Tonic Water 338

FEATHERWEIGHT
Tuna 238

FERRARA
Pasta 157
Olive Oil 307

FESTIDA
Salsa 356

FI-BAR
Bars 126

FIDDLE FADDLE
Caramel Corn 109

FIFTY 50
Cookies 126

FILIPPO BERIO
Olive Oils 307

FINFISH 223, 224

FINN CRISP
Dark w/Caraway 142

FIRESIDE
Fig Bars 126

FISHER BOY
Fish 224

FIVE ALIVE
Frozen Concentrate
Citrus Beverages 342

FLANNAGAN'S
Krrrrisp Kraut 175

FLAVOR TREE
Hot N' Spicy Mix 109
Party Mix 109
Sesame Chips 109
Sour Cream & Onion
Sesame Sticks 109

FLEISCHMANN'S
Canola Choice 295
Egg Beaters 243
Margarines 295
Move Over Butter 295

FLEUR-DE-LAIT
Cream Cheese 191

FLORIDA GOLD
Orange Juice 342

FOOD FOR LIFE
Low Fat Carrot Nut Muffins 87

FORMAGG
Mozzarella Cheese 191

FOUNTAIN SHAKE
Drink Mixes 349

FRANCO AMERICAN
Pasta and Sauces 259

FRANK'S
Kraut Juice 352
Stewed Tomatoes 175

**FRANKENMUTH POULTRY
COMPANY**
Chicken 215

FREEZER PLEEZER
Frozen Desserts 326

FREEZER QUEEN
Entrées 263

FRESCA
Soft Drinks 338

FRESHLIKE
Canned Vegetables 175, 176
Frozen Vegetables 171

FRIEDA'S
Tofu — 252

FRIENDSHIP
Cottage Cheese — 191

FRIGO
Cheese — 191

FRITO LAY
Baked Lays — 109
Baked Tostitos — 109
Chee-tos — 109
Chester's — 109
Dips and Salsas — 356
Doritos — 109, 110, 142
Fritos — 110
Funyons — 110
Lays Potato Chips — 110
Munchos — 110
Rold Gold Pretzels — 109, 110
Ruffles Potato Chips — 110
Santitas — 110
Sun Chips — 110
Taco Bell Tortilla Chips — 110
Taco Bell White Corn Chips — 110
Tortilla Thins — 110
Tostitos — 110, 111
Wavy Lays — 111

FROZEN DESSERTS
All Brands — 323

FROZEN FRUITSTICK
Frozen Desserts — 327

FRUIT DRINKS WITH ADDED SUGAR
All Brands — 340

FRUITS
Canned — 182
Dried — 185
Fresh — 181

FRUIT JUICE (no added sugars)
All Brands — 340

GARDEN OF EATIN
California Bakes — 111
Snack Chips — 111
Whole Wheat Naan — 76

GARDETTO'S
Pretzel Mix — 111
Snak-ens — 111

GATORADE
Iced Tea Cooler — 347
Sport Drink — 351

GEISHA
Canned Fruits — 183

GENERAL FOODS
Coffee Mixes — 349

GENERAL HENRY
Fruit Bars — 126

GENERAL MILLS
Cereal — 96
Cheerios Snack Mix — 111

GHIRARDELLI
Hot Chocolate — 349

GIRALDA
Olive Oil — 308

GIRARD'S
Salad Dressings — 313

GOGURT
Gogurt — 205

GOLD MEDAL
Cake Mix — 69
Cookie Mix — 69
Fudge Brownie Mix — 69
Muffin Mix — 62
Pizza Crust Mix — 62

GOLD MINE
Bullets — 327

GOLDEN GRAIN
Macaroni & Cheese — 157

GOLDEN TEMPLE
Cereal — 97

GOOD HEARTH
Bread — 76

GOOD HUMOR
Frozen Desserts — 327

GOOSE
All Parts — 215

GORTON'S
Fish — 224, 225

GOTEBORGS
Dinosaurs Chocolate
Cookies — 126

GOURMET JOSE
Salsa — 356

GRAINFIELDS
Cereal — 97

GRAINS
All Brands — 151

GRANDMA SHEARER'S
Potato Chips — 111
Tortilla Chips — 111

GREAT HARVEST BREAD CO.
Bread — 76

GREAT LAKES
Enriched White Bread — 76

GREAT PLAINS
American Meal — 76
Whole Grain Bread — 76

GRECIAN DELIGHT
Gyros — 263

GREEN GIANT
Baked Beans — 248
Canned Vegetables — 176
Create A Meal — 263
Frozen Vegetables — 171, 172
Pasta Accents — 263
Rice Originals — 151
Sliced Mushrooms — 176

GREENFIELD
Air Popped Popcorn — 111
Healthy Foods — 126

GROBBEL'S
Gourmet Corned
Beef Brisket — 209

GUILTLESS GOURMET
Dips and Salsas — 356
Baked Tortilla Chips — 111, 112

GUILTLESS LOW-FAT
Cookies — 126

GUINEA
All Parts — 215

HAAGEN DAZS
Frozen Desserts — 327

HABITANT
Soup — 282

HAIN
99% Fat Free Soups — 282
Black Turtle Beans — 248
Chick Peas — 248
Eggless Mayonnaise — 317
Fat Free Crackers — 142
Fat Free Mini Popcorn
Rice Cakes — 112
Fats and Oils — 308
Honey Grahams — 142
Margarine — 295
Rice Cakes — 112

HAMBEENS
Soups — 282

HANOVER
Baked Beans — 248
Chick Peas — 248
Kidney Beans — 248

HARRIS
Crab Meat — 238

HARRY'S
Sourdough Pretzels — 112
Whole Wheat Honeys — 112

HAWAIIAN PUNCH
Punch — 342
Typhoon Blasters — 342

HBO
Microwave Popcorn — 112

HEALTH VALLEY
100% Cereal — 97
100% Natural Bars — 126
Baked Beans — 248
Breakfast Bars — 126
Fast Menu Vegetarian
Cuisine — 259
Fat Free Bakes — 126
Fat Free Dessert Bars — 127
Fat Free Caramel Corn Puffs — 112
Fat Free Cheese Puffs — 112
Fat Free Chocolate — 127
Fat Free Corn Puffs — 112
Fat Free Crackers — 142
Fat Free Graham Crackers — 142
Fat Free Healthy Tarts — 127
Fat Free Soy Moo — 200
Fruit and Nut Bars — 127
Fruit Lites — 97

Healthy Chips	127	
Healthy Tarts	127	
Jumbo Fruit Cookies	127	
Oat Bran Jumbo fruit Bars	127	
Soups	283, 284	
Vegetarian Cuisine	248	

HEALTHY CHOICE
Cereals	97
Cheese	191
Egg Product	243
Entrée Sauces	364, 365
Franks	232
Frozen Desserts	327, 328
Lunchmeats	231, 232
Meals and Entrées	263, 264, 265
Sausage	232
Soups	284

HEARTLAND
Granola	97
Iron Kettle Baked Beans	248

HEBREW NATIONAL
Bologna	232
Franks	232

HEINZ
Fancy Tomato Juice	352
Homestyle Gravy	365
Vegetarian Beans	248

HENRI'S
Salad Dressings	313

HERB MAGIC
Fat Free Dressings	314

HERB'S
Pasta	157

HEREFORD
Corned Beef	232

HERSHEY
Chocolate Drinks	347
Free Pudding Packs	332
Lowfat Milk in Drink Boxes	199

HI-C
Fruit Drink	342

HICKORY FARMS
Nacho Cheese Sauce	356

HIDDEN VALLEY RANCH
Party Dips	356
Salad Dressings	314

HILLSHIRE FARM
Lunchmeats	232
Sausage	232

HIRES
Root Beer	338

HELLMAN'S
Sandwich Spreads	317

HODGSON MILL
Bread Mix	62
Cornbread and Muffin Mix	62
Cracked Wheat Cereal	98
Jalapeno Cornbread mix	62
Muffin Mix	62

Oat Bran	98
Pancake Mix	62
Veggie Bow	157
Wheat Bran	98
Wheat Germ	98
Whole Wheat Pasta	158

HOLLYWOOD
100% Natural Carrot Juice	352
Fats and Oils	308

HOLSUM
Bread	76
Sof-Buns	76

HOME PRIDE
Buttertop	77

HOMEMADE
Frozen Desserts	328

HORIZON
Yogurt	205

HORMEL
Chili	259
Kid's Kitchen	259
Lasagna & Beef	260
Light & Lean 97 Boneless Ham	211
Light & Lean 97 Turkey	215
Lunchmeats	232, 233
Noodles & Chicken	260
Pasta and Sauce	259
Pepperoni Slices	232
Sandwiches	265
Scalloped Potatoes	162
Scalloped Potatoes-Ham	260
Smoked Pork Chops	211
Soups	284
Spaghetti and Meatballs	260
SPAM	232
Vienna Sausage	233

HOSTESS
Assorted Donuts	87
Brownie Bites	127
Choco-licious	127
Cup Cakes	127
Frosted Donettes	87
Fruit Pies	127
Ho Hos	127
King Dons	127
Lights	127
Muffins	87
Powdered Donettes	88
Sno Balls	127
Suzy Q's	127
Twinkies	127

HOT POCKETS
Sandwiches	265

HOUSE OF FLAVORS
Ice Creams	328

HUNT'S
Big John's Beans n Fixins	248
Canned Tomatoes	176
Dips and Salsas	356, 357
Entrée Sauces	365
Snack Packs	332

Tomato Juice	352
Homestyle Chili Fixin's	248
Peaches in Heavy Syrup	184

HYGRADE'S
Bacon	233
Ball Park Franks	233
Grill Master Franks	233
Hot Dogs	233
Lunchmeats	233

I CAN'T BELIEVE IT'S NOT BUTTER
Spreads	295

IBC ROOT BEER CO.
Root Beer	338

ICE MOUNTAIN
Spring Water	347

ICELAND WATERS
Kippered Herring	238

IDAHO
Idaho Spuds Mashed Potatoes	162

IDAHOAN
Mashed Potatoes	162
Potato Mixes	162

IMPERIAL
Vegetable Oil Spreads	295

INDIAN SUMMER
100% Apple Juice	342
Cosmic Cooler Fruit Drink	342

INLAND VALLEY
Shimply Shreds Potatoes	172

INSTANT COFFEE
All Brands	348

INSTANT RICE
All Brands	151

INSTANT TEA
All Brands	348

INTERNATIONAL BAZAAR
Crab Meat	238
Hearts of Artichokes	176
Kipper Snacks	238
Olive Oil	308
Sliced Kiwi in Syrup	184

INTERNATIONAL DELIGHT
Creams	301

ITALICA
Olive Oil	308

J.R. SIMPLOT
Hashbrown Shreds	172

J.T.M.
Beef Patties	210

JACK RABBIT
Beans	249

JACOBSEN'S
Snack Toast	142

JAMAICAN
Flavored Soda	338

JARDINE'S
Crackers	142

JAYS
100% White Corn
  Crispy Rounds 112
100% White Corn
  Restaurant Style 112
Hot Stuff Potato Chips 112
O-Ke-Doke Popcorn 113
Potato Chips 113
Tortilla Chips 113

JEFFERSON
Lunchmeat 233

JELL-O
Gelatins and Puddings 332, 333
No Bake Cheesecake Mix 69
No Bake Dessert 69

JENNIE O
Lunchmeat 233

JENOS
Crisp 'n Tasty Pizza 265

JIF
Peanut Butters 291

JIFFY
Baking Mix 62
Brownie Mix 69
Buttermilk Biscuit Mix 62
Cake Mix 69
Muffin Mix 62
Pie Crust Mix 69
Pizza Crust Mix 62

JIFFY POP
Glazed Popcorn Clusters 113
Popcorn 113

JIMMY DEAN
Flapsticks 88
Sausage 233

JOAN OF ARC
Beans 249

JOGGING IN A JUG
Sport Drink 351

JOHNSONVILLE
Sausage 233, 234
Table for Two Meals 260

JONES DAIRY FARM
Canadian Style Bacon 234

JOSEPH'S
Middle East Style 77

JUICYFUL
100% Apple Juice 342
Drink Boxes 342

KA-ME
Rice Crunch Crackers 142

KABOODLES
Egg Noodles 158

KANE
Bean Threads 151

KANGAROO
No Pocket Pita 77
Pocket Bread 77

KASHI
Breakfast Pilaf 98
Medley 98
Puffed 7 Grains and Sesame 98

KAUKAUNA
Dips and Salsas 357
Lite 50 Port Wine Cheese 192

KAVLI
Whole Grain Crispbread 142

KEEBLER
Chacho's 113
Cookies 128
Crackers 143
Deluxe Grahams 128
E.L. Fudge 128
Graham Selects 143
O'Boisies 113
Pizzarias 113
Pretzels 113
Ripplin's 113
Salsa Verde 357
Tato Wilds Criss Cross 113
Tato Wilds Tato Skins 113

KELLOGG'S
Cereal 98
Croutettes Stuffing Mix 163
Eggo Minis 88
Eggo Waffles 88
Low Fat Pop-Tarts 88
NutriGrain Cereal Bars 128
Pop-Tarts 88
Pop-Tarts Minis 128
Rice Krispies 128

KEMPS
Frozen Desserts 328

KEN & ROBERT'S
Veggie Burger 252
Veggie Pockets 265, 266

KEN'S
Salad Dressings 314

KETTLE KRISP
Toffee Caramel Popcorn 113

KID CUISINE
Meals 266

KING'S
Hawaiian Bread 77
Hawaiian Rolls 77

KITCHEN CUPBOARD
Croutons 163

KLEEN-MAID
Enriched Bread 77

KLEEN-MAID
Soft Buns 77

KLONDIKE
Ice Cream Bars 328

KNORR
Dessert Mixes 69
Pilaf 151

KNOTT'S BERRY FARM
Salad Dressings 314

KNOX
Unflavored Gelatin 333

KNUDSEN
Cottage Cheese 192
Premium Real Sour
  Cream Dip 357
Sour Creams 302
Yogurt 205

KOALA
Flavored Fruit
  Juice Beverage 338

KOEGEL
Frankfurters 234
Lunchmeats 234
Viennas 234

KOEPPLINGER'S
Bread 77
Hamburger Buns 77
Hot Dog Buns 77
Stuffing Mixes 163

KOEZE'S
Peanut Butters 291

KÖLLN
Cereal 98
Crispy Oats 98

KOOL-ADE
Drink Mixes 349
Bursts 342
Koolers 342

KOWALSKI
Franks 234
Lunchmeat 234
Sausage 234

KOZY SHACK
Pudding and Flan 333

KRAFT
Cheese 192
Dips 357
Egg Noodle Dinner 158
Handi Snacks 143
Light Pasta Salad 158
Macaroni & Cheese 158
Macaroni & Cheese Dinner 158
Rotini & Cheese 158
Salad Dressings 314, 315
Sandwich Spreads 317
Shells & Cheese 158
Spaghetti Dinner 158
Touch of Butter 295
Velveeta Rotini & Cheese 158
Velveeta Shells & Cheese 158

KREMA
Peanut Butters 291

KRETSCHMER
Toasted Wheat Bran 98
Wheat Germ 98

KRINOS
Tahini 291

KRUNCHERS
Potato Chips 113

KRUSTEAZ
Belgian Waffle Mix	63
Biscuit Mix	63
Cinnamon Swirl	
French Toast	88
Honey Cornbread and	
Muffin Mix	63
Muffin Mix	63
Pancake & Waffle Mix	63
Pancake Mix	63
Pancakes	88

KUDOS
Bars	128

KUNER'S
Black Beans	249
Canned Vegetables	176

L.B. JAMISON'S
Flavored Soup Base	284

L'ESPRIT DE CHAMPAGNE
Dried Cherries	186

LA CHOY
Egg Rolls	266

LA CROIX
Sparkling Mineral Water	338

LA FAMOUS
Dips and Salsas	357

LA FRONTERIZA
Flour Tortillas	88

LA MARTINIQUE
Salad Dressings	315

LA PREFERIDA
Beans	249
Extra Long Grain	
Enriched Rice	152
Olive Oil	308

LA ROSA
Pasta	158

LA VICTORIA
Dips and Salsas	357

LA YOGURT
Sabor Latino Yogurt	206
Yogurt	206

LACTAID
Milk	199

LAMB
All Cuts	210

LANCE
Crackers	143
Van O Lunch	129

LAND O FROST
Lunchmeats	234

LAND O LAKES
Butter	297
Cheese	193
Cocoa Classics	349
Country Morning Blend	295
Margarine	296
Sour Creams	302
Vegetable Oil Spreads	296

LARD
All Brands	309

LAUGHING COW
Cheese	193

LAURA'S LEAN BEEF
All Cuts	210

LAWRY'S
Chicken 'n Rice	152
Nacho Rice	152
Salad Dressings	315
Santa Fe Rice	152

LE SUEUR
Small Young Peas	176

LEAN POCKETS
Sandwiches	266

LENDER'S
Bagels	88

LEON'S
Pita Bread	77

LESS
Breads	78
Hamburger Buns	78

LIBBY'S
Canned Fruits	184
Country Gravy	365
Fruit Nectar	342
Juicy Juice	342
Morning Classics	261
Pumpkin Pie Mix	69
Solid Pack Pumpkin	333

LIBERTY GOLD
Pineapple Juice	343

LIFE SAVERS
Flavor Pops	328

LIFESTREAM
Cereal	99
Crackers	143

LIGHT N' FLUFFY
Egg Noodles	158

LIGHT N' LIVELY
Cottage Cheese	194
Kidpack Lowfat Yogurt	206
Sour Creams	302
Yogurt	206

LIGHTLIFE
Meat Alternatives	252, 253
Savory Seitan	253
Tofu Pups	253
Wonderdogs	253

LIGUORI
Macaroni Products	158

LINDA McCARTNEY'S
Pasta Meals	266

LIPTON
Golden Saute	152, 158
Pasta & Sauce	158
Rice and Sauce	152
Soups	284
Tea Mixes	350
Teas	347

LITTLE CROW
Coco Wheats	99
Popcorn Oil	308

LITTLE DEBBIE
Cakes	129
Coffee Cake	89
Cookies	129
Crackers	144
Dessert Bars	129
Donut Sticks	89
Pies	129
Rolls	129

LLOYDS
Chicken Fillet	215

LONDON'S
100% Pure Orange Juice	343
Cottage Cheese	194
Frozen Desserts	328

LORIVA
Fats and Oils	308

LOTTE
Koala Yummies	129

LOUIS RICH
Franks	234
Lunchmeat	234, 235
Turkey	215

LOUISE'S
Low Fat Popcorn	114
Low Fat Potato Chips	114
Low Fat Tortilla Chips	114

LU
Cookies	129

LUIGI'S
Real Italian Ices	328

LUMBER JACK
Breads	78
Lumber Camp Style Buns	78

LUND'S
Swedish Pancake Mix	63

LUNDBERG
Elegant Rice Pudding	334
One Step Entrée	152

LUPITA
Tortillas	89

LUZIANNE
Etoufee Dinner	152
Gumbo Dinner	152
Jambalaya Dinner	152
Shrimp Creole Dinner	152

MACKINAW MILLING CO.
Bread	78

MAGGI
Spaetzle	159

MAHATMA
Extra Long Grain	
Enriched Rice	152
Red Beans w/Rice	152
Saffron Yellow Rice	152
Wild Rice w/Seasonings	152

MALT-O-MEAL
Cereal 99

MAMA MARY'S
Pizza Crust 89

MAMA TISH'S
Original Italian Ices 328

MAMA'S
Cookies 129, 130
Oyster Crackers 144

MAMMA BELLA
Garlic Bread 78

MAMMA RIZZO'S
Marinara Italian Sauce 365

MANISCHEWITZ
Angel Food Cake Mix 69
Bagel Chips 114
Bagel Shaped Pretzels 114
Cereal 99
Chocolate Chocolate
  Cake Mix 69
Chocolate Chunk
  Macaroons w/Cherry Bits 130
Matzo 144
Mom's Helper Cupcake Mix 69
Mom's Helper Fudgey
  Gooey Brownie Mix 69
Muffin Mix 63
Passover Gold Matzo
  Crackers 114
Passover Gold Pasta 159
Passover Gold Pizza Mix 63
Passover Gold
  Salad Dressing 315
Potato Pancake Mix 63
Premium Gold Matzo 144
Rocky Road Macaroons 130
Soups 284, 285
Sponge Cake Mix 69
Tam Tam Crackers 144

MANN'S
Broccoli Cole Slaw 170
Sunny Shores
  Vegetable Medely 170

MAPLE GROVE FARMS
Pancake Mix 63
Salad Dressings 315

MARANTHA
Nut Butters 291

MARGARET HOLMES
Beans 249

MARIE CALLENDER'S
Croutons 163
Meals 266, 267
Peach Cobbler 328

MARIE'S
Dips 357
Salad Dressings 315

MARQUÉE
Diet Cola 338
Soda 338
Sparkling Water Beverage 338

MARRAKESH EXPRESS
Cous Cous 153

MARS
Frozen Desserts 328

MARTHA WHITE
Bix Mix 63
Brownie Mix Chewy Fudge 69
Buttermilk Corn Bread Mix 63
Deep Pan Pizza Crust Mix 63
Flapstax 63
Grits 99
Legumes 252
Muffin Mix 63
Pizza Crust Mix 63
Spud Flakes 162

MARTINELLI'S
100% Apple Cider 343
100% Apple Juice 343

MARY KITCHEN
Corned Beef Hash 260
Roast Beef Hash 260

MARZETTI
French Onion Dip 357
Salad Dressings 315

MASTER OLD COUNTRY
Crackers 144

MAVERICK RANCH
Beef 210

MAXWELL HOUSE
Cappio 347
Cappuccino Mixes 350
Iced Cappuccino 347

MAYACAMAS
Just Enough Soups 285

MAYPO
Instant Oatmeal 99

MAZOLA
Cooking Spray 309
Corn Oil 308
Right Blend 308

MCARTHUR
Frozen Desserts 329

MCCAIN
Junior Juice 343

MCCLEARY'S
Elite Quality Caramel Corn 114
Elite Quality Tortilla Chips 114

MCCORMICK
Best O Butter 297

MCKENZIE'S
Garden Fresh Mixtures 172

MEADOW GOLD
Sweetened Condensed
  Milk 200

MELODY FARMS
100% Pure Orange Juice 343
Buttermilk 199
Chocolate Milk 199
Cottage Cheese 194
Creams 302

Frozen Desserts 329
Fruit Drinks 343

MENDOCINO PASTA CO.
Pasta 159

MERKT'S
Cheese Spread 194

MERRITT FOODS COMPANY
Bomb Pop Jr. 329

MEXICAN
Salsa Chunky Style 357

MEYENBERG
Evaporated Goat Milk 200

MI-DEL
100% Whole Wheat
  Honey Grahams 144

MICELI'S
Ricotta Cheese 194

MICHAEL SEASON'S
40% Less Fat Potato Chips 114
Corn Tostados 114
Party Mix 114
Potato Bakes 114
Pretzels 114
Shape Ups 114
White Corn Tortilla Chips 114

MICHAELENE'S
Gourmet Granola 99

MICHELINA'S
International Recipes 267
Meals 267

MICHIGAN
Cottage Cheese 194

MICRO MAGIC
Microwave French Fries 172

MICRO SHAKE
Frozen Desserts 329

MIKE'S ORIGINAL
Frozen Desserts 329

MILKHOUSE CHEESE
American Singles 194

MILLSPRING
Bagels 89

MINUTE MAID
All Natural Drink Boxes 343
Frozen Concentrate 343
Fruit Juices 343
Fruit Punch 343
Lemonade 343
Orange Soda 339

MINUTE
Rice 153
Tapioca 334

MISSION
Tortillas 89

MISTIC
Sparkling Water Beverage 339
Spring Water Iced Tea 347

MOCHA MIX
Frozen Desserts 329

MOHAWK VALLEY
Limburger Cheese 194
MOLLUSKS
All Types 224
MOLLY MCBUTTER
Butter Substitutes 297
MOM'S CHOICE
Cheeseburger
Macaroni Dinner 159
Lasagna Dinner 159
Stroganoff Dinner 159
MONDO
Fruit Squeezers 343
MORI-NU
Tofu 253
MORNINGSTAR FARMS
Egg Product 243
Meat Alternatives 253
MOTHER'S
Cereal 99
Popped Corn Cakes 115
Rice Cakes 115
Whole Wheat Fig Bars 130
MOTT'S
100% Juice Boxes 343
100% Pure Apple Juice 343
Applesauce 184
Clamato 352
Prune Juice 343
MOUNTAIN DEW
Soft Drinks 339
MOUNTAIN HIGH
Honey Light 206
Yogurt 206
MOUNTAIN TOP
Apple Pie 322
MOVE OVER BUTTER
Vegetable Oil Spreads 296
MOXIE
Sodas 339
MR. PHIPPS
Pretzel Chips 115
Tater Crisps 115
Tortilla Crisps 115
MR. TURKEY
Franks 235
Lunchmeat 235
Sausage 235
Turkey 215
MRS. ALISONS
Cookies 130
MRS. BUTTERWORTH'S
Cinnamon Sweet Rolls 89
Dinner Rolls 78
Enriched White
Frozen Bread Dough 78
Pancake Mix 63
MRS. GRASS
Soup Mix 285

MRS. PAUL'S
Fish 225
MRS. SMITH'S
Desserts 322
MRS. T'S
Pierogies 267
MRS. WEISS
Kluski 159
MUDPIE
Veggie Burger 253
MUELLER'S
Pasta 159
MUIR GLEN
Entrée Sauces 365, 366
Ground Peeled Tomatoes 176
MURRAY
Graham Crackers 144
Low Fat Cookies 130
MUSSELMAN'S
Apple Juice 343
Apple Juice Box 343
Applesauce 184
MW POLAR
Shrimp, Oysters,
Clams, Crab Meat 238
NABISCO
Cereal 99, 100
Cookies 130, 131
Crackers 144, 145
Easy Cheese 194
Honey Maid Graham
Cracker Crumbs 69
Mister Salty Pretzels 115
Mr. Salty Fat Pretzel Chips 115
Ritz Snack Mix 115
ROYAL Cheesecake 69
ROYAL Gelatins
and Puddings 334
ROYAL No Bake Pie Mix 69
Snackwell's Pies 322
Toastettes 89
NANCY'S
French Baked Quiche 267
NAPA VALLEY
Gourmet Salsa 357
NATURAL GRAINS
Bread 78
NATURAL OVENS
Bagels 89
Bread 78
Muffins 89
NATURALE 90
Natural Soda 339
NATURALLY LIGHT
Cooking Sprays 309
NATURALLY YOURS
No Fat Sour Cream 302
NATURE VALLEY
Granola Bars 131

NATURE'S CHOICE
Granola Bars 131
Real Fruit Bars 131
NATURE'S FAVORITE
Apple Chips 115
NATURE'S HARVEST
Stuffing Croutons 163
NATURE'S PATH
Cereal 100
NAUTILUS
Lite 'n Luscious Lunch 260
NAYONAISE
Salad Dressing 315
NEAR EAST
Couscous Moroccan Pasta 159
Curry Rice Mix 153
Falafel Mix 253
Long Grain and Wild Rice 153
Pilaf Mix 153
Spanish Rice Mix 153
Taboule Wheat Salad Mix 153
NESCAFE
Drink Mixes 350
NESTEA
Drink Mixes 350
Teas 348
NESTLE
Cookie Dough 137
Drink Mixes 350
Frozen Desserts 329
Quik 199
Sweet Success Snack Bars 131
NEW MILL
Kluski 159
NEW MORNING
Fruit-E-O's 100
NEW YORK
Bagel Chips 115
Garlic Bread 79
NEW YORK FLATBREADS
Low Fat Flatbreads 89
NEWLYWEDS
English Muffins 89
NEWMAN'S OWN
Entrée Sauces 366
Popcorn 115
Pretzels 116
Salad Dressings 316
Salsa 358
NILE SPICE
Soups 285
NISHIKI
Sushi Rice 153
NO YOLKS
Cholesterol Free
Egg Noodle Substitute 159
NORTH CASTLE
Jarlsberg Cheese Chips 116

NORTHERN KING	
Cooked Shrimp	225
NORWEIGAN	
Jarlsberg	194
NUTELLA	
Creamy Hazelnut Spread	291
NUTRA-FIG	
Figs	186
NUTTY BUDDY	
Chocolate Nut	
Sundae Cones	329
O.T.C.	
Crackers	145
OBIE'S COOKIE JAR	
Cookie Mixes	69
OCEAN SPRAY	
100% Grapefruit Juice	343
Cran-Raspberry	343
Cranapple	344
Cranberry Juice Cocktail	344
Cranberry Sauces	184
Drink Boxes	344
Juice Drinks	344
Lemonade	344
Mauna Lai Fruit Drink	344
Pink Grapefruit	
Juice Cocktail	344
Reduced Calorie Drinks	344
Refreshers	344
Ruby Red	344
Ruby Red and Tangerine	344
Ruby Red Grapefruit Juice	344
OLD DUTCH	
Sweet & Sour Dressing	316
OLD EL PASO	
Dips and Salsas	358
Refried Beans	249
OLD EUROPEAN STYLE	
Farmers Cheese	194
OLD FAMILY RECIPE	
Salad Dressings	316
OLD FASHIONED	
Instant Egg Nog Mix	350
OLD LONDON	
Melba Snacks	145
Melba Toast	145
Restaurant Style Croutons	163
OLD MONK	
Olive Oil	308
OLD ORCHARD	
Four Seasons	
from Concentrate	34
Frozen Concentrate	344
OLD TYME	
Cola Champagne	339
Jamaican Style	
Ginger Brew	339
Park Avenue Punch	339
OLD FASHIONED FOODS	
Cheese	194

OLIO SASSO	
Olive Oil	308
OLIVIERI	
Italian Pizza Shell	89
ORE IDA	
Frozen Chopped Onions	172
Frozen Potatoes	172
Onion Rings and Ringers	173
OREGON	
Canned Fruits	184
OREGON FARMS	
Carrot Cake	322
ORGANIC VALLEY	
Cheese	194
ORIGINAL LADY COOKIES	
100% Natural	131
ORLEANS	
Shrimp	238
Oysters	238
Clams	238
Kipper Snacks	238
ORTEGA	
Dips and Salsas	358
Refried Beans	249
ORVILLE KENT	
Chilled Selections	
Fruit Salad	182
ORVILLE REDENBACHER	
Gourmet Popcorn	116
Redden Budders	116
Smart-Pop	116
Popcorn Oil	308
OSCAR MAYER	
Bacon	235
Franks, Hot Dogs, Weiners	235
Healthy Favorites	236
Lard	310
Lunchmeat	235, 236
OSTRICH	
All Parts	216
OSTRICH	
Salami	236
OVALTINE	
Drink Mixes	350
OVEN FRESH	
Bread	79
Bread Crumbs	164
Buns	79
PABLO'S	
Dips and Salsas	358
PACE	
Dips and Salsas	358
PACIFIC GRAIN	
No Fries	116
Nuttry Rice Cereal	100
Nutty Rice	100
PACIFIC SNAX	
Popcorn Shaped Rice	116

PACKERS PRIDE	
Canned Cherries	184
PAM	
Cooking Sprays	309
PANNI	
Potato Dumpling Mix	162
PAPETTI'S	
Egg Product	243
Healthy Morn	
Egg Substitute	243
Pizza	268
PARAMOUNT	
Non Fat Lavash Bread	79
Pita Bread	79
PARISIAN	
Sourdough Sandwich Rolls	79
PARKAY	
Margarine	296
Vegetable Oil Spreads	296
PARMALAT	
Long Life Half & Half	302
Milk	199
PASTA	
All Brands	155
PASTA DEFINO	
No Boil Lasagna	159
PASTA LABELLA	
Pasta	159
PASTORELLI	
Pizza Sauce	366
PASTRIES	
All Brands	85
PATIO	
Burritos	268
PATRICK CUDAHY	
Realean Ham	211
PAVITCH	
Raisins	186
PAVONE	
Pepperoni	236
PEARSON	
Cole Slaw Salad Mix	170
PEEK FREANS	
Assorted Creme	131
Biscuits	131, 132
Coffee Creme	131
PENNSYLVANIA DUTCHMAN	
Mushrooms	176
PEPPERIDGE FARM	
Gravy	366
Bread	79, 80
Buns	79, 80
Butter Crescents	89
Butter Thins	145
Cookies	132, 133
Croissant Crust Pizza	268
Desserts	322
English Muffins	89
Goldfish	116, 146

Goldfish Party Mix	116
Hearty Wheat Crackers	145
Nutty Deluxe	146
Rolls	79
Snack Sticks	116
Soups	285
Stuffing Mixes	164

PEPSI
Soft Drinks	339

PERFECTION DELI
Old World Rye Bread	80
Rolls	80
Super Sub Buns	80

PERRIER
Mineral Water	339

PET INC.
Evaporated Milk	200

PET-RITZ
Cream Pies	322

PETER PAN
Peanut Butters	291

PHEASANT
All Parts	216

PHILADELPHIA
Cream Cheese	195

PICTSWEET
Frozen Vegetables	173
Stir-Fry Mixes	173

PILLAR ROCK
Red Salmon	238

PILLSBURY
All Ready Pizza Crust	89
Biscuits	89
Bread Machine Mix	63
Brownie Mix	70
Bundt Cake Mix	70
Cake Mix	70
Cookie Dough	137
Cornbread Twists	89
Crusty French Loaf	80
Deluxe Bar Mix	70
Deluxe Brownie Mix	70
Farina	100
Fudge Brownie Dough	137
Hot Roll Mix	63
Hungry Jack Biscuits	90
Hungry Jack Mixes	63
Hungry Jack Potato Mixes	162
Lovin' Lites	70
Pillsbury Plus Cake Mix	70
Pipin' Hot Loaf	80
Quick Bread Mix	63
Reduced Fat Chocolate	
Chip Cookie Dough	137
Rolls	89
Soft Breadsticks	89
Streusel Swirl	70
Teddy Bears	137
Toaster Strudel	90

PINE CONE
Canned Tomatoes	176

PIONEER
Biscuit & Baking Mix	64

PLANTERS
Cheez Snacks	116
Peanut Oil	308

PLEVALEAN
Burger Patty	210

PLUM ROSE
Bacon	236

POLAND SPRING
Sparkling Spring Water	339

POLLY-O
Nonfat Ricotta Cheese	195

POMPEIAN
Olive Oil	308

POPCORN KERNELS
All Brands	105

PORK
All Cuts	211

POST
Cereal	100

POSTUM
Hot Beverage Mixes	350

POW-WOW
Puffs	116

POWER BAR
Power Bar	133

POWERADE
Sport Drink	351

PREGO
Entrée Sauces	366

PRIME TIME
Microwave Popcorn	117

PRINCE
Pasta	159

PRINGLES
Potato Crisps	117
Ridges	117
Right Crisps	117

PRITIKIN
Entrée Sauces	366
Hearty Hot Cereal	100
Rice Cakes	117
Salad Dressings	316
Soups	286
Whole Wheat Spaghetti	160

PROGRESSO
Beans	249
Bread Crumbs	164
Canned Vegetables	177
Entrée Sauces	366, 367
Olive Oils	308
Soups	286

PROMISE
Margarines	296
Vegetable Oil Spreads	296

PURE SPRING WATER
All Brands	346

PURITY FARMS
Ghee Clarified Butter	297

QUAIL
All Parts	216

QUAKER
Cereal	101
Corn Cakes	117
Granola Bars	133
Quick Barley	153
Rice Cakes	117
Toasted Oatmeal Waffles	90

QUALITY HEARTH
Stuffing Mixes	164

QUARK
Spreadable Cheese	195

QUEST
2 Calorie Quest	339

QUIBELL
Sparkling Spring Water	339

QUICK EGGS
Egg Product	243

QUINLAN
Pretzels	117

R W FROOKIE
Cookies	133
Cool Fruit Freezers	329
Crackers	146
Frisps	117

RABBIT
All Parts	216

RACCONTO
Olive Oils	308
Pasta	160

RAGU
Entrée Sauces	367

RALSTON
Cereal	101
Chex Mix	117

RANDALL
Beans	249

RANGER LUKE'S
7J Ranch Texasalsa	358

RATH BLACK HAWK
Breakfast Beef	236
Hickory Smoked Bacon	236
Hot Dogs	236
Polska Kielbasa	236
Smoked Sausage	236

READ
German Potato Salad	162
Three Bean Salad	249

REAL DAIRY
Sour Cream	302

REBER
Butter Beans	249

RED BARON
Deep Dish Singles	268
Oven Stuffs	268

RED GOLD
Tomato Juice 352

RED OVAL FARMS
Crackers 146

REDDI WIP
Whipped Toppings 302, 303

REESE
Anchovies, Clams,
Sardines, Snails 238
Canned Vegetables 177
Croutons 164
Tapioca 334

REESE'S
Peanut Butter Ice Cups 329
Peanut Butters 291

RHODES
Pizza Dough and
Italian Bread 90
Raisin Bread Dough 90
Whole Wheat Texas Rolls 90

RICE DREAM
Frozen Desserts 329
Non-Dairy Beverage 200, 201

RICE-A-RONI
1/3 Less Salt Mixes 153
Fast Cook Side Dishes 160
Pasta Roni 160
Rice Mixes 153, 154

RICELAND
Extra Long Grain
Enriched Rice 154

RICESELECT
Rice 154

RICH N' READY
Punch 344

RICH'S
Coffee Rich Creams 302
Bread Dough 80
Roll Dough 90

RIPPIN' GOOD
Cookies 133

RO-TEL
Canned Tomatoes 177

ROBB ROSS
Salad Dressing 316

ROJO'S
Salsa Ranchero 358

ROLAND
Sardines 238

ROMAN MEAL
Bread 80
Corn Cakes 117
Rice Cakes 117

ROMANCE
Entrée Sauces 367
Pasta 160

RONZONI
Macaroni Products 160

ROSETTO
Ravioli 268
Salad & Soup Tortellini 268

ROTANELLI'S
Cannelloni 268
Manicotti 268

ROTHBURY FARMS
Croutons 164

ROYAL
Brownie Rounds 133
Cakes 133
Cookies 133

ROYAL CROWN COLA
Diet Rite Cola 339
RC Cola 339

ROYAL SELECT
Apple Juice 344

RS
Olive Oils 308

RUBSCHLAGER
Cocktail Bread 80

RW KNUDSEN
Fruit Beverages 344
Fruit Floats 344
Fruit TeaZer 339
Sport Drink 351
Vegetable Juices 352
Vita Juice 344

RY-KRISP
Natural Ry-Krisp Crackers 146

RYVITA
Whole Grain Crisp Bread 146

S & W
Baked Beans 250
Canned Fruits 185
Canned Vegetables 177
Salad Dressings 316

SACO
Easy Ceasar Salad Kit 170
Sassy Spinach 170
Buttermilk 199

SACRAMENTO
Vegetable Cocktail 352

SALERNO
Cookies 133, 134
Crackers 146
Graham Crackers 146
Graham Cracker Crumbs 70
Salsa Crisps 146

SANALAC
Nonfat Dry Milk 199

SAN GIORGIO
Pasta 160

SANS SUCRE
Cheesecake Mousse Mix 70

SANTA BARBARA OLIVE CO.
Pasta Sauce 367

SANTA CRUZ NATURAL
Organic Orangeade 344

SANTE
Creme Fraiche 302

SANWA
Ramen Pride soups 287

SAPPORO
Ichiban 154

SARA LEE
Coffee Cake 90
Desserts 322, 323
Premium Bagels 90

SARGENTO
Cheese 195, 196
Dips and Salsas 358
MooTown Snackers 117, 134

SAVINO
Sorbets 330

SCHAFER'S
Hillbilly Old
Fashioned Bread 80

SCHOONER
Fish 225

SCHWEPPES
Beverages 339

SEA HARVEST
Cape Capensis Loins 225

SEA SIDE
Beans 250
Mixed Vegetables 177

SEAGRAMS
Beverages 340

SEALTEST
Cottage Cheese 196
French Onion Dip 358
Frozen Desserts 330
Sour Creams 302

SEAPAK
Fish and Shrimp 225
Shrimp Sensations 268

SEASONS
Anchovies, Sardines 238

SECOND NATURE
Egg Product 243

SENECA
Frozen Concentrate 345

SEVEN SEAS
Salad Dressings 316

SEYFERT'S
Cheese Twistees 118
Pretzel Rods 118

SHARI'S BISTRO
Soups 287

SHASTA
A Sante Sparkling Waters 340
Plus - 10% Juice Beverage 345
Soft Drinks 340
Sport Drink 351
Spree All Natural Soda 340

SHEDD'S SPREAD
Country Crock Spreads 296
Willow Run
Soybean Margarine 296

SHOTGUN WILLIE'S
Picante Sauce 358

SILVER AWARD
Pasta 160

SILVER FLOSS
Sauerkraut 177

SINATRA'S
Entrée Sauces 367

SINGLETON
Shrimp 238

SKINNY
Corn Chips 118

SKIPPY
Peanut Butters 292

SMART BEAT
Cheese 196
Margarine 296
Nonfat Mayonnaise
Dressing 318

SMART CHOICE
Fruit Snacks 118

SMART TEMPTATIONS
Dips and Salsas 358, 359
No Oil Tortilla Chips 118
Salad Dressings 316

SMARTFOOD
Popcorn 118

SMUCKER'S
Fat Free Apple Dip 359
Peanut Butters 292

SNACK APPEAL
95% Fat Free Snacks 118
Fat Free Pretzels 118

SNACK TIME
Potato Chips 118

SNAPPLE
Bottled Drinks 345, 348

SNICKERS
Ice Cream Bars 330

SNYDER'S OF HANOVER
Potato Chips 118
Pretzels 118, 119
Snack Mix 118

SOHO
Soda 340

SONOMA
Marinated Dried Tomatoes 178

SORRENTO
Cheese 196

SOVEX
Good Shepherd 101
Oat Bran Hot Cereal 101

SOY BOY
Meat Alternatives 253

SPEAS FARM
Apple Juice 345

SPECIAL EDITION
Salad Nuggets 164

SPECTRUM NATURALS
Canola Mayonnaise 318
Oils 309

SPICE ISLANDS
Quick Meal Soups 287

SPIRIT OF NORWAY
Kipper Snacks 239
Sardines 238, 239

SPRITE
Soft Drinks 340

SQUAB (Pigeon)
All Parts 216

SQUIRT
Ruby Red 340
Squirt 340

STARBURST
Lowfat Frozen
Yogurt Snacks 330

STARKIST
Charlie's Lunch Kit 260
Tuna 239

STELLA D'ORO
Cookies 134

STELLA
Ricotta 196

STEPHEN'S
Hot Beverage Mixes 351
Rootbeer 340

STILLWELL
Frozen Select Fruits 182

STOKELY'S
Stewed Tomatoes 177
Tomato Sauce 367

STONYFIELD FARM
Frozen Yogurts 330
Sour Creams 302
Yogurt 206

STOUFFER'S
Creamed Spinach 173
Escalloped Apples 182
Homestyle 269, 270
Lean Cuisine 269, 270
Lean Cuisine
Lunch Express 269, 270
Meals and Entrées 269, 270
Welsh Rarebit Sauce 367

STOVE TOP
Stuffing mixes 164, 165

STROH'S
Frozen Desserts 330

SUCCESS
Rice 154

SUMMER SONG
100% Fruit Juice Blends 345

SUN MAID
Dried Fruits 186
English Muffins 90
Raisin Oatmeal Cookies 134

SUNBELT
Banana Nut Granola 102
Five Grain Muesli 102
Fruit & Nut Granola 102

SUNKIST
Diet Sunkist 340
Frozen Juice Concentrate 345
Fruit Rolls 119
Sunkist 340

SUNSHINE
Bite Size Shredded Wheat 102
Cheez-it 119, 146
Cinnamon Grahams 147
Cookies 134, 135
Crackers 147
Graham Cracker Crumbs 70
Old San Francisco
Style Pretzel Pieces 119
Shredded Wheat 102

SUNSWEET
Dried Fruits 186
Prune Juice 345
Ready to Serve Prunes 185

SUPERIOR DAIRY
Frozen Desserts 330

SUPERPRETZEL
Soft Pretzels 120
Softstix 120

SUTTER HOME
Entrée Sauces 367

SWANSON
Breakfast Blasts 261
Chicken 239
Fun Feast Meals 270, 271
Great Starts 261
Great Starts-Budget 261
Hungry-Man Meals 271
Meals 270, 271
Sauces 260
Soups 287

SWEET 'N LOW
Cake Mix 70

SWEET NOTHINGS
Frozen Desserts 330

SWEET ROLLS
All Brands 85

SWEET SUE
Broths 287

SWEETHOME FARM
Cereal 102

SWEETZELS
Ginger Snaps 135

SWIFT PREMIUM
Brown 'N Serve Sausage 236
Dried Beef 236

Pizza Size 'Peperoni' 236
Turkey Roast 216

SWISS MISS
Hot Beverage Mixes 351

T. ABRAHAM'S
Crispy-O's Cereal 102

T. MARZETTI'S
Salad Dressings 316
Dips 359

TABATCHNICK
Soups 287

TACO BELL
Dips and Salsas 359
Refried Beans 250

TAJ CUISINE OF INDIA
Side dishes 271

TAMPICO
Citrus Punch 345

TANG
Drink Mix 351

TASTE O'SEA
Cod Fillets 225

TASTEE
Apple Chips 119

TASTY TOMATO
Premium Spaghetti Sauces 367

TASTYKAKE
Butterscotch Krimpets 135
Creamies 135
Kandy Kakes 135
Tasty Too 135

TAYSTEE
Eights Enriched Buns 80
Golden Split Top 80

TCBY
Frozen Yogurt 330
Yogurt 206

TENDER TOASTS
Crackers 147

TERRA
Terra Chips 119

TERRAZZA
Legume Side Dishes 160

TEXSUN
Pink Grapefruit Juice 345

THANK YOU
Canned Fruits 185
Cut Asparagus 177
Dips 359
Pudding and Pie Filling 334

THE ALLENS
Canned Vegetables 177
Legumes 250
Shoestring Potato Sticks 119

THE BUDGET GOURMET
Light and Healthy
Entrées and Dinners 272
Meals and Entrées 272, 273
Side Dish Vegetables 173

Side Dishes 272
Special Selections 272

THE FAT FREE GOURMET
Baked Potato Corns 119
Baked Tortills Chips 119
Sourdough Pretzels 119

THE HUDSON BAY MILLING CO.
Bread 80, 81
English Muffins 90

THE SPICE HUNTER
Soups 287

THE TURKEY STORE
Gobble Stix 236
Sausage 236
Turkey Products 216

THE UNIVERSITY OF MICHIGAN
M-Fit Muffin 90

THOMAS'
Bagels 90
English Muffins 91

THOMSON BERRY FARMS
Salad Dressing 317

THORN APPLE VALLEY
Corned Beef Brisket 210
Golden Classic Ham 211
Lunchmeat 236
Sausage 237
Spiral Sliced Ham 237

TIGER'S MILK
Light Bar 135
Nutrition Bar 135
Tiger Crunchie 135
Tiger Sport Bar 135

TINA'S
Burritos 273

TIRRENO
Olive Oil 309

TOAST'EM
Toaster Fruit Pastries 91

TODAY'S MENU
Veggie Pattie 253

TOFUTTI
Frozen Desserts 330

TOMBSTONE
Pizzas 273

TONY'S
Pizzas 273

TOTINO'S
Party Pizza 273
Pizza Rolls 274

TOUFAYAN
Breadsticks 81
Snuggles Hot Dog Buns 81

TRADEWINDS
Teas 348

TRAPPEY'S
Beans 250

TREE SWEET
Fruit Juices 345

TREETOP
Crispy Apple Chips 119

TRIX
Pops 330

TROPICANA
Fruit Juices 345, 346

TRYSON HOUSE
Cooking Sprays 309

TURKEY
All Parts 216

TWINLAB
Sport Drink 351

TWIX
Cookie Bars 135

TYSON
Chicken 216
Franks 237
Ham Loaf 211
Healthy Portion
Meals and Entrées 274
Lunchmeat 237
Meals and Entrées 274

ULTRA SLIM FAST
Bars 135, 136
Cheese Curls 119
Cookies 135, 136

UNCLE B'S
Bakery Bagels 91

UNCLE BEN'S
Rice 154
Rice Mixes 154
Specialty Blends 154

UNCLE DAVE'S
Entrée Sauces 368

UNDERWOOD
Spreads 239

UNITED DAIRY FARMERS
Frozen Desserts 331

UTZ
Hard Pretzels 119

V8
Vegetable Juices 352

VALET
Ice Creams 331

VALLEY FRESH
Chicken 239

VALSUGANA
Instant Polenta 154

VAN CAMP'S
New Orleans Style
Red Kidney Beans 250
Pork and Beans 250
Spanish Rice 154
Fish 'N Fries 274
Fish and Shrimp 225

VEAL
All Cuts 211, 212

VEG ALL
Canned Vegetables 178

VEGETABLES
- Canned 173-178
- Dried 178
- Fresh 169-170
- Frozen 170-173

VENISON
- All Parts 217

VENUS
- Fat Free Crackers 147

VERNORS
- Soft Drinks 340

VERYFINE
- Fruit Juices 346

VIC'S
- Gourmet Popcorn 119

VIGO
- Beans and Rice 250
- Mexican Style Rice Dinner 154
- Olive Oil 309
- Spinach Pasta Tortellini
  w/Cheese 274

VIRGIL'S
- Root Beer 340

VISTA
- Double Fudge Cremes 136
- Soup & Oyster Crackers 147

VOORTMAN
- Cookies 136

VRUIT
- Fruit Juices 346

WACKY MAC
- Wacky Mac 161

WALDON FARMS
- Salad Dressings 317

WALKERS
- Shortbread Cookies 136

WASA
- Crispbread 147

WATERMAID
- Enriched Rice 155

WEETABIX
- Whole Wheat Cereal 102

WEIGHT WATCHERS
- Apple Chips 120
- Breakfast On-The-Go! 91, 261
- Cheese 196
- Cooking Sprays 309
- Crunchy Snacks 120
- Drink Mixes 351
- Entrées 274, 275
- Frozen Desserts 331
- Fruit Snack 120
- Low Fat Muffins 91
- Margarine 296
- Mayonnaise 318
- Microwave Popcorn 120
- Nonfat Milk 199
- Salad Dressings 317
- Smart Ones Entrées 274

Smart Options
- Pasta Sauce 368
- Smart Snackers 120, 136
- Ultimate 90 Yogurt 206

WELCH'S
- Fruit Juice Bars 331
- Fruit Juices 346
- Sparkling Soda 340

WESSON
- Cooking Spray 309
- Oils 309

WEST END
- All Natural Soda Brew 340

WEST VIRGINIA BRAND
- Bacon 237
- Ham 211, 237

WESTBRAE NATURAL
- Canned Beans 250
- Chocolate Chip Classics 136
- Cookie Jar Classics 136
- Mayonnaise 318
- Pasta 161
- Rice Cakes 120
- Vitasoy Non-Dairy
  Beverages 201
- Westsoy Non-Dairy
  Beverages 201

WESTERN
- Salad Dressings 317

WHEATENA
- Hi Fiber Wheat Cereal 102

WHITE CASTLE
- Hamburgers and
  Cheeseburgers 275

WHITE HOUSE
- Applesauce 185

WHITE KERNEL
- Popcorn 120

WHITE RICE
- All Brands 151

WHITE SWAN
- Marachino Cherries 185

WHITE WAVE
- Dairyless Yogurt 206
- Meat Alternatives 253

WHOLESOME ACCENTS
- Lowfat Cookies 137
- Almond Mylk 201
- Garden Burger 253
- Garden Dogs 253
- Garden Sausage 254
- Garden Veggie Burger 254

WILD RICE
- All Brands 151

WILDERNESS
- Apple Juice 346
- Applesauce 185

WILEY'S
- Precious Purple Hull Peas 250

WIN SCHULER'S
- Bar-Scheeze 196

WISE
- Lowfat Pretzel Stixs 120
- Potato Chips 120

WISH-BONE
- Salad Dressings 317

WISPRIDE
- Cheese 196

WOLFF'S
- Kasha Roasted Buckwheat 155

WOLFGANG PUCK'S
- Pizza 275

WONDER
- Bread 81
- Crouton & Stuffing Mix 165
- English Muffins 91
- Soft Wraps 91

WORLD CAFE
- Egg Rolls 275
- Sanchos 275

WORLD CLASSICS
- Cookies 137

WORTHINGTON
- Meat Alternatives 254
- Natural Touch Chili 260
- Natural Touch Meat
  Alternatives 254
- Wham Vegetable
  Protein Roll 254

WUNDERBAR
- Frozen Dessert 331

WYLER'S
- Broths 288

YODER'S
- Sour Creams 302

YOOHOO
- Chocolate Flavored Drink 348

YOPLAIT
- Frozen Dessert 331
- Yogurt 206

YU SING
- Egg Roll Snacks 275
- Entrées 275

YUBI
- Yogurt 206

YVES VEGGIE CUISINE
- Meat Alternatives 254

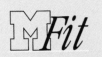

ORDER FORM

Make check payable to:
The University of Michigan Medical Center

Mail to:
The University of Michigan Medical Center
M-Fit Supermarket Program
P. O. Box 363
Ann Arbor, MI 48106-0363

Phone: 1-800-433-**MFit**
E-mail address: community.nutrition@umich.edu

❏ Please send me

____ copies of the *M-Fit Grocery Shopping Guide* $18.95 each _____

____ copies of the *High Fit—Low Fat Cookbook* $14.95 each _____

____ copies of the *High Fit—Low Fat Vegetarian Cookbook* $14.95 each _____

Michigan Residents, add 6% sales tax _____

+ $4.00 shipping and handling (for 1st book only) _____

+ $1.00 shipping & handling for each additional book _____

TOTAL _____

Name _____

Address _____

City _____

State _____ Zip _____

Daytime Phone _____

Deliver to: (if different address)

Name _____

Address _____

City _____

State _____ Zip _____

My payment is by:

   ❏ Check   ❏ Money Order   ❏ Visa   ❏ Mastercard

Credit Card Number (all digits) _____

Expiration Date _____

Signature: _____
(required if using credit card)

Prices subject to change without notice

Take a Minute and Help Us Help You

The University of Michigan Medical Center would like to continuously improve *The M-Fit Grocery Shopping Guide* to better suit your needs. We want to know how *The M-Fit Grocery Shopping Guide* has influenced your food choices. Please take a few minutes to answer the following questions.

After using *The M-Fit Grocery Shopping Guide* for at least one month, how do you rate the following statements on a scale from 1 to 10?

		Disagree									Agree

1. *The M-Fit Grocery Shopping Guide* helps me make heart-healthy food choices.
    1 2 3 4 5 6 7 8 9 10

2. *The M-Fit Grocery Shopping Guide* is easy to use.
    1 2 3 4 5 6 7 8 9 10

3. As a result of purchasing *The M-Fit Grocery Shopping Guide*:

    a. I more often choose foods because they are found in the green "Best Choice" or in the yellow "Acceptable Choice" columns.
        1 2 3 4 5 6 7 8 9 10

    b. I continue to choose foods in the red "Occasional Choice" column.
        1 2 3 4 5 6 7 8 9 10

    c. I choose foods in the red "Occasional Choice" column less often.
        1 2 3 4 5 6 7 8 9 10

4. I strongly recommend *The M-Fit Grocery Shopping Guide* to others.
    1 2 3 4 5 6 7 8 9 10

5. Are you currently following any special diet?   No   Yes

    If yes, which of the following (circle all that apply):

    low fat – low cholesterol – low salt – weight reducing – vegetarian – diabetic –

    other (specify): _____

6. I use *The M-Fit Grocery Shopping Guide* to make heart-healthy choices in the following food categories (circle all that apply):

Breads	Frozen Meals	Snack Foods
Cereals	Margarine	Vegetables
Cheese	Meats	Vegetable Oils
Desserts	Milk	Other (specify):
Fruits	Salad Dressings	_____

Please return this survey with your name and address.
To receive a $5 coupon towards your next *Guide* or cookbook mail order, check here. ❏

DO NOT STAPLE
TAPE HERE

Fold Here

- -

BUSINESS REPLY MAIL
FIRST-CLASS MAIL PERMIT NO. 1100 ANN ARBOR, MI

POSTAGE WILL BE PAID BY THE ADDRESSEE

University of Michigan
M/FIT SUPERMARKET PROGRAM
PO BOX 363
ANN ARBOR MI 48106-9847

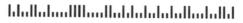